food science and nutrition

SECOND EDITION

Sunetra Roday

Principal
Maharashtra State Institute of Hotel Management and
Catering Technology, Pune

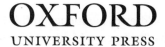

OXFORD
UNIVERSITY PRESS

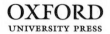

OXFORD
UNIVERSITY PRESS

Oxford University Press is a department of the University of Oxford.
It furthers the University's objective of excellence in research, scholarship,
and education by publishing worldwide. Oxford is a registered trademark of
Oxford University Press in the UK and in certain other countries

Published in India by
Oxford University Press
YMCA Library Building, 1 Jai Singh Road, New Delhi 110001, India

First Edition published in 2007
Second Edition published in 2012
Eighth impression 2016

ISBN-13: 978-0-19-807886-9
ISBN-10: 0-19-807886-2

Typeset in Garamond
by Pee-Gee Graphics, New Delhi
Printed in India by Manipal Technologies Ltd., Karnataka 576104

Dedicated to
My loving mother Smt. Sudha A. Shrouti
on her 86th birthday
and
My father Late Colonel A.W. Shrouti
whose fond memories I will forever cherish

Preface to the Second Edition

Food Science and Nutrition assimilates and applies knowledge that is based on the disciplines of biology, chemistry, and nutrition. The subject concerns itself with various aspects of food, beginning with the various components of food and ending with aspects related to consumption such as menu planning and balanced diets. Some of the sub-disciplines of food science include food microbiology, food preservation, sensory analysis, and food chemistry.

There have been major changes in the Indian consumer's lifestyle and eating habits over the past decade. There is an emerging awareness among consumers about the relationship between food selection and wellness along with a desire to experience new products. The continued growth of the food sector has presented the industry with challenges in meeting the increasing demand for products that are both nutritionally sound and high in quality.

It is heartening to note that the first edition of the book has been well accepted by both students and faculty members. This new edition has been prepared based on user feedback and the changes in the business environment since the first edition was published in 2007.

The aim of this text has been and remains the same—to provide students with a wide range of basic principles and practices in the subject area, thus enabling them to apply their knowledge efficiently in the hospitality as well as health care sector.

About the Book

Although the first edition was designed both as an introduction to the subject and as a textbook for students of the 'B.Sc in Hospitality and Hotel Administration' course offered by the National Council for Hotel Management and Catering Technology, New Delhi, the book has also proved useful to students pursuing a course in home science. Based on feedback from faculty members, a need to expand the coverage of the book was felt. Therefore, the book now becomes a complete and exhaustive textbook for students of home science too.

Two new chapters and many new topics have been added to ensure adequate coverage of latest trends and make the book useful for students pursuing a course in home science or hospitality studies.

In addition, six original chapters have been revised to include the latest examples and trends in the food and beverage industry. Illustrations have been updated and augmented to add interest to the text.

As in the last edition, each chapter in the book is designed with a focus on the learning objectives. Key terms are explained at the end of every chapter. Simple illustrations, formulae, and reactions are added to portray concepts. Review questions are listed at the end of each chapter. A concise summary to highlight the main points is given for every chapter.

Key Features

- Completely matches the National Council for Hotel Management & Catering Technology (NCHMCT) syllabus
- Emphasizes the importance of sensory as well as chemical properties of food
- Provides ample examples, review questions, analytical thinking exercises, and reference charts and tables

New to the Second Edition

Based on changing trends as well as the invaluable feedback received from reviewers, users, industry professionals, and academicians, this edition now includes the following:

- Chapter 6 on Fruits and Vegetables discusses the various kinds of fruits and vegetables as well as the structure and natural plant pigments present in them. The chapter goes on to discuss the role of fruits and vegetables in our diet and the measures to retain the bright, attractive pigments when fruits and vegetables are processed.
- Chapter 10 on Food Microbiology introduces the reader to microorganisms that are of significance to the food industry. Both useful and harmful microbes that are of special importance to the food industry have been discussed. An introduction to hygienic handling measures of food items to prevent contamination, spoilage and spread of foodborne disease has been briefly covered along with factors that affect and control the growth of microorganisms.
- New sections on cereals and cereal products, nuts and oilseeds, special protein supplements, prebiotics, probiotics, and more.
- Colour plates depicting various nutrient sources.

Extended Chapter Material

The following additions have been made in the food science section:

- Chapter 4 on Carbohydrates has a new section on cereals and cereal products that are available in the market today.
- Chapter 5 on Proteins includes pulses as a vegetarian source of protein and the effect of steeping, sprouting, and cooking on pulses.

- Chapter 7 on Fats and Oils introduces readers to popular oils and also has a new section on nuts and oilseeds.
- Chapter 8 on Flavour has an additional section on spices and herbs.
- Chapter 11 on Food Processing and Preservation has a new section on the different additives used in the food industry.

The following additions have been made in the nutrition component:

- Chapter 14 on Introduction to Nutrition has two new topics added, namely factors affecting food intake and food habits, and various ways in which nutrients can be classified.
- Chapter 16 on Proteins in Nutrition has a new topic on special protein supplements for individuals who are health and fitness conscious.
- Chapter 18 on Water has an additional section on beverages.
- Chapter 22 on Balanced Diet discusses various food pyramids and the latest concept of the food plate.
- Chapter 25 on New Trends in Nutrition highlights different nutraceuticals, such as prebiotics and probiotics, and their role in maintaining health.

Coverage and Structure

The text is divided into two sections: (1) *food science* and (2) *nutrition*. The section on food science now comprises 13 chapters that cover scientific principles and their applications in the preparation of food and commercial food products. New commodities and processes which are of relevance have been included. This section concentrates on the composition, structure, and behaviour of food in relation to pre-preparation, cooking, packaging, and storage relevant to catering operations.

Chapter 1 and 2 introduce students to the basic concepts of food science. Colloidal systems in foods are covered in Chapter 3. Carbohydrates and proteins are discussed in Chapters 4 and 5, respectively. Chapter 6 on Fruits and Vegetables discusses the structure and natural plant pigments as well as the role of plants in human diet.

Chapter 7 on Fats and Oils discusses concepts such as rancidity, reversion, refining, winterization, and more. The various aspects as well as the use of flavours in food preparation are discussed in Chapter 8. Chapter 9 discusses types of browning reactions and the role of browning in food preparation.

Chapter 10 introduces the reader to microorganisms of significance to the food industry. Chapter 11 discusses the objectives of food processing, methods of food preservation, and the effect of processing on food constituents. While methods of food evaluation are covered in Chapter 12, new trends in foods have been discussed in Chapter 13.

The section on nutrition comprises 12 chapters related to nutrients and planning of diets for sustaining a healthy lifestyle. Crucial issues such as weight control, eating disorders, and lifestyle-related diseases are included in this section. Dietary guidelines for prevention of deficiency and problems related to excessive consumption have been covered.

Chapter 14 introduces readers to the concept of nutrition. The classification as well as dietary sources of carbohydrates are discussed in Chapter 15. Chapter 16 introduces students to classification and functions of proteins. Fatty acids, antioxidants, saturated fatty acids, cholesterol, and more are discussed in Chapter 17 on Lipids.

Chapter 18 explains the various functions of water as well as the concept of water balance. While Chapter 19 discusses the various types of vitamins, Chapter 20 discusses the classification and general functions of minerals. Forms of energy, energy requirements, energy balance, etc. are discussed in Chapter 21 on Energy Metabolism.

Chapter 22 discusses the various aspects of a balanced diet and Chapter 23 introduces students to menu planning and mass food production. Diet therapy and various types of modified diets are discussed in Chapter 24 on Modified Diets. Chapter 25 discusses the new trends in nutrition including the nutritional evaluation on new products and the significance of nutritional labelling.

Sunetra Roday

Acknowledgements

Many people from the industry and academia have helped me in successfully completing this book and I am grateful for their contributions. It is practically impossible to name them all but I would specially like to mention a few.

I am grateful to Dr S.K. Mahajan, Director of Technical Education, Maharashtra State, Mumbai and Mr D.N. Shingade, Joint Director of Technical Education, Pune, for their inspiration and encouragement.

I owe an immense debt of gratitude to my daughter, Dr Neha Saraf, for her invaluable contribution towards the section on nutrition and to my son, Vikrant Roday, for providing all technical assistance.

I would also like to thank my colleagues, support staff, and students for their suggestions, contributions, and help.

I am greatly indebted to my husband and entire family for putting up with impossible hours and schedules.

I extend my sincere thanks to the editorial and production staff of the publisher.

I am also thankful to Mr Varinder Singh Rana, Lovely Professional University, Punjab; Ms Smritee Raghubalan, Garden City College, Bangalore; and Prof. Ruchita Verma, ITM Institute of Hotel Management, Mumbai for their valuable feedback.

I hope that this revised edition with its enhanced content will be more useful to the students and faculty of both hotel management and home science. I shall be happy to receive feedback on this new edition at sunetraroday@gmail.com.

Sunetra Roday

Preface to the First Edition

The provision of food and beverages is one of the oldest services associated with the hospitality industry. The food services industry has evolved and has come full circle. The need for providing nutritious meals for balanced overall development has acquired greater significance in the past few decades.

Eating out is no longer the occasional special event to be celebrated where people indulge. It has become a way of life. We are forced to eat out or order take-away meals due to work patterns, education, or social commitments. The number of people depending on food service providers for meeting their daily nutritional requirement is increasing at a rapid pace, making it necessary for professionals in the hospitality sector to be able to offer healthy choices on the menu to the customers.

Food science and nutrition has gained added significance with an increase in the number of lifestyle-related diseases, such as high blood pressure, atherosclerosis, heart diseases, diabetes mellitus, and obesity. Food manufacturers are introducing new products keeping these diseases in mind. A need was felt for a book designed specially for students in hospitality-related courses that addresses all the basic issues of food science and nutrition. Keeping this aspect in mind, I decided to write this book.

Food Science and Nutrition is designed both as an introduction to the subject and as a textbook for 'Principles of Food Science and Nutrition' for students of the 'B.Sc. in Hospitality and Hotel Administration' course offered by the National Council for Hotel Management and Catering Technology, New Delhi.

The students who join catering courses have little or no background in food science. They need a textbook that relates to what they practice in practical sessions. They find science difficult to comprehend and time-consuming to study.

From my experience of teaching the subject to students of catering, I have developed a text that concentrates on those aspects of food science and nutrition of particular relevance to the catering industry.

The text is divided into two sections: (1) food science and (2) nutrition.

The section on food science comprises 11 chapters that cover scientific principles and their applications in the preparation of food and commercial food products. New commodities and processes which are of current relevance have been included. This section concentrates on the composition, structure, and behaviour of food in relation to pre-preparation, cooking, packaging, and storage relevant to catering operations.

The section on nutrition comprises 12 chapters pertaining to nutrients and planning of diets for maintaining good health throughout the life cycle. Weight control, eating disorders, and lifestyle-related diseases are included. Dietary guidelines for prevention of deficiency and problems related to excessive consumption have been covered.

Each chapter in the book is designed with a focus on the objectives. Key terms are explained at the end of the chapter. Simple illustrations, formulae, and reactions are added to portray concepts. Review questions are listed at the end of each chapter. A concise summary to highlight the main points is given for every chapter.

Today's consumers ask questions about the nutritional value and health benefits of food. They are aware of the role the diet may play in maintaining and promoting good health. This makes it imperative for the food service provider to understand the fundamentals underlying food science and nutrition and put theory into practice.

Reader's views and comments are most welcome and will be appreciated.

Sunetra Roday

Features of the Book

Learning Objectives
Each chapter begins with learning objectives that focus on learning and the knowledge you should acquire by the end of the chapter.

Well-labeled illustrations
Each chapter is interspersed with numerous illustrations that supplement the explanation in the text.

Tables
All chapters contain tables that provide an outline of the topics discussed in the chapter.

Table 16.4 Recommended protein allowances for Indians

Group	Particulars	Body weight (kg)	Protein (g/day)
Man	Adult	60	60
Women	Adult	50	50
	Pregnancy		+15
	Lactation (0–6 months)		+25
	(6–12 months)		+18
Infants	0–6 months	5.4	2.05 g/kg
	6–12 months	8.6	1.65 g/kg
Children	1–3 years	12.2	22
	4–6 years	19.0	30
	7–9 years	26.9	41
Boys	10–12 years	35.4	54
	13–15 years	47.8	70
	16–18 years	57.1	78
Girls	10–12 years	31.5	57
	13–15 years	46.7	65
	16–18 years	49.9	63

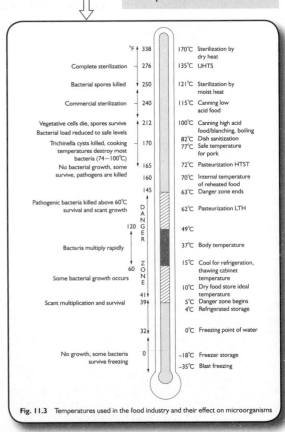

Fig. 11.3 Temperatures used in the food industry and their effect on microorganisms

SUMMARY

Fats, oils, and fat-like substances belong to a group collectively known as lipids. Lipids of importance in human nutrition include simple fats and oils such as butter, cooking oils, phospholipids, lipoproteins, and cholesterol. Simple fats which constitute 98 per cent of dietary fats are made up of glycerol and three fatty acid molecules. Food fats or triglycerides are mixed triglycerides with saturated, monounsaturated, or polyunsaturated fatty acids. Two fatty acids which are polyunsaturated, namely linoleic and linolenic acid, are essential as they cannot be synthesized by the body and must be present in the diet. They belong to omega-3 and omega-6 fatty acids which are essential for maintaining the integrity of cell membranes and lowering blood cholesterol levels.

Summary
The summary at the end of each chapter draws together the main concepts discussed within the chapter. This will help you to reflect and evaluate important concepts.

Key Terms
All important terms have been explained at the end of each chapter as key terms. This will help you to retain all the new terms that you have learnt in the chapter.

KEY TERMS

Anaemia A condition in which number of RBCs or haemoglobin content of blood is reduced.

Antagonist A substance that interferes with the action of another substance.

Antioxidant A substance naturally present or added to a product to prevent its breakdown by oxygen.

Carotene Reddish orange colour pigment in yellow/orange/red fruits and vegetables and green leafy vegetables which include α-, β-, and γ-carotenes and cryptoxanthin.

β-carotene A fat-soluble carotenoid pigment which is present in plants and is a precursor of vitamin A.

Cheilosis Swollen, cracked, and red lips.

Co-enzyme A substance that must be present along with an enzyme for a specific reaction to occur.

Collagen Intercellular cementing substances which is protein matrix of cartilage, connective tissue, and bone.

Glossitis Inflammation of the tongue.

REVIEW EXERCISES

1. How does an emulsifying agent stabilize an emulsion? Explain briefly.
2. What is the main difference between a solution, colloidal dispersion, and a suspension?
3. Explain the following terms:
   (a) Reverse sol   (d) Suspensoid
   (b) Osmosis   (e) Aerosal
   (c) Stabilizer
4. What is a foam? Which food constituent helps in strengthening and stabilizing a foam? Explain giving suitable examples.
5. Explain the four main colloidal systems prominent in food, stating the phases and giving relevant examples for each.
6. Classify food emulsions and name the natural emulsifying agent present in mayonnaise.

Exercises
Each chapter contains a series of exercises that enhance learning and can be used for review and classroom discussion.

Fill in the blanks

1. The basic building blocks of proteins are called _____.
2. Cereals are deficient in amino acid _____ and pulses are deficient in amino acid _____.
3. In a protein, the amino acids are linked together by _____ linkages.
4. The essential amino acid _____ is converted to niacin in the human body.
5. The quality of protein depends upon the _____ and _____ of amino acids present in them.

ASSIGNMENT

Visit a local supermarket or grocery store and read the label for ingredients on any four of the following ready-to-cook/ready-to-serve convenience foods:

1. Breakfast cereals
2. Multigrain biscuits
3. Infant foods
4. Other foods

List the different cereals used in preparing the same and correlate the choice of cereal with nutrients present in them.

Brief Contents

Detailed Contents

Part Two   Nutrition

List of Colour Plates

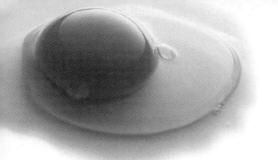

PART ONE

Food Science

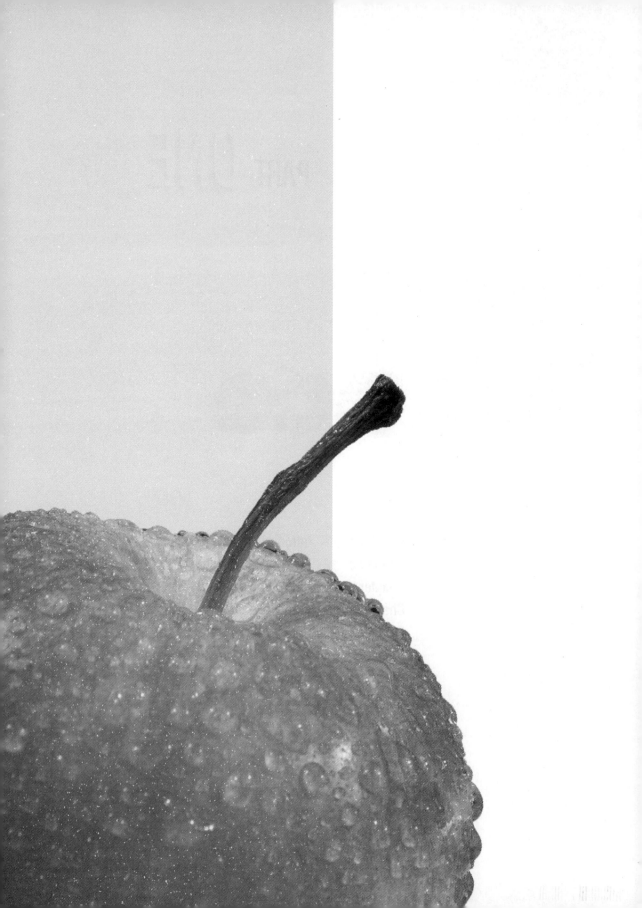

CHAPTER 1

Introduction to Food Science

LEARNING OBJECTIVES

After reading this chapter, you should be able to
- appreciate the importance of food science to a caterer in the context of the processed food revolution
- understand the relationship of food science to food chemistry, food microbiology, and food processing
- appreciate the role of convenience foods in our day-to-day life
- define the term food science and know the types of changes which take place in food

INTRODUCTION

The food industry, be it the processing industry or the catering industry, is one of the largest and most needed industry in the world today fulfilling one of our three basic needs, i.e., food. Its growth rate is phenomenal, growing by leaps and bounds to provide three square meals to our rapidly increasing population and keeping pace with the ever-changing demands of the people.

The developments in the food industry can be traced back to surplus food which needed to be preserved for a rainy day. Food preservation is not a new phenomenon. Our forefathers understood the basic principles underlying food preservation and practised them using natural ingredients and the forces of nature, such as sunlight and ultraviolet (UV) rays, till newer and more scientific methods were developed.

Improvement in equipment and machinery has made it possible to increase the capacity of food processing plants greatly. The shelf life of perishable foods has increased dramatically with the invention of the refrigerator and the use of dry ice.

With the advent of the wheel, surplus food was transported several hundred miles. As early as in 1850, milk was transported by special milk trains and tank trucks over a distance of several hundred miles with negligible loss in quality. Food which was perishable was moved thousands of miles before it was processed, stored, and consumed.

Over the past few decades, the food industry has witnessed a significant change. The market has witnessed a flood of food commodities, superior in quality and available all year round. Ice cream filled cones and nuts in ice cream retaining their crunch, fresh milk stored on the shelf for months, and crisp croutons in a ready to serve cream soup are a few marvels of food science and technology. With these advances in science and technology, the consumer has an unlimited choice of meals to choose from all year round.

The aesthetic value of food is important. To be able to offer the consumer quality cuisine, basic knowledge of food science and its applications is necessary. Every food handler should know the composition, structure, and behaviour of food and the changes that take place during cooking, holding, and storage as well as what happens to the food once it is consumed, i.e., its digestion, absorption, and metabolism in the human body.

The study of food is today accepted as a separate discipline called food science.

Definition   Food science is a systematic study of the nature of food materials and the scientific principles underlying their modification, preservation, and spoilage.

To understand food science, the basic concepts of physics, chemistry, mathematics, and biology and their applications, i.e., biochemistry, microbiology, and food technology, are necessary in order to prepare, package, store, and serve wholesome, high quality products.

All foods are chemical compounds which undergo various chemical reactions at all stages from production to consumption. These reactions are based on the laws of chemistry. Many processes used while preparing food involve physical changes apart from chemical changes.

Matter exists in three states: solid, liquid, and gas.

In general, as the temperature is increased, a pure substance will change from solid to liquid and then to a gas, without change in chemical composition. However, many organic compounds will decompose, undergoing various chemical reactions, rather than a change of state when temperature is raised.

Many foods are complex mixtures of chemical substances. In processed foods, additives are added to improve colour, texture, flavour, etc., and these additives are also chemical compounds. It undergoes further chemical changes during storage, cooking, processing as well as in the human body during digestion of food by action of chemical substances.

Physical aspects of food such as the various food systems are of colloidal dimensions. Food is subjected to various physical conditions during preparation and storage which affect its quality such as temperature and pressure changes.

Food chemistry is the science that deals with the composition, structure, and properties of food, and with chemical changes that take place in food. It forms a major part of food science and is closely related to food microbiology. The chemical composition of food dictates which microorganisms can grow on it and the changes which take place in the food because of their growth. The changes may be planned and desirable or may result because of contamination, causing disease, i.e., causing food poisoning and food infection or just spoiling the food rendering it unfit for consumption. Microorganisms have basic growth requirements, namely food, moisture, temperature, time, osmotic pressure, pH, and the presence or absence of oxygen.

Food chemistry and food microbiology are intimately related to food processing because the processes to which food needs to be subjected to improve its taste, texture, flavour, and aroma depend on its composition and ingredients. The time and temperature for food processing depend not only on the chemical composition of food but on its microbial load and the type of packaging to be used.

The growing public demand for meals away from home has made the problem of serving safe wholesome food more critical and challenging. This makes it imperative for food handlers to understand and implement the basic principles of the food science to enable them to prepare and serve high quality products over extended lunch hours.

NEED FOR CONVENIENCE FOODS

Rapid urbanization and changes in social and cultural practices have modified the food habits of the community. Industrial development in Indian cities has compelled labour from villages to migrate to cities in search of employment. It is estimated that within the next five years, half the world's population will be living and working in urban areas. Increase in buying power and long hours spent away from home commuting to work places, make convenience foods a necessity in every home.

The ever-increasing market for convenience foods, be it tinned, canned, chilled, frozen, or preserved, presents a whole array of complex operations in food processing. This weaning away from the traditional fare of yesteryears provides a tremendous and urgent challenge to the food industry—serving safe, attractive, and nutritious food that is wholesome and bacteriologically safe and conforms with quality standards.

The urban workforce does not have the time or inclination to follow the traditional recipes and prefers picking up packed, clean, and reasonably priced meals rather than returning home from work and doing domestic chores.

Most food consumed in developed countries is in the form of *convenience foods*. Convenience foods are foods that require little labour and time to prepare. A packet of frozen green peas is a convenience food since it requires no shelling. A packet of whole wheat flour is also a convenience food as it has already been milled. A packet instant idli mix is more of a convenience food, and 'ready to eat' or 'heat and eat' foods, such as chicken *keema matar* or canned *palak paneer*, are most convenient since they need no further cooking.

Many different types of convenience foods are available in the market today. The speed and efficiency of cooking and service increases dramatically with the use of convenience foods, giving the caterer, homemaker, or working professional more time to devote to other activities. The convenience food revolution is possible because of a wide variety of chemicals which are added to food not only to preserve it but to enhance its overall quality. These numerous chemicals, tested and permitted by law to be added to food are called *food additives*.

Today, convenience foods are being specially packed for caterers and are available in large catering packs. Manufacturers of specialized food supplies pack food so that it fits into standard catering equipment, e.g., catering packs that fit into vending machines. The caterer can choose between smaller packs and larger packs that are economical.

Convenience foods need to be handled with care because one source of infection can contaminate thousands of pre-packed items. Take-away meals should not be kept for a long time, hygiene should be practised in processing plants, and time and temperature control should be observed during storage. Leftover contents in large catering packs should not be stored in the open.

Convenience foods help by saving considerable time and effort. However, the cost of convenience foods compared to home-prepared foods should be considered before purchase. Some foods may not be costlier while others may work out to be expensive. For people who have to rush home from work and prepare a meal, such foods purchased on the way home or stacked in the deep freezer are not only time-saving but also convenient.

Convenience foods vary widely in their palatability, nutrient content, and cost. The consumer can choose from a bewildering display of snacks, soups, sauces, fruit chunks and juices, desserts, meat, and vegetable preparations and gravies in the ready-to-eat and ready-to-cook form. They need to be warmed up in a microwave before they are served.

Canned foods, commercially prepared chapattis, snacks both sweet and savoury, main course, vegetable preparations, soups, gravies, sauces, breakfast cereals, bakery items, deep frozen foods, dry ready mixes, etc., are not only time saving but convenient to cook and store.

Thus, food science covers all aspects of food, from the properties of food materials and influences of all factors affecting food, beginning from growing the food to harvesting or slaughter, i.e., all stages from the farm to the table, from raw food till it is consumed such as processing, nutritive value, shelf life, novel sources of food, fabricated food and food analogs, conservation and reuse of resources to make more food.

A study of food science and nutrition will be of benefit to all food professionals.

SUMMARY

The food industry is a fast-growing industry that applies the principles of food science and technology to offer the consumer a wide array of fresh and processed foods to meet their nutritional needs, wants, and budget. These foods are available under different brand names, all year round in delectable flavours and assorted preparations.

The aesthetic value of food is an important criterion in its acceptability. Every food handler should be aware of the composition, structure, and behaviour of food and what happens to it during processing and after consumption. The systematic study of food is called food science. All foods are chemical compounds and undergo physical as well as chemical changes. The various food systems are of colloidal dimensions and various physical conditions, such as temperature and pressure, affect its quality.

Food science is intimately related to food chemistry, food microbiology, and food processing. To understand this, the basic concepts of physics, chemistry, mathematics, and biology are necessary.

The growing demand for meals away from home has made the problem of serving safe and wholesome food critical and challenging. With rapid urbanization and changes in food habits and lifestyles, and increase in the number of couples who have little time has caused a shift in focus from farm-grown fresh foods to partially or totally processed convenience foods. These foods require little labour and time to prepare and are useful to caterers and homemakers. The shelf life and acceptability of these foods are enhanced by the use of permitted additives. The consumer can choose from a wide range of ready-to-cook and ready-to-eat foods.

KEY TERMS

Additives   All material added to food to improve its shelf life, colour, flavour, texture, taste, and quality such as flavouring agents, antioxidants, and preservatives.

Convenience foods   Processed foods in which much pre-preparation/preparation has already been done by the manufacturer, e.g., frozen green peas, breakfast cereals, and canned foods.

Dry ice   Solid carbon dioxide having temperature of $-79°C$ and used to refrigerate foodstuffs being transported.

Food microbiology   A study of bacteria, yeasts, and moulds, and their harmful and useful effects on food and its consumption.

Food science   A study of the physical and chemical constituents of food and the scientific principles underlying their modification, preservation, and spoilage.

Food technology   Application of the principles of food science to the preservation, processing, packaging, storage, and transportation of food materials.

REVIEW EXERCISES

1. What changes has the food industry witnessed in the last century?
2. Why is knowledge of the principles of food science necessary for a catering professional?
3. What do you understand by the term convenience foods? What foods does it include? Give suitable examples from your daily life.
4. Do you think convenience foods are necessary? Justify your answer giving suitable examples.

CHAPTER 2

Food Science Concepts

LEARNING OBJECTIVES

After reading this chapter, you should be able to
- appreciate the importance of understanding the basic concepts in physics, chemistry, and biology
- interpret the weights and measures in recipes
- weigh and measure ingredients accurately
- understand and define the relevant terms that play an important role in food preparation
- understand the applications of these concepts in the food industry
- know the meaning of food rheology

INTRODUCTION

Weights and measures are set standards which are used to find the size of substances. To obtain a high-quality product and carry out a profitable business, accurate weighing and measuring of all ingredients is essential.

BASIC SI UNITS OF LENGTH, AREA, VOLUME, AND WEIGHT

The SI or International System of measurement is used universally for measurement of matter. In this system, prefixes such as 'deci', 'centi', and 'milli', and units such as 'litre', 'gram', 'metre', and derived units such as 'joule' and 'pascal' are used.

Prefixes represent numbers or numerical quantities symbolized by letters.

$$\text{mega} = M = 1,000,000 = \text{one million}$$
$$\text{kilo} = k = 1,000 = \text{one thousand}$$
$$\text{deci} = d = 1/10 = \text{one tenth}$$

centi = c = 1/100 = one hundredth

milli = m = 1/1,000 = one thousandth

micro = μ = 1/1,000,000 = one millionth

Measurement of Length

The unit for measuring length is the metre (m).

Length is measured using a measuring tape or ruler.

One thousand metres (1,000 m) = one kilometre (km)

A metre is divided into hundred parts. Each part is called a centimetre (cm).

1 metre (m) = 100 centimetres (cm)

Each centimetre is made up of ten smaller parts called millimetre (mm).

1 centimetre = 10 millimetres (mm)

The simplest instrument for measuring length is a scale or ruler measuring one metre, or a measuring tape.

Measurement of Volume

Volume and capacity is measured in litres. A litre is made up of 10 decilitres (dl). Each decilitre is made up of 10 centilitres (cl). A centilitre is made up of 10 millilitres (ml), which means that a litre is made up of one thousand millilitres (1,000 ml).

Most measuring cups and jugs are marked in millilitres and litres. The capacity of cups and spoons are listed below.

1 tablespoon = 15 ml

1 teaspoon = 5 ml

1 breakfast cup = 240 ml

1 coffee cup = 100–120 ml

1 teacup = 150–180 ml

1 water glass = 280–300 ml

The volume of solids that is not greatly affected by water can be measured by the water displacement method. Solids are immersed in the displacement can and the volume of water displaced, equal to the volume of the solid, is noted.

The seed method is used to measure the volume of cake and bread. A large tin box is filled to the brim with seeds and the volume of seeds required to fill the box is measured in a measuring cylinder. The cake of which the volume is to be measured is placed in the empty tin and covered with seeds. The volume of seeds remaining after covering the cake is equal to the volume of the cake.

Measurement of Weight or Mass

Weight is the pull experienced on the body by the earth's force of gravity. Mass is the amount of matter contained in a known volume of substance. Mass always remains constant but

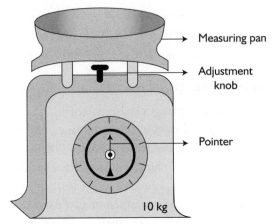

Fig. 2.1 Single pan weighing scale

weight may change in different parts of the world because the force of gravity varies from place to place.

Weight is measured on a weighing scale (see Fig. 2.1). The kilogram is the unit for measuring weight and is made up of one thousand smaller parts called grams.

$$1 \text{ kilogram (kg)} = 1{,}000 \text{ grams (g)}$$

Each gram is further divided into one thousand smaller parts called milligrams (mg).

$$1 \text{ g} = 1{,}000 \text{ mg}$$

Each milligram is further divided into 1,000 micrograms (μg).

$$1 \text{ mg} = 1{,}000 \text{ } \mu\text{g}$$

From the above we conclude that

1 kg = 1,000,000 mg and a measure of 1 ppm means 1 mg in 1 kg of a substance.

DENSITY

Density is the relationship between the weight and volume of a substance expressed as

$$\text{Density} = \frac{\text{weight in kg}}{\text{volume in m}^2}$$

It is expressed in kilograms per cubic metre and is used to compare the heaviness or lightness of different foods.

A fruit cake has a greater density as compared to a sponge cake. The density of liquids is measured in g/cm^3. Water has a density of 1 g/cm^3.

Relative Density

Relative density (RD) is the ratio of the mass of a known volume of a substance to the mass of the same volume of water. It tells us the number of times the volume of a substance is heavier or lighter than an equal volume of water. If the RD of a volume of lead is 11, it means that it is eleven times as heavy as an equal volume of water.

$$\text{Relative density} = \frac{\text{mass or weight of a substance}}{\text{weight of equal volume of water}}$$

A hydrometer is used to measure the relative density of different liquids. It is made up of a weighted bulb with a graduated stem calibrated to measure the relative density of the liquid directly. The liquid is kept at room temperature and the hydrometer is allowed to float in the liquid. The depth to which it sinks is read on the graduated stem. Hydrometers are specifically calibrated to measure the RD of different liquids used in the catering industry.

Saccharometers are used to determine the concentration of sugar solutions, denoted in degrees Brix. A 75 per cent sugar solution is called 75 degrees Brix.

Salinometers are used to determine the RD of brine or sodium chloride solutions used for canning vegetables or pickling ham.

Lactometers are used for checking the purity of milk. Addition of water or removal of cream affects the RD and is depicted on the graduated scale on the stem. The scale is marked 1.00 to 1.04. 'W' denotes RD of water, 'M' denotes pure milk, and 'S' denotes skim milk.

Alcoholometers are used to test the RD of alcoholic beverages. It is used to check the number of degrees proof or ethanol content of wines, beers, and spirits, and whether it has been diluted.

Refractometers (see Fig. 2.2) are used to measure the sugar or total solids in solution (TSS) while preparing jam, syrups, etc. They measure the refractive index of light reflected through the solution.

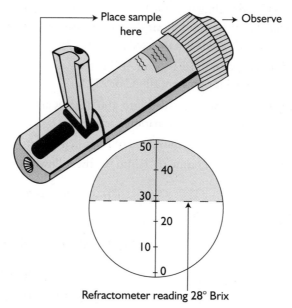

Refractometer reading 28° Brix

Fig. 2.2   A refractometer

Besides checking the purity of milk, ethanol content of alcoholic beverages, strength of salt solution, and concentration or stage of 'doneness' for sugar syrups and preserves such as jam, sauce, and candied fruit, the other applications of RD are

- testing eggs for freshness when eggs are dipped in a 10 per cent salt solution, fresh eggs sink and stale eggs float because of a large air space caused by staling;
- determining the lightness of cakes; and
- choosing potatoes for boiling and frying potatoes that have a low RD should be boiled, while those that have a high RD should be baked or fried.

TEMPERATURE

Heat is a form of energy needed to carry out work. Energy is the capacity for doing work. Energy is present in two forms:

1. Potential energy or stored energy, such as the energy stored in a bar of chocolate
2. Kinetic energy or active energy in motion, such as when a person is walking

Energy is present in many forms. Heat is one form of energy. Solar energy, electrical energy, and chemical energy are some of the others.

Heat energy is measured in units called joules and the energy present in food is measured in kilocalories. One kilocalorie is made up of 1,000 calories.

$$1 \text{ kilocalorie (kcal)} = 4.2 \text{ kilojoules (kj)}$$

$$1 \text{ calorie} = 4.2 \text{ joules}$$

Temperature refers to the relative hotness or coldness of a substance compared with melting ice at 0°C and boiling water at 100°C. Thermometers are used to measure temperature.

Temperature is measured either in the Celsius or centigrade scale (°C) or in the Farenheit scale (°F). Each scale has two fixed points:

1. Melting point of ice (0°C or 32°F)
2. Boiling point of water (100°C or 212°F)

The Celsius scale is divided into 100 degrees and the Farenheit scale into 180 degrees. The Celsius scale is the international scale.

Conversion of Farenheit scale to Celsius scale

To convert temperature in °F into °C, the following formula is used

$$(\text{°F} - 32) \times \frac{5}{9} = \text{°C}$$

To convert 212°F into °C

$$(212\text{°F} - 32) \times \frac{5}{9} = \overset{20}{\cancel{180}} \times \frac{5}{\cancel{9}^{1}}$$

$$= 20 \times 5 = 100\text{°C}$$

so $212\text{°F} = 100\text{°C}$

The conversion of imperival units to metric equivalents are given in Table 2.1.

TABLE 2.1   Conversion of imperial units to metric equivalents

	Non-metric units	Metric units
Length	1 inch (in)	2.5 centimetres (cm)
	1 foot (ft)	30.5 centimetres (cm)
	39.4 inches (in)	100 centimetres (cm)or 1 metre
	1 mile	1.6 kilometres
Volume	1 pint	568 millilitres (ml)
	1 gallon	4.5 litres (l)
	1.8 pints	1 litre (l)
Weight	1 ounce (oz.)	28.4 grams (g)
	1 pound (lb)	454 grams (g)
	2.2 pounds (lb)	1 kilogram (kg)
Energy	1 kilocalorie (kcal)	4.2 kilojoules (kJ)
	1 calorie (cal)	4.2 joules (J)
Temperature	32°Fahrenheit (F)	0°Celsius (C)
	212°Fahrenheit (F)	100°Celsius (C)
Area	1 square inch (sq. in)	6.45 square centimetres (sq. cm)
	1 square foot (sq. ft)	929 sq. cm
	1 square mile	2.59 sq. km

TYPES OF THERMOMETERS

Most thermometers (see Fig. 2.3) are mercury in glass thermometers with different temperature ranges depending on their purpose. Some common thermometers are:

1. Sugar or confectionery thermometers (40°C to 180°C)
2. Dough testing thermometers (10°C to 43°C)
3. Meat thermometers with a special spike which can be pierced into meat and a round dial to record temperature
4. Refrigeration thermometers filled with red coloured ethanol (−30°C to −100°C)

POTENTIAL HYDROGEN or pH

When an acid is diluted with water, it dissociates into hydrogen ions and acid radical ions.

$$HCl = H^+ + Cl^-$$

Hydrochloric acid   Hydrogen ion   Chloride ion (acid radical)

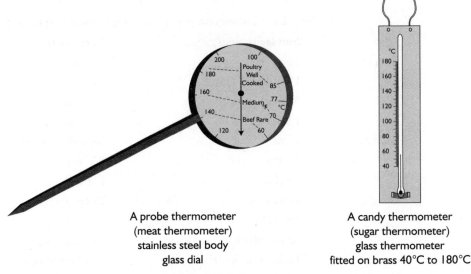

A probe thermometer
(meat thermometer)
stainless steel body
glass dial

A candy thermometer
(sugar thermometer)
glass thermometer
fitted on brass 40°C to 180°C

Fig. 2.3 Thermometers

The term pH (hydrogen ion concentration) is used to express the degree of acidity or alkalinity of a food. It is defined as the negative logarithm to base 10 of the hydrogen ion concentration, i.e., higher the hydrogen ion concentration, lower will be the pH and vice versa. Some foods, such as fruits, contain organic acids and have an acid reaction while others such as milk are neutral. Bakery products leavened with baking powder, have an alkaline reaction. Pure water is pH 7 or neutral.

The pH scale of pH 0 to pH 14 (see Fig 2.4), i.e., from extremely strong acids to extremely strong alkali is used to describe the acidity or alkalinity of food.

A reading between pH 1 to pH 6.5 indicates acidic food while pH 7.5 to pH 14 indicates alkaline food (see Table 2.2). The pH of a solution can be measured electrically using the pH metres or it may be measured colorimetrically using pH papers which change colours according to the pH.

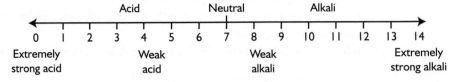

Fig. 2.4 The pH scale

Buffers

They are defined as solutions that can resist a change of pH on addition of acids or alkalis but within limits. These solutions are made up of a weak acid and one of its salts or a weak base and one of its salts.

TABLE 2.2   pH values of some common foods

pH	pH value	Food
Strongly acidic	2.0	Vinegar
	2.3	Lime juice
	2.7	Pickles
	3.0	Apples
	3.7	Orange juice
Mildly acidic	4.0	Fruit cake
	4.3	Tomato
	4.6	Banana
	5.0	Bread
	5.4	Spinach
	5.5	Potatoes
	6.0	Peas
	6.2	Butter chicken
	6.4	Salmon
	6.5	Milk
Neutral	7.0	Chocolate
Mildly alkaline	8.0	Egg white
	9.0	Soda bread

When hydrogen ions (H^+) or hydroxide ions (OH^-) are added, they can be absorbed by these systems without altering the pH of the resulting solution. Common buffers are

1. Acetic acid and sodium acetate mixture
2. Citric acid and sodium citrate mixture

Buffering action is very important in the human body and in food. The salts of calcium, phosphorus, sodium, and potassium function as buffers and maintain the pH of milk at a constant level of 6.5.

Applications of pH

1. Preparation of jam—The pectin in jam and marmalade does not form a gel until the pH is lowered to 3.5. If fruit used for making these preserves does not contain sufficient acid, small amounts of citric acid should be added.
2. Retaining bright green colour in green vegetables—Green vegetables tend to get discoloured when cooked. Green colour can be retained by adding a pinch of sodium bicarbonate to the cooking liquor but B complex vitamins and vitamin C gets destroyed in an alkaline medium.
3. Food digestion—pH of the gastrointestinal juices affects our digestive process. The pH of gastric juice is strongly acidic, between 1 and 2, and aids in digestion of food in the stomach while a mildly alkaline pH, between pH 7 and 8, is needed to complete digestion in the intestine.

4. Texture of cakes—A significant change in texture is observed with a change in pH while baking cakes. Low pH gives a fine texture and high pH gives a coarse texture to the cake crumb.
5. pH of dough—In bread making, compressed yeast is used for fermentation. During fermentation, yeasts convert simple sugars to ethyl alcohol and carbon dioxide.
   (a) Ethyl alcohol takes up oxygen and forms acetic acid
   (b) Carbon dioxide dissolves partially in water to form carbonic acid
   (c) Chemical yeast food, i.e., ammonium sulfate and ammonium chloride if used produce sulphuric acid and hydrochloric acid respectively

All these acids lower the pH of the dough from pH 6.0 to pH 4.5. This change in pH makes the dough less sticky and more elastic.

IMPORTANT TERMINOLOGIES, THEIR DEFINITION AND RELEVANCE

Boiling Point

Boiling is the use of heat to change a substance from a liquid to a gas. The change takes place throughout the body of the liquid at a definite temperature.

Like the melting point, the boiling point of a pure substance is always constant. It changes if impurities or dissolved substances are present or by changes in atmospheric pressure. Pure water boils at 100°C.

Applications of boiling point

1. Boiling vegetables in salted water increases the boiling point above 100°C.
2. In sugar cookery, the boiling points of sugar solutions is noted at various stages so that fondant, fudge, toffee, and caramel can be prepared.

Boiling under pressure   When atmospheric pressure is lowered, water boils at a lower temperature of 70°C. At hill stations, the atmospheric pressure is low so temperature is also lower and food takes longer time to cook. When pressure is increased, e.g., below sea level or boiling in a pressure cooker, water boils at higher temperatures and cooks food faster.

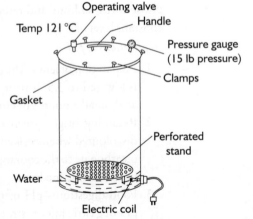

Fig. 2.5   An autoclave

Applications of boiling under pressure

1. Food is cooked in pressure cookers to reduce cooking time to one-fourth of ordinary cooking time as water boils at a higher temperature under pressure.
2. Autoclaves are used for sterilization by moist heat under pressure at 121°C and 15 lb pressure for 20 minutes (see Fig. 2.5).

Evaporation

Evaporation is a change of state from liquid to gas which takes place continuously from the surface of a liquid.

Volatile liquids vaporize easily, e.g., petrol and acetone.

Non-volatile liquids, such as oils, evaporate very gradually. Evaporation is faster when there is breeze and low humidity in the air as well as a large surface area and high temperature.

Applications of evaporation

1. Bread and cake if left uncovered, hardens and becomes stale because of loss of moisture. This can be prevented by storing food in covered tins.
2. Cooking in shallow uncovered pans will cause greater evaporation and are used for preparing mawa from milk.
3. Milk powder is prepared by dehydration or spray drying in which water from milk is removed by circulating hot air.

Melting Point

Melting or fusion is the change of state from a solid to a liquid.

The temperature at which a solid melts and turns into a liquid is called its melting point. The melting point of fats depends on the percentage of saturated long chain fatty acids present in it.

The melting point for any chemical is fixed and is used to measure the purity of a substance. It is lowered by adding other substances.

Melting point of fats

Vanaspati	37–39°C
Butter	36°C
Lard	44°C
Tallow	48°C
Coconut oil	26°C

Applications of melting point

1. Ice has a melting point of 0°C. If adequate sodium chloride is added to ice, the melting point falls to −18°C. This lowering of melting point is used in the setting of ice cream.
2. Fat is removed from adipose tissue of animals by a process called rendering, which is based on the melting point. Boiling water or dry heat is used to liberate the oil from the fat cells.

Corn oil temperatures

Frying	180–195°C
Smoke point	232°C
Flash point	330°C
Fire point	363°C

TABLE 2.3 Smoke point of some common fats

Oil	Smoke point (°C)
Corn oil	232
Cotton seed	236
Soya bean	243
Ground nut	243
Butter	201
Lard	222
Beef dripping	163

Smoke point   When fats and oils are heated strongly above frying temperature, they decompose and a stage is reached at which it emits a visible thin bluish smoke. This temperature is called the smoke point (see Table 2.3).

The temperature varies with different fats and ranges between 160 and 260°C. The bluish vapour is because of the formation of acrolein from overheated glycerol. Acrolein has an acrid odour and is irritating to the eyes. The effect of high temperature on fat is shown in Fig. 2.6.

The smoking point is lowered by the following factors:

1. Presence of large quantities of free fatty acids
2. Exposure of large surface area while heating
3. Presence of suspended food particles

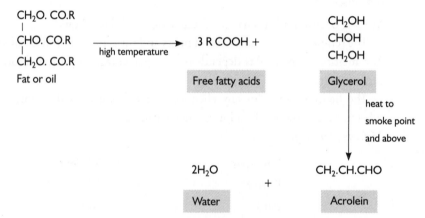

Fig. 2.6   Effect of high temperature on fat

Flash point   This is the temperature at which the decomposition products of fats and oils can be ignited, but will not support combustion. The flash point varies with different fats and ranges between 290 and 330°C.

Fire point   This is the temperature at which the decomposition products of fats and oils support combustion. It ranges between 340 and 360°C for different fats. The oil or fat may catch fire and burn.

The smoke point, flash point, and fire point are lowered by the presence of free fatty acids.

Normal frying temperature for most oils is 180–195°C. The smoke point is 25–40°C above normal frying temperature. The application of smoke point is in frying foods. Fats and oils used for deep fat frying should have a high smoke point. Moist foods should be coated well before frying as moisture present in food tends to hydrolyse the fat and increase the free fatty acids present.

Surface Tension

Surface tension is a force experienced on the surface of a liquid. It is caused by cohesion, i.e., a force that causes the molecules of a substance to be attracted to one another.

The molecules of a liquid that are below the surface are pulled by cohesive forces from all directions. But the molecules at the surface behave differently because they are only pulled downwards or sideways. This downward or sideways attraction causes a constant pull on the surface molecules which makes the liquid behave as if it is covered by a thin elastic film. For example, the surface of water can support needles if they are placed carefully.

Because of surface tension, drops of liquid take a spherical shape, which has the smallest possible surface area, e.g., dew drops.

Surface tension causes liquids to rise in a thin tube (capillary tube) when the tube is dipped in liquid. This property of liquids is important in many food systems and in the action of detergents.

Surface tension is also defined as the force of attraction which exists between liquid and solid surfaces.

Applications of surface tension

1. Addition of detergent to liquids reduces the surface tension of water and the surface attraction between the fibre and greasy stain, and allows the soil to be removed from the fabric.
2. Release agents help prevent the paper lining the tin from sticking to the cake. They contain silicone compounds.
3. Silicones have a property of lowering the surface tension and is added to wood polishes to allow the polish to spread easily.
4. Non-stick cookware is coated with polytetrafluoroethane plastic or silicone to prevent attraction between the food and pan.

Osmosis

Osmosis is the passage of water from a weak solution to a stronger solution through a semi-permeable membrane.

When raisins are soaked in a cup of water for sometime, the raisins swell because water from the cup enters the raisins. Similarly, if raisins are placed in a concentrated sugar solution, they shrivel up after some time because water from the raisins passes into the sugar solution because of osmosis.

Plant and animal cell membranes act as semi-permeable membranes and selectively permit water and electrolytes to enter or leave the cell.

Applications of osmosis

1. Osmosis plays an important role in food processing and preservation to retain the original shape and size of canned fruits in syrup and of vegetables in pickles.
2. The freshness of fruits and vegetables depends on the osmotic pressure in the cells. Salads lose their crisp crunchy texture and become limp if salt and sugar is sprinkled much in advance. Lettuce leaves can be revived by immersing them in chilled water.

Humidity

Humidity refers to the presence of water vapour in the air. Water vapour is produced by respiration of plants and animals, evaporation from food during cooking and from water bodies, from rain during the monsoons, etc.

In catering establishments, moisture in the air is quite high because of large volumes of steam from boilers, from cooking food, from dishwashers and laundry processes, and respiration and perspiration of people in a confined area.

A humid atmosphere causes discomfort, headache, and tiredness.

The humidity of the air is measured with the help of a hygrometer. This instrument depicts the percentage of water vapour in the air. It is a ratio between the amount of water vapour which air could hold and what it actually holds at the same temperature. Humidity of 60–70 per cent is considered normal and does not cause discomfort or undue spoilage of food.

Applications of humidity

1. Spoilage organisms multiply and spores germinate at high moisture levels in the atmosphere.
2. Humidity needs to be controlled in air-conditioned rooms along with ventilation and heating which is done by humidifier water sprays which maintain 60–70 per cent humidity.
3. Processed foods are prevented from drying up by adding substances with hygroscopic properties called humectants. Glycerine and sorbitol are used as humectants in jam.

FOOD RHEOLOGY

It is the science of measuring forces, which are needed to deform food materials or to study the flow properties of liquid foods. It deals with the viscous behaviour of a system.

Solid food can be chopped up, ground, minced, sliced, torn apart, or broken while it is being prepared or eaten. The texture is determined when we chew food and it is described as crisp, tough, chewy, creamy, sticky, spongy, etc.

Liquid foods are fluid or viscous. Viscosity is defined as the resistance of a liquid to flow. It is measured by an instrument called a viscometer. This property of a liquid is seen in batters, sauces, syrups, etc.

Compression   It is the pressure needed to squash foam or spongy foods to find out their freshness or tenderness. The compressimeter or tenderometer is used to measure the lightness of a product.

Adhesion   Adhesive gum-like properties give stickiness to food which sticks to the teeth when chewed, such as toffee. Breaking strength of dry foods, such as spaghetti, biscuits, and potato wafers, are measured by applying a load till the product breaks.

Shearing   It is the force needed to cut or slice through meat, vegetables, fruits, etc., and indicates the toughness of a food. Penetrometers measure the force needed to penetrate a food such as jelly, cooking fat, canned and fresh fruits, and vegetables.

Rigidity   It is the property of those substances which do not flow, e.g., baked custard and cake. Rigid substances show either elastic property or plastic property.

Elastic substances   These substances do not flow, but flow when force is applied. However, when the force is removed it regains its original shape, e.g., sponge cake.

Elasticity   It is the property which permits a substance to change its shape when a force is applied to it and to come back to its original shape once the force is removed, provided the force applied is within elastic limits.

Applications of elasticity

1. The stretching power of the dough can be tested before baking. The extensibility of flour is due to gluten formed in flour. Over kneading of dough results in decreased elasticity.
2. Dough improvers are chemicals added to improve or strengthen the elasticity of bread dough.
3. Addition of malt flour gives a softer-textured dough because of the enzymes present in malt.

Plastic substances   These substances resist flow to a certain point, but beyond that point they flow, i.e., they become plastic in nature.

Plasticity is an important property of margarine. A plastic fat is one which can be creamed as well as forms a thin sheet or layer in dough when the dough is rolled out, e.g., flaky pastry.

 SUMMARY

A knowledge of basic physical, chemical, and biological sciences is needed by all students studying catering. Today, the SI or International System of measurement is used universally for measuring matter. The unit for measuring length is the metre and for volume, it is the litre. Weight is measured in kilograms and may change from place to place because of the force of gravity or the pull of the earth. Density is the relationship between weight and volume of a substance while relative density is the mass of a known volume of a substance divided by the mass of the same volume of water. The hydrometer is used to measure the relative density of different liquids and is specifically calibrated to measure the relative density of different substances. The lactometer is used to test the purity of milk, the saccharometer is used to measure the concentration of sugar solutions, alcoholometers are used to check the degrees proof, and salinometers to check the relative density of brine.

Energy is present in many forms such as heat, solar, electrical, and chemical. Heat is measured in joules. Temperature is measured in degrees Farenheit and degrees Celsius, the potential hydrogen (pH) is used to express the degree of acidity or alkalinity of a food. A pH between 1 and 6.5 is acidic and above 7.5, it is basic or alkaline. Pure water has a pH of 7, which is neutral.

Buffers help in maintaining the pH of foods at a constant level.

Many other terminologies are relevant and need to be known and their applications understood by the caterers.

KEY TERMS

Acrolein   A substance formed when glycerol from fat is heated at high temperatures which is irritating to the eyes and the respiratory tract.

Hygroscopic   Readily absorbing water, such substances are used as drying agents, e.g., silica gel and calcium chloride.

Relative humidity   Method of measuring the moisture present in air relative to saturation at the same temperature.

Rendering   The process of removal of fat from the fat cells of adipose tissue of animals by dry heat method.

Silicone   Organic compounds of silicon used on non-sticking wrapping paper.

REVIEW EXERCISES

1. Define the following terms:
   (a) Viscosity
   (b) Osmosis
   (c) pH
   (d) Smoke point
   (e) Relative density
2. Give scientific reasons why:
   (a) Food takes longer time to get cooked at high altitudes
   (b) Fat used for deep fat frying should have a high smoke point
   (c) The weight of a substance changes when weighed in different parts of the world
   (d) Fresh eggs sink and stale eggs float in water
   (e) Small amount of citric acid is added while making jelly preserve.
3. List the main factors which affect the rate of evaporation.
4. What does surface tension mean? Give two examples to explain this term.
5. How would you determine the density of a bread roll?
6. Convert the following measurements:
   (a) 2200 kcal into kJ
   (b) 37°C into °F
   (c) 90°F into °C
   (d) 5 ft 6 inches into cm
   (e) 8 ozs into ml

CHAPTER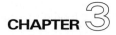

Colloidal Systems in Foods

LEARNING OBJECTIVES

After reading this chapter, you should be able to
- appreciate the importance of the physical quality of products as a caterer and as a consumer
- understand the close relationship between various processes and food quality
- define and differentiate between the various food systems
- understand the principles underlying these food systems
- know the factors which affect the stability of these systems
- appreciate the importance of these systems in obtaining high-quality products
- classify food into these systems

INTRODUCTION

Food served in catering establishments can be divided into two broad categories, namely intact edible tissues and food dispersions. Sliced pineapple, diced vegetables, and fish fillets are examples of intact tissues. However, most food preparations are subjected to different processes before they are brought to the table. Large masses of food may be subdivided into smaller particles by processes, such as mincing, grinding, pulping, and homogenizing, and ingredients may be mixed in different ways, such as beating, cutting and folding, blending, whipping, stirring, and emulsifying, converting the intact tissue into complex dispersions. The kind of process food is subjected to will have a bearing on the final quality of the product.

A well-baked cake, where ingredients have been mixed correctly and a heavy-collapsed cake may have the same chemical composition and nutritive value, but the latter will have no market because its physical qualities, i.e., its volume, texture, and appearance do not meet acceptable standards. These standards are of utmost importance to both the caterer and the consumer, and an understanding of the principles underlyling food dispersions is necessary for caterers to prepare high-quality products.

CONSTITUENTS OF FOOD

Apart from water, food is mainly composed of three main groups of constituents, namely carbohydrates, proteins, fats, and their derivatives. Along with these constituents, minerals, vitamins, organic acids, pigments, enzymes, flavouring substances, and other organic constituents are present in varying amounts in different foods. These constituents give food their structure, texture, colour, flavour, and nutritive value. To the caterer and consumer, the physical appearance is as significant as its chemical composition.

Foods are mixtures or dispersions of two or more types of substances. These substances are present as particles of various sizes. Depending on the particle size or size of the molecule in the mixture, these substances may be classified as a true solution, a colloidal dispersion, or a coarse suspension.

True Solution

It is composed of two parts: the solute which is the dissolved substance and the solvent which is the substance in which the solute is dissolved. In a true solution, ions or molecules smaller than one millimicron are dissolved in a liquid. They contain varying amounts of ions or molecules of dissolved substances depending on the temperature of the solvent and on the solute. Solutions may be unsaturated, saturated, or supersaturated. They have the smallest particle size of the three types of dispersions. A solution is homogenous, i.e., alike in all parts, e.g., sugar syrup and brine.

Suspension

Suspensions are dispersions of coarse particles in a liquid. The particles are large and require continuous agitation to keep them dispersed. When agitation ceases, these coarse suspended particles settle down because of force of gravity. When the mixture is stirred, the suspension is formed again. In a suspension, the particle size is larger than one micrometre or micron, e.g., starch and cold water paste. Many dispersions in food contain substances which are larger than one micron in size.

Colloidal Systems

Between the particle sizes of the solutions and those of suspensions, lies the area of colloidal systems. The particles are large enough to impart to the system some properties different from those found in true solutions, but small enough so that they do not separate out on standing. Colloidal systems deal with dispersions of a definite size, since it is the size of the particles in the colloidal range that impart the specific and characteristic properties to the system. Table 3.1 shows the size of dispersed particle based on the type of system.

TABLE 3.1 Size of dispersed particle

S. no.	Type of system	Size of particle
1.	True solution	Upto one millimicron
2.	Colloidal dispersion	One millimicron up to one micrometre
3.	Coarse suspension	More than one micrometre

Colloidal dispersions are characterized by particles ranging between one millimicron (0.001 μm) and 100 millimicrons (0.1 μm) with maximum size of up to one micrometre (μm) in diameter.

$$\text{One micrometre (micron) } (\mu m) = 10^{-3} \text{ mm or } 1/1{,}000 \text{ mm}$$
$$10^{-4} \text{ cm or}$$
$$10^{-6} \text{ m}$$
$$\text{One millimicron } (m\mu) = 10^{-3} \mu m \text{ or } 1/1{,}000 \mu m$$

There is no distinct line of demarcation. Particles approaching the limits of the size of one zone may show properties of two zones. For example, sugar exhibits both crystalloid and colloidal properties in food systems. The properties exhibited by colloidal particles around 1 mμ in size are different from those of particles around 0.1 μm in size, e.g., crystalline candies have an organized crystalline structure while amorphous candies such as fondant lack an organized crystalline structure.

The gluten particles of hydrated flour proteins have colloidal dimensions but gluten particles of cake and pastry flours are more dispersed or of smaller size than those of bread flours. This is one reason for the different results obtained in cakes when bread flour is used instead of cake flour.

All colloidal dispersions or colloidal systems have two phases: a continuous phase and a discontinuous or dispersed phase. The continuous phase extends throughout the system and surrounds the dispersed phase completely. Proteins, carbohydrates, and fats exist in foods as particles of colloidal dimensions. The system is a colloidal system as long as the particle size of the dispersed phase is within colloidal dimensions. Colloidal systems may be a combination of solid, liquid, or gas as the continuous or dispersed phase.

In food, the following colloidal systems are of importance.

1. *Sol* Colloidal dispersion of a solid dispersed in a liquid.
2. *Gel* Colloidal dispersion of a liquid dispersed in a solid.
3. *Emulsion* Colloidal dispersion of a liquid dispersed in a liquid.
4. *Foam* Colloidal dispersion of a gas dispersed in a liquid.
5. *Solid foam or suspensoid* Colloidal dispersion of a gas dispersed in a solid.

Dispersions may be simple or complex. In a simple dispersion, a colloid may consist of a solid dispersed in a liquid, e.g., when gelatin is dissolved in warm water, a simple dispersion called a sol is formed. Mayonnaise is an example of a complex dispersion since it is an emulsion, a sol, and a foam combined in one. Milk is another example of a complex dispersion, i.e., more than one phase is dispersed in a liquid. Milk is a solution of lactose in water, an emulsion of fat in water, and a sol as milk protein is dispersed in water.

Colloidal particles have different characteristics. Some are attracted to water and are called *hydrophilic* or water loving. They get hydrated easily. Others repel water and are called *hydrophobic* or water hating. These different characteristics are seen because of the difference in chemical composition of the compounds. In certain substances, a part of their structure is hydrophobic, while other parts are hydrophilic. Those parts or functional groups that are attracted to water are called *polar groups*. Examples of polar groups are the organic acid group or COOH group in proteins, the aldehyde or CHO group in carbohydrates, etc. *Non-polar* groups are hydrophobic, e.g., carbon chains, –C–C–C–C–, and cyclic structures, ⬡, which are seen in organic compounds.

Organic substances which have both polar and nonpolar groups are useful as emulsifying agents in food emulsions as part of their molecule is attracted towards the dispersed phase and part towards the continuous phase.

STABILITY OF COLLOIDAL SYSTEMS

The stability of a colloidal system depends on two factors.
1. The charge on the colloidal particle
2. A layer of water that is tightly bound to the molecule

Charge on the colloidal particle   As the surface charge on the colloidal particle is similar, like charges repel and the particles do not get attracted or join together. This helps in keeping the system stable. When the charge is neutralized, the colloidal particles flocculate and separate out.

Layer of water   Water is present in food in two distinct physical states: free water and bound water. Part of the water present in food which can act as a solvent is free water and has flow properties. The rest of the water is bound water which is closely combined with starch or protein by hydrogen bonding and influences the physical properties of food. Many colloidal systems are hydrophilic and attract a layer of water around them. The layer of water acts as an insulation and keep the colloidal system stable.

TYPES OF COLLOIDAL SYSTEMS IN FOOD

The type of colloidal systems in food (see Table 3.2) are discussed below.

Sol

In this system, solids of colloidal dimensions are dispersed throughout a liquid. Solids form the dispersed phase and liquids the continuous phase. The viscosity of sols may range from liquid, e.g., skim milk to extremely viscous, e.g., tomato ketchup which barely flows. The viscosity of the sol will depend on the concentration of solid and the temperature of the sol. The higher the concentration of solid in a sol, the more viscous the sol. The viscosity of a sol can be adjusted by adding more liquid.

TABLE 3.2 Types of colloidal systems in food

Name of colloidal system	Dispersed phase	Continuous phase	Examples
Sol	Solid	Liquid	Skimmed milk Soups Gravy Pouring custard
Gel	Liquid	Solid	Caramel custard Curd Jam Jelly
Emulsion	Liquid	Liquid	Butter Mayonnaise Salad dressing Whole milk
Foam	Gas	Liquid	Whipped egg white Whipped cream
Solid foam/ Suspensoid	Gas	Solid	Baked meringue Cake Fluffy omlette Set whipped gelatin
Aerosol	Solid	Gas	Smoke for flavouring

Irrespective of the viscosity, in a sol, the solid is always distributed throughout the sol and does not settle at the bottom. Protein in milk remains dispersed because of the like electrical charges on the surface of the protein molecule, which repel each other. When the charge on the dispersed protein molecules is neutralized by addition of acid, protein flocculates and separates out as is seen while preparing paneer.

Pectin remains dispersed because of its hydrophilic nature. It attracts a layer of water that is tightly bound to the pectin molecule by hydrogen bonding. All sols have flow properties. They flow more readily at higher temperatures than at a lower one. Sometimes a sol may change into a gel when the system is viscous and there is a drop in energy level, e.g., during cooling. The solids start associating with one another and form a three-dimensional meshwork in which the liquid is trapped. Milk, cream soups, pouring custard, béchamel sauce, and gravy are commonly used sols in the kitchen.

Gel

A gel is a colloidal system in which liquid forms the dispersed phase and solid forms the continuous phase. It is also called a reverse sol. A gel does not flow. Some of the liquid is adsorbed on the surface of the solid molecules and is called bound water. Because of this bound liquid, the gel has structure. The remaining liquid is trapped in the solid three-dimensional meshwork of the gel. As compared to a sol, the concentration of solid is higher in a gel.

A food gel consists of a continuous phase of interconnected particles or macromolecules in which liquid is dispersed. The rigidity, elasticity, and brittleness of the gel depends on the type and concentration of the solid or gelling agent, the pH, salt content, and temperature, e.g., pectin does not form a gel unless the pH is acidic.

The gelling agent may be a polysaccharide such as cornflour in blancmange, a protein such as albumin in caramel custard or complex colloidal particles such as calcium caseinate in curds. Gums, pectins, and gelatin can form gels even at low concentrations.

When a gel is stored for sometime or becomes stale, there is a reduction in gel volume. The liquid which was entrapped in the three-dimensional meshwork of the gel is expelled from the interstitial spaces and the gel shrinks. This condition is called syneresis or weeping gel. Syneresis is seen in baked custards, moulded desserts, and curds. Free liquid may also be released if the gel structure is cut, e.g., in curds, whey separates out when the set gel is cut or disturbed.

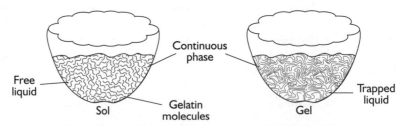

Fig. 3.1   In a gelatin sol, gelatin forms the dispersed phase.
On cooling, gelatin forms the continuous phase

Sols and gels are reverse colloidal systems and many can be changed from one type to another. Many gels are first sols which on cooling form gels provided the concentration of solids is adequate (see Fig. 3.1).

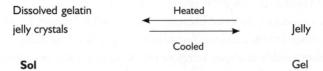

When a sol is converted into a gel, the energy levels fall. This is seen during the cooling process. The solids in the dispersed phase move with difficulty through the continuous phase and ultimately associate with one another by forming secondary bonds. When the dispersion is cold enough, permanent bonds form, which can hold the liquid in the solid meshwork. A gel is formed which differs from a sol because it is apparently solid and is capable of holding its shape when served.

Emulsion

An emulsion is a colloidal dispersion of tiny droplets of one liquid suspended in another. In this colloidal system, liquids form the dispersed as well as the continuous phase. One liquid is dispersed as droplets in another liquid. For an emulsion to form, agitation or shaking the two liquids is necessary till they are well mixed. Emulsions form only when the two liquids are immiscible in each other, e.g., oil and water. The liquid with the higher surface tension forms small droplets or the dispersed phase. When an emulsion is formed the dispersed liquid has a much larger surface area as compared to the two liquids as separate layers (see Fig. 3.2).

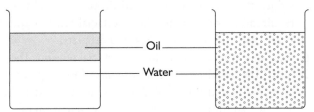

Fig. 3.2   Surface area of oil as a layer and as an emulsion
(note the increase in surface area)

Food emulsions are of two types:

1. Oil in water emulsion or O/W emulsion in which the droplets of oil are dispersed in water, e.g., mayonnaise and milk.
2. Water in oil emulsion or W/O emulsion in which droplets of water are dispersed in oil, e.g., margarine and butter.

Emulsions may also be classified on the basis of stability as follows:

1. Temporary emulsions, e.g., French dressing
2. Semi-permanent emulsions, e.g., milk
3. Permanent emulsions, e.g., mayonnaise, homogenized milk

An emulsion is more viscous than the liquids that form the emulsion. Vinegar and oil when seen individually are very fluid, but when they are agitated together to make the emulsion mayonnaise the mixture becomes viscous.

In a temporary emulsion, the droplets that form the dispersed phase tend to coalesce as they bump into one another and form larger droplets till the emulsion breaks or separates into oil and water.

In food emulsions, the water phase may also contain water-soluble constituents of milk, fruit juice, cooked starch paste, whole egg, vinegar, or lime juice as well as salts and other water-soluble compounds. The oil phase may contain a blend of different fats and oils and fat-soluble compounds.

Theory of emulsification

1. During the process of emulsification, the main step is to break down the bulk liquid into small droplets and then stabilize the emulsion.
2. In a stable emulsion, the droplets remain dispersed. Due to interfacial tension, there is a tendency for droplets to coalesce and separate out. The interfacial tension is lowered by the addition of emulsifiers. Emulsifiers are surface active agents which lower the interfacial tension, i.e., the tension at the interface of two immiscible liquids.

3. The dispersed droplets which are of colloidal dimensions tend to form spherical structures in the continuous phase.

4. To prepare a stable emulsion, it is necessary to reduce the size of the droplets, prevent their coalescing, and increase their surface area.

5. Mechanical aids, such as beaters, stirrers, homogenizers, and colloid mills, help to reduce the size of the dispersed droplets, thereby increasing surface area. Energy is required to work against the interfacial tension and allow the continuous phase to stretch out and cover the dispersed droplets.

6. Emulsifiers are used to reduce interfacial tension. They get adsorbed at the interface.

7. In an O/W emulsion, e.g., mayonnaise, the non-polar group of the emulsifier is oriented towards the oil droplet (salad oil) and is adsorbed in the outermost layer of the droplet. See Fig. 3.3 for the diagrammatic representation of the orientation of an emulsifying agent in an O/W emulsion.

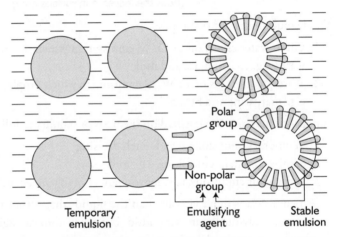

Fig. 3.3 Diagrammatic representation of orientation of emulsifying agent in an O/W emulsion

8. The polar group of the emulsifier is oriented towards the continuous phase of water (vinegar, lime juice, water from egg) surrounding the oil droplet.

9. The molecules of emulsifier surround the droplet completely forming a monomolecular layer of emulsifier (lecithin) around the droplet.

10. The oil droplet is thus protected by a film consisting of three layers, namely
    (a) the outermost layer of oil molecules
    (b) a layer of emulsifier
    (c) the innermost layer of water
    This protective film/layer prevents two oil droplets from coalescing when they collide.

11. Emulsions are further stabilized by the electric charge.

12. The ingredients used should not be chilled. Warm ingredients emulsify sooner as they are more fluid and spread or split into droplets faster.

13. The consistency of an emulsion ranges from liquid to a plastic solid.

Stability of an emulsion

The stability of an emulsion depends on the following factors:

1. The presence and type of emulsifying agent present
2. The amount or concentration of the emulsifying agent
3. The size of the droplets in dispersed phase
4. The ratio of oil and water used
5. The viscosity of the continuous phase

The presence and type of emulsifying agent present   The most important factor which determines the stability of an emulsion is the presence of an emulsifying agent. The emulsifying agent may be present naturally in one of the ingredients, e.g., lecithin is a natural emulsifying agent present in egg yolk or the emulsifying agent may be added to the emulsion.

An emulsifying agent is a compound containing both polar and non-polar groups and is thus attracted to both phases of the emulsion at the interface. The polar groups are oriented towards the water phase and the non-polar groups pull the molecule of the emulsifying agent towards oil. The emulsifier forms a layer at the interface which coats the surfaces of the dispersed droplet completely.

The droplets do not touch each other and coalesce because of the protective layer of the emulsifying agent. The emulsion formed becomes stable and does not separate out into two separate layers because of the presence of the emulsifying agent.

The type of emulsion formed will also depend on the emulsifying agent used, and whether the polar or non-polar group on the emulsifying agent is stronger.

If the non-polar group is stronger, the emulsifying agent is more strongly attracted to oil. The surface tension of oil is reduced and water will form droplets or the dispersed phase. The emulsion formed will be a W/O type of emulsion.

The amount or concentration of the emulsifying agent   The amount of emulsifier present in the emulsion should be sufficient to coat the dispersed droplets completely. The emulsifier forms a layer at the interface, which is monomolecular in thickness. The droplets do not touch each other and coalesce because of the protective layer of emulsifying agent around each droplet. Addition of extra emulsifying agent does not have any beneficial effects. If the emulsifier is insufficient, all droplets will not be coated or protected and stability of the emulsion is affected.

The size of the droplets in dispersed phase   Mechanical aids, such as beaters, homogenizers, and colloid mills, help to reduce the size of the droplets dispersed, i.e., increase their surface area. The smaller the size of the dispersed droplets, the more stable the emulsion. A large droplet represents a lower energy state than two small droplets and has less stability. Homogenized milk is a stable emulsion as the size of the fat droplets are reduced.

The ratio of oil and water used   The ratio of oil and water used or the ratio of dispersed phase to the continuous phase is important. The continuous phase should stretch out and cover the dispersed droplets completely. For this, proper mixing, shaking, or beating of the emulsion is necessary.

The viscosity of the continuous phase   The viscosity of the continuous phase is an important factor. A viscous continuous phase will prevent the droplets of the dispersed phase from moving freely, bumping into one another, and coalescing.

Substances that increase the viscosity of a colloidal system are called stabilizers. They do not orient themselves at the interface as an emulsifier, but reduce the speed with which the dispersed droplets move. As viscosity increases, the collision between droplets decreases and the droplets remain dispersed for a fairly long time. Examples of stabilizer are starch, sugar, gelatin, gums, finely powered spices, carboxy methyl cellulose, sodium alginate, pectin, etc. The addition of stabilizer alone is not enough to prevent the breakage of an emulsion.

Temporary emulsions have very little emulsifying agent or stabilizer present and are fluid systems. The dispersed droplets move and bump into one another and coalesce. This emulsion separates out on standing in a short while.

Formation of stable emulsions is of utmost importance in the food industry. A broken emulsion loses its viscosity, cannot be spread, and gives the product an unappetizing curdled appearance. Broken emulsions affect the texture and consistency of the final product.

Sometimes stable or permanent emulsions may break due to high changes in temperature like heating and freezing, e.g., Hollandaise sauce curdles at high temperatures and mayonnaise may break if frozen due to ice crystal formation.

Egg yolk contains a phospholipid lecithin which is a good emulsifying agent and forms O/W emulsions. Lecithin contains fatty acids as the hydrophobic group, and phosphate and choline as the hydrophilic group. Caseinogen, a protein found in milk acts as a natural emulsifying agent. Glycerly monostearate (GMS) is added as an emulsifier in ice creams. Mayonnaise is a stable emulsion because of lecithin in the egg yolk.

The most widely used natural emulsifiers are lecithins present in egg yolk and extracted from soya beans, which is more economical.

Synthetic food emulsifiers most commonly used are mono- and diglycerides. A common example is glyceryl monostearate or GMS. Mono- and diglycerides have one or two fatty acids attached to glycerol. The free groups of glycerol are hydrophilic, while fatty acids are hydrophobic giving good emulsifying properties.

Some of the other emulsifying agents are stearyl tartarate, lactic acid monoglyceride, polyoxyethylene monostearate, etc.

Some common food emulsions

1. *Milk and cream*   O/W emulsion stabilized by phospholipids and protein caseinogen
2. *Butter and margarine*   W/O emulsion containing approximately 80 per cent fat. Butter is stabilized by caseinogen and margarine is stabilized by GMS

3. *Egg yolk* O/W emulsion. It is a good emulsifier as it contains lecithin
4. *Hollandaise sauce* O/W emulsion stabilized by egg yolk
5. *Salad dressings*
    (a) *Mayonnaise* O/W emulsion stabilized by egg yolk. Not less than 65 per cent oil by weight. Synthetic emulsifiers may be added like mono- and diglycerides of fatty acids, e.g., GMS.
    (b) *French dressing* O/W emulsion may be temporary or permanent emulsion
6. *Gravies, sauces, cream soups* O/W emulsions contain high percentage of water stabilized with refined flour
7. *Choux pastry* O/W emulsion stabilized by egg
8. *Batters* O/W emulsion stabilized by flour and egg
9. *Ice cream* O/W emulsion stabilized by caseinogen, GMS, alginates, gums/ gelatin.

Foams   A foam is a dispersion of gas bubbles in a liquid or semi-solid phase. In this colloidal dispersion, gas forms the dispersed phase and liquid is the continuous phase. Foams are of two types:

1. Gas in liquid
2. Gas in solid

In food systems, the continuous phase is usually a liquid with added solids or changed to a solid by heating, e.g., beaten egg white and sugar foam is a gas in liquid dispersion. When it is baked, it becomes a gas in solid dispersion, e.g., meringue.

The liquid or semi-solid walls are elastic in stable foams and separate the gas bubbles from each other. The gas bubbles range in size from 1 μm to several centimetres.

To form a foam, energy is required to overcome the surface tension of the liquid and stretch it into thin films, which surround bubbles of gas. Liquids which form foams easily have a low vapour pressure and low surface tension.

The presence of solid matter increases the stability of a foam. When egg white, cream, or gelatin is whipped into a foam, the protein which collects at the air–water interface gets denatured or coagulated by the energy used for whipping and helps in making the foam stable.

Whipped cream forms stable foam because of the following reasons.

1. Proteins get denatured and become firmer.
2. Butter fat and other milk solids present in cream increase the viscosity giving the foam a fine texture.
3. Cream which has been aged is more concentrated and gives a better foam.

In homogenized cream, the fat is split into very fine particles, reducing its whipping properties. For a stable light textured foam of good volume, adequate mechanical agitation is necessary. At the same time, care should be taken to avoid over beating or converting cream into butter.

Foams used in cookery include egg white, egg yolk, gelatin, and cream. They contribute towards lightness, volume, and texture of the product.

The caterer should understand that most of the food materials which are used or prepared in the kitchen are a combination of various colloidal systems. Since the colloidal state depends on particle size, it is important to understand the methods and ingredients used in food preparation that influence degree of dispersion.

1. Mechanical stress to which food has been subjected to before and during production, such as grinding, beating, and homogenizing, affects dispersion. Grinding of cereals, stirring of custard to prevent clumping, and beating of curdled custards reduces the size of the particles and increases dispersion. Homogenization of milk is a mechanical means of increasing the dispersion of fat globules.

2. Increasing the temperature may bring about greater or lesser dispersion. When milk is heated, dispersion of fat globules in milk increases. When proteins are heated, coagulation takes place, which decreases the degree of dispersion.

3. The addition of acid to milk causes casein to clot and decreases the dispersion. Alkalies bring about greater dispersion of cellulose and pectin in fruits and vegetables during cooking, making them mushy.

4. Amount of water present or the concentration of solids in a sol or gel influences gel formation. If water is present in excess, it will increase dispersion and prevent setting.

5. Enzymes may cause increased or decreased dispersion of foods. The proteinase enzyme in flour increases the dispersion of gluten. Clotting of milk on addition of rennin is an example of decreased dispersion of protein.

Milk, butter, margarine, cream, curd, doughs and butters, soufflés and desserts, soups, sauces and gravies, etc., are all examples of colloidal systems. Many of these are multiphase food systems, which have two or more discontinuous phases dispersed in a continuous phase.

SUMMARY

Food products are generally multiphase systems in which solids, liquids, and gases are finely distributed during manufacture to give the finished product the desired structure and quality. The physical qualities in terms of volume, texture, appearance, and stability are as important as the chemical constituents present in food. The basic principles underlying food dispersions must be understood by the caterer to prepare high-quality products.

Each type of processing or method of mixing and the ingredients used affect the quality of the finished product. Apart from intact tissues of food, the caterer has to deal with solutions, suspensions, and colloidal dispersions, such as sols, gels, emulsions, and foams, which are of colloidal dimensions. These systems impart special characteristics to food.

Colloidal systems are stabilized by the charge on the surface of the colloidal particles which being alike, keeps the molecules apart. Hydrophilic colloids are stabilized by a layer of water which is adsorbed on the surface of the colloidal particles, preventing attraction between colloids.

Sols, gels, emulsions, and foams are common food systems which the caterer has to prepare. Very often, more than a single system is encountered in foods. Many factors affect the degree of dispersion in these systems such as mechanical agitation, heat, water, enzymes, and pH.

KEY TERMS

Bound water   Water that is bound to other substances and can no longer flow or act as solvent.

Colloidal dispersion   A two-phase system which has particles of 0.001 μm and 1 μm dispersed in the continuous phase.

Emulsifying agent   A compound which stabilizes an emulsion by orienting itself at the interface of the two phases of an emulsion. An emulsifying agent contains both polar and non-polar groups in its molecule.

Gums   Complex carbohydrate of plant origin made up of galactose and other sugars or sugar derivatives.

Homogenization   A mechanical process in which milk is forced through tiny apertures under pressure so that fat globules are reduced in size and do not separate out as cream.

Immiscible   That which cannot be mixed together.

Interfacial tension   The difference between the attractive forces acting on the molecules within the two liquids.

Lecithin   Phospholipid present in egg yolk which is an effective emulsifying agent and is commercially obtained from soya bean.

Permanent emulsion   An emulsion containing adequate emulsifying agent so that it remains intact during normal handling.

pH   The measure of the acidity or alkalinity of a substance.

Rennin   An enzyme from calves' stomach that forms a curd when added to milk.

Stabilizer   A substance which prevents an emulsion from breaking by increasing the viscosity of the continuous phase and preventing coalescing of droplets in dispersed phase.

Supersaturated solution   True solution containing more solute than can be normally dissolved at that temperature.

Surface tension   Attraction between molecules at the surface of a liquid.

Syneresis   Oozing of liquid from a gel when cut or allowed to stand.

Temporary emulsion   A fluid emulsion which has very little emulsifying agent and separates out into two distinct layers when agitation ceases.

Vapour pressure   Pressure exerted as molecules of a liquid attempt to escape and vapourize.

REVIEW EXERCISES

1. How does an emulsifying agent stabilize an emulsion? Explain briefly.
2. What is the main difference between a solution, colloidal dispersion, and a suspension?
3. Explain the following terms:
   (a) Reverse sol   (d) Suspensoid
   (b) Osmosis   (e) Aerosal
   (c) Stabilizer

4. What is a foam? Which food constituent helps in strengthening and stabilizing a foam? Explain giving suitable examples.
5. Explain the four main colloidal systems prominent in food, stating the phases and giving relevant examples for each.
6. Classify food emulsions and name the natural emulsifying agent present in mayonnaise.

Fill in the blanks

1. Foams contribute to the _____ and texture of many food products.

2. The formation and stability of a foam depend on the _____ and _____ of the liquid being whipped.

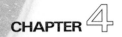

Carbohydrates

LEARNING OBJECTIVES

After reading this chapter, you should be able to
- describe the chemical nature of carbohydrates
- classify carbohydrates and know their sources
- understand the structure and functions of different carbohydrates in processed foods
- know the changes that take place when heat is applied to starch mixtures
- learn more about cereals and cereal products
- distinguish between sugars and non-nutritive sweeteners
- understand factors which affect the texture and consistency of starch-based products
- appreciate the role of carbohydrates in the food industry

INTRODUCTION

Food is composed of three main constituents, namely carbohydrates, proteins, and fats and their derivatives. In addition to these constituents, inorganic mineral elements and diverse organic compounds, such as vitamins, pigments, flavouring compounds, enzymes, and acids, are also present. The percentage of water is large in certain foods. The variation in structure, texture, colour, flavour, and nutritive value is because of the varying proportions and arrangements of these constituents.

A knowledge of these constituents, their properties, and reactions with other constituents is necessary for a person who processes, serves, and stores food.

Carbohydrates are present in various forms in the food we cook, and processed food which we purchase and form the bulk of our diet. They are available in the market in the natural form, processed form, or modified form as an additive in many different products.

Before we study the types of carbohydrates, it is necessary to understand their basic structure.

Definition   Carbohydrates are polyhydroxy aldehydes or polyhydroxy ketones, or substances that yield such compounds on hydrolysis. Carbohydrates are organic compounds made up of carbon, hydrogen, and oxygen. They are called carbohydrates because hydrogen and oxygen are present in the same proportion as found in water, i.e., 2:1.

$$C_6H_{12}O_6 \qquad C_{12}H_{22}O_{11} \qquad (C_6H_{10}O_5)_n$$

Glucose Table sugar Starch

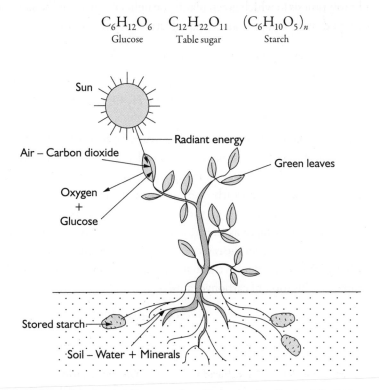

The glucose formed is converted into starch and stored as food in the following parts of the plant

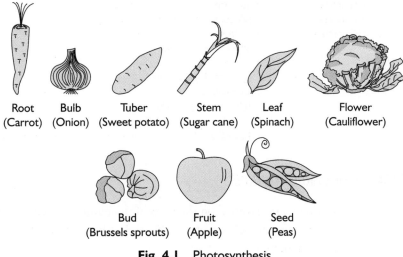

Root	Bulb	Tuber	Stem	Leaf	Flower
(Carrot)	(Onion)	(Sweet potato)	(Sugar cane)	(Spinach)	(Cauliflower)

Bud
(Brussels sprouts)

Fruit
(Apple)

Seed
(Peas)

Fig. 4.1 Photosynthesis

The chlorophyll present in plants can harness the light energy from the sun and convert it to chemical energy (Fig. 4.1). This is accomplished by a complex process known as photosynthesis in which green plants use light energy from the sun, water from the soil, and carbon dioxide from the air to manufacture carbohydrates.

$$6CO_2 + 6H_2O + \underset{\text{(from sunlight)}}{\text{Energy}} \xrightarrow{\text{chlorophyll}} \underset{\substack{\text{Glucose} \\ \text{(chemical energy)}}}{C_6H_{12}O_6} + 6O_2$$

$$\underset{\text{Glucose}}{nC_6H_{12}O_6} \xrightarrow{\text{green plants}} \underset{\text{Starch}}{(C_6H_{10}O_5)_n} + nH_2O$$

Glucose cannot be stored on a large scale. So it is converted to starch with the removal of water and stored in various parts of the plant. In cereal grains and potatoes, carbohydrate is stored as starch. In bananas, mango, and sugar beets, it is stored as sugar. Tender green peas and maize contain carbohydrate in the form of sugar, which is converted to starch as the seeds mature. However, the reverse is seen in fruits. Immature fruits contain starch, which changes to sugar as the fruit ripens. Irrespective of the form in which it is stored, carbohydrates represent the reserve energy for the plant. The various parts of the plant where carbohydrate is stored form the main source of carbohydrate in diet. Figure 4.2 discusses the simple classification of carbohydrates.

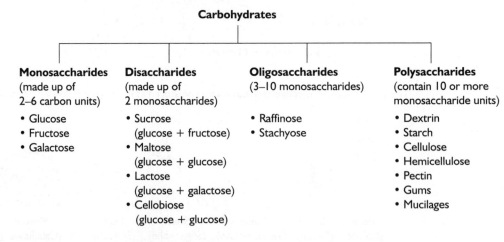

Fig. 4.2   Simple classification of carbohydrates

CLASSIFICATION OF CARBOHYDRATES

Carbohydrates are classified on the basis of the number of sugar units or saccharide units, which are present in their structures (Fig. 4.3). Only natural carbohydrates of significance have been elaborated.

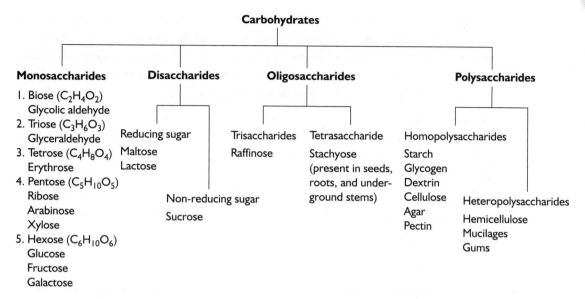

Fig. 4.3 Classification of carbohydrates based on saccharide or sugar units

Monosaccharides

These are the simplest forms of carbohydrates found in nature. Three monosaccharides are of importance in human nutrition. They are glucose, fructose, and galactose. These simple sugars are made up of a six-carbon chain or ring to which hydrogen and hydroxyl (OH) groups are attached. All hexoses contain the same number and kinds of atoms and have the formula $C_6H_{12}O_6$. They differ from one another because of the arrangement of different atoms around the carbon chain. Because of the difference in structure, they have different properties and vary in their degree of sweetness. These are the chemical building blocks or units from which all other carbohydrates are built.

Glucose   It is the most important of all the monosaccharides as it is the primary carbohydrate used by the body. Glucose is the sugar which is absorbed into the blood stream after carbohydrates are digested in the body. It is also known as dextrose. Glucose is available in powder and liquid form.

Fructose   It is the sweetest of all sugars and is also known as fruit sugar because it is found in fruits and honey. In the human body, it is converted to glucose and oxidized as a source of energy. It is also called levulose.

Galactose   It is found in combination with glucose in the disaccharide lactose in milk. This sugar is converted to glucose in the human body.

Disaccharides

These are double sugars composed of two monosaccharides linked together with the removal of a molecule of water. The disaccharides which are of importance in the diet are sucrose, maltose, and lactose. Their general formula is $C_{12}H_{22}O_{11}$.

Sucrose   Sucrose is the name given to the sugar which we use daily. It is prepared from sugar cane and sugar beet. It is the most common of all the disaccharides. It is present in some fruits and vegetables, and forms a substantial part of the diet of children and adults because of the increase in consumption of junk foods, processed foods, and fast foods. Sucrose is made up of one unit of glucose and one unit of fructose.

Lactose   It is the sugar present in milk. It is made up of one unit of glucose and one unit of galactose. It is the least sweet of all the sugars and is easily fermented to lactic acid by lactic acid bacteria while preparing curds and cheese. Lactic acid, which is formed from lactose, helps in setting curds and curdling milk.

Maltose   It is formed when whole grains are sprouted and in the commercial preparation of malt from starch. In the body, maltose is formed during digestion of starch. It is composed of two units of glucose.

Oligosaccharides

They are composed of three to ten monosaccharide units linked to each other by the removal of a molecule of water. They are not as common in food as the mono-, di-, and polysaccharides, but are formed during breakdown of starch into simpler sugars, e.g., raffinose and stachyose. They are present in pulses.

Polysaccharides

These are complex carbohydrates made up of 100–2,000 glucose units linked to each other in a chain or branched form. The number of glucose units, their arrangement, and linkage to one another influence the properties of the polysaccharides.

Starches   They form approximately half the dietary carbohydrates which are consumed. They are present in abundance in cereals, pulses, tapioca, *sago*, roots, and tubers.

Glycogen   This is also called animal starch as it is the form in which the animal body stores carbohydrates as a reserve source of energy. One-third of the glycogen is stored in the liver and two-thirds is stored in the muscles. Approximately 340 g of glycogen is stored in the body. This store is sufficient to meet the energy needs for less than a day. However, animal liver or muscle is not a source of glycogen in the diet as it is immediately converted to lactic acid when the animal is slaughtered.

Dextrin   This is formed in the first stage of starch breakdown either by enzymes during digestion, or by the action of dry heat on starch during toasting bread or browning flour. The very long chains of starch are split into shorter chains called dextrins. Dextrin is sweeter and more soluble than starch. This is the reason why bread or chapatti tastes sweeter when it is chewed for a longer time.

Dietary fibres   They are made up of many glucose units. The structure of cellulose differs from starch because the glucose units in cellulose form a different linkage as compared to starch.

STRUCTURE OF CARBOHYDRATES

The structure of carbohydrates can be represented in two ways:

1. A cyclic or ring structure
2. A three-dimensional structure.

Figure 4.4 discusses the formation of disaccharide sucrose with the elemination of a molecule of water.

Cyclic or ring structure

A six-membered ring of glucose

A five-membered ring of fructose

$-H_2O$

Sucrose

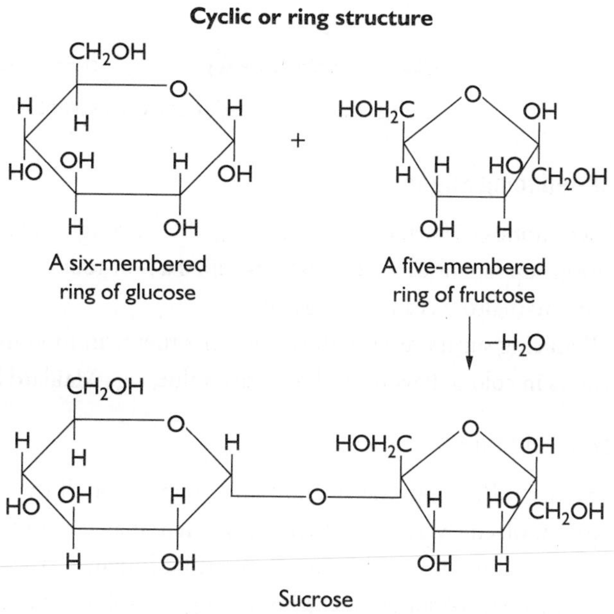

Fig. 4.4 Formation of disaccharide sucrose with the elimination of a molecule of water

Reducing Sugars

They are sugars that possess free aldehyde or ketone groups (Fig. 4.5). All monosaccharides are reducing sugars.

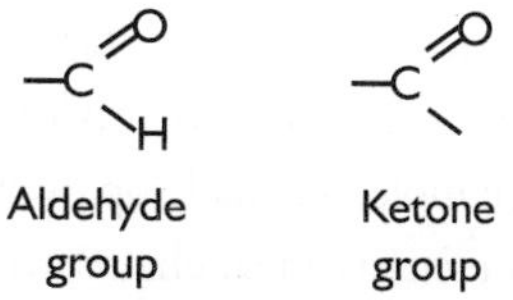

Aldehyde group

Ketone group

Fig. 4.5 Aldehyde and ketone groups

See Fig. 4.6 for the three-dimensional structure of sugars.

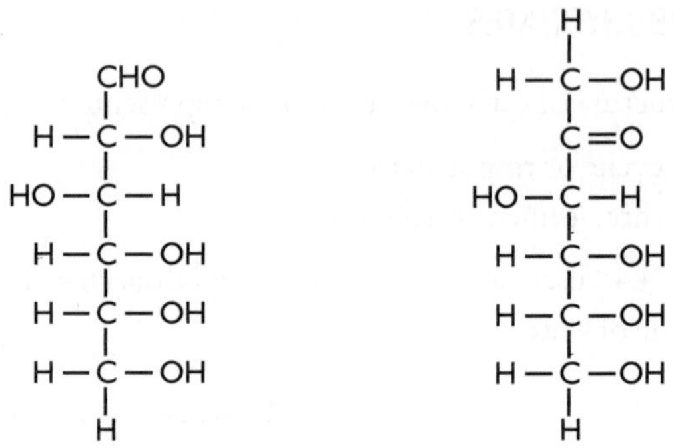

$$
\begin{array}{cc}
\text{CHO} & \text{H} \\
| & | \\
\text{H—C—OH} & \text{H—C—OH} \\
| & | \\
\text{HO—C—H} & \text{C=O} \\
| & | \\
\text{H—C—OH} & \text{HO—C—H} \\
| & | \\
\text{H—C—OH} & \text{H—C—OH} \\
| & | \\
\text{H—C—OH} & \text{H—C—OH} \\
| & | \\
\text{H} & \text{H} \\
\text{D-Glucose, an aldehyde sugar} & \text{D-Fructose, a ketone sugar}
\end{array}
$$

Fig. 4.6   Three-dimensional structures of sugars

Non-reducing Sugar

When monosaccharides are linked together through their aldehyde or ketone group and these groups are not free, the sugar is called a non-reducing sugar. Sucrose is a non-reducing sugar and maltose is a reducing sugar.

Reducing sugars react with other constituents in food like amino acids and bring about changes in colour, flavour, and nutritive value, e.g., Maillard browning (refer Chapter 9).

Polysaccharides

Dextrins   These are the smallest and simplest of all the polysaccharides. The size of the dextrin molecule varies widely, but it is much smaller than that of starch. They are composed of glucose units linked by 1,4-a-glucosidic linkages. They are formed by dry heating or acid hydrolysis of starch. Dextrins are slightly soluble, have a mild sweet taste, and limited thickening ability.

Some important polysaccharides in food are made up of only glucose units linked together by α or β glucosidic linkages.

Starch

Starch is found in most parts of a plant as a reserve store of carbohydrate. It is usually present in the seed and root in large amounts. Cereals contain approximately 70 per cent, pulses 60 per cent, and potatoes 22 per cent starch. Starch consists of long chains of glucose units present in two forms: amylose and amylopectin.

Amylose is a large molecule made up of 200 or more glucose units linked by 1,4-α-glucosidic linkages. They are present as linear chains, which can bond to each other by hydrogen bonds and form a gel. Amylose does not have a sweet taste, is slightly soluble, has good thickening ability, and represents 20–30 per cent of the total starch in most grains. The glucose units in amylose are linked to each other by elimination of a molecule of water at each linkage. Starches from various sources differ in their amylose content.

Amylopectin, like amylose, is made up of glucose units only (see Fig. 4.7). Two types of linkages are seen in amylopectin — 1,4-α-glucosidic linkages as in amylose and occassional 1,6-α-glucosidic linkages, resulting in a very large branched polysaccharide. The 1,4 linkages form a straight chain of 15–30 glucose units after which a 1,6 linkage occurs resulting in cross-linking and a complex branched structure. The molecules of amylopectin is very large, and because of its branched structure is sparingly soluble, not sweet, and is the predominant form in the starch granule with low gelling ability.

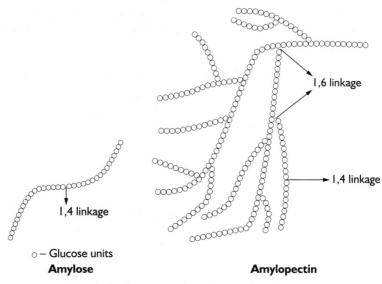

Fig. 4.7   Structure of amylose and amylopectin

See Table 4.1 for the difference between amylose and amylopectin.

Table 4.1   Difference between amylose and amylopectin

Amylose	Amylopectin
1. It is a linear polymer, which contains glucose units in α 1,4 linkages	1. It is a branched polymer of glucose units in α 1,4 and α 1,6 linkages
2. Molecular weight is less than amylopectin	2. Molecular weight is four times that of amylose
3. Good thickening power	3. Lesser thickening power as compared to amylose
4. Capable of forming gels because of linear form	4. No gel formation because of branched structure

The relative proportion of amylose and amylopectin in starches are of considerable importance because both forms have different behaviour in cooked starch products.

As glucose produced during photosynthesis is bulky, it is condensed to form starch, which is more concentrated. This starch is deposited in an orderly manner in the form of granules.

The starch granules are made in the leucoplasts within the cytoplasm of the cell. Each granule is made up of concentric layers of amylopectin molecules interspersed with amylose molecules. Amylose and amylopectin molecules are deposited as tightly coiled polymer chains in the starch granule in an organized manner.

Starch granules are densely packed with amylose and amylopectin. Each type of starch has a characteristic shape by which it can be microscopically identified (Table 4.2). The size varies from a few microns to 100 microns.

TABLE 4.2 Characteristic shape and size of starch granules

S. no.	Starch	Description	Granule
1	Potato	Large granules shaped like mussel shells	
2	*Sago*	Large elliptical granules	
3	Wheat	Mixture of large dish shaped + small granules	
4	Corn	Polygonal cells	
5	Tapioca	Small round or oval granules	
6	Oats	Small oval granules	
7	Rice	Very small polygonal granules	

Tapioca, the root starch from cassava, has small round or oval granules.

Sago starch granules are elliptical in shape and larger than potato starch granules. Potato starch granules are large and shaped like mussel shells.

Corn starch granules are polygonal in shape.

Wheat starch has two types of granules: small spherical granules and large disk-shaped granules.

Rice starch granules are polygonal in shape but very small in size.

Cereal starches, such as that of corn, rice, wheat, oats, *sago*, and tapioca are used as thickening and gelling agents. Genetic research and plant breeding have enabled us to develop starches containing 100 per cent amylopectin. These starches are called waxy starch and they do not form a gel. Starch with high amylose has also been developed. Such starches form hydrogen bonds very easily because of amylose and are used to make thin edible films to wrap candies. Figure 4.8 classifies various types of starches.

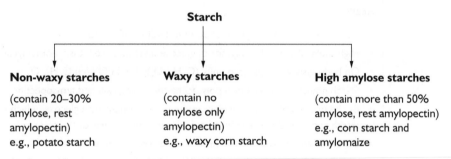

Fig. 4.8   Classification of starches

The Starch Granule

- Starch is stored as granules within leucoplasts in plant cells.
- Each type of starch has different shapes and sizes of granules.
- Amylose and amylopectin are closely packed in an orderly manner in the granule in two regions.
- The amorphous region contains mostly amylopectin arranged randomly.
- In the crystalline region, both amylose and amylopectin are arranged in a definite manner.
- Crystalline and amorphous areas alternate with each other.

Figure 4.9 provides a diagrammatic arrangement of amylose and amylopectin in a starch granule.

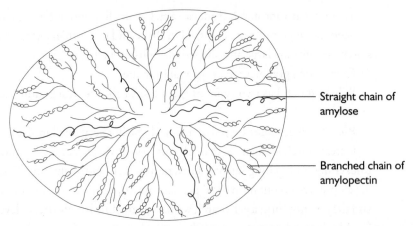

Straight chain of amylose

Branched chain of amylopectin

Fig. 4.9   Diagrammatic arrangement of amylose and amylopectin in a starch granule

---

Starch

- General formula $(C_6H_{10}O_5)_n$ value of n is 400–4,000 units
- High molecular weight polymer of glucose units only, i.e., it is a homoglycan
- On hydrolysis yields glucose units $(C_6H_{10}O_5)_n + n\,H_2O \rightarrow n\,C_6H_{12}O_6$
- Starch granules contains two polysaccharides—amylose and amylopectin
- By the process of photosynthesis, green plants manufacture glucose, which is converted to starch and stored in the form of granules in various parts of the plant
- Starch is present as granules within leucoplasts in plant cells.

Effect of cooking on starch

Gelatinization and viscosity   When starch granules are mixed with cold water, they do not dissolve, but form a suspension. When the water is heated, the granules begin to swell. The heat energy breaks the hydrogen bonds in the starch granules and facilitates the entry of water into the granules (Fig. 4.10). At the same time, some amylose from the granule leaches into the cooking water. The temperature at which the granules swell is called the gelatinization temperature and is characteristic for each starch.

The starch chains in the granules absorb moisture and begin to uncoil from their tightly packed configuration. The size of the granule increases as more and more water enters. The water in the granule gets bonded to amylose and amylopectin. The mixture becomes viscous and translucent after continuous heating. The increase in viscosity is due to the water bonded to starch and increase in size of starch granule as well as reduction in free water in the mixture. Swollen grains find it difficult to move past each other, adding to the viscosity of the mixture. This process of swelling of the starch grains and formation of viscous starch pastes is called gelatinization.

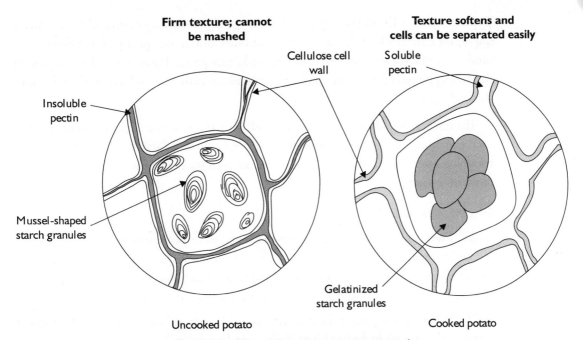

Fig. 4.10   Effect of cooking on potato starch

Factors which affect the property of starch as a thickening agent

Mixing and stirring   When starch is used as a thickening agent in soups or custards, it should be dispersed completely to prevent unequal swelling or lumps forming in a starch thickened product. This can be achieved by either of the following methods:

1. Mixing well with a cold liquid
2. Mixing with melted fat to coat starch particles
3. Mixing with another dry ingredient

Once the starch is dispersed, continuous stirring is necessary till gelatinization is complete. Stirring of hot starch pastes prevents lumps and sticking of gelatinized starch to the sides and bottom of the pan. Excessive stirring of the starch paste can break the starch granules, releasing amylose and amylopectin into the liquid resulting in a less viscous product.

Temperature   Starch pastes gradually thicken with increase in temperature from 52°C to 65°C. The starch granules continue to swell and amylose leaches out of the granule. Shorter amylose molecules have more solubility. As the temperature approaches 90–100°C, some granules may burst and fragment.

Continuous heating decreases the viscosity of starches as granules which reach their maximum volume implode and result in thinning of starch pastes. When cool, it may thicken again.

Type of starch   The thickening ability, texture, and translucency during gelatinization are important criteria which determine the palatability and overall quality of starch-thickened products. Different starches have different thickening power. Potato starch has the greatest thickening power, followed by waxy starches, tapioca, corn, rice, and wheat which has least thickening power.

The texture should ideally be smooth and not stringy or mucilaginous. Root starches, such as tapioca and potato, are more mucilaginous than cereal starches. They are also more translucent when gelatinized. Of all the starches, corn starch is the best thickening agent in terms of texture.

Effect of added ingredients

Sugar   When sugar is added to a starch-thickened paste, because of its hygroscopic nature it competes with starch for water needed for gelatinization. Gelatinization temperature is higher when sugar is an added ingredient and time taken for gelatinization is longer. Sugar reduces the viscosity and strength of the gel. It increases translucency.

Acid   When starch paste is heated with an acid, such as lime juice, at a pH below 4, starch molecules are hydrolysed into slightly smaller molecules. Acid hydrolysis results in thinning of the starch paste as smaller molecules move freely in the paste. If acid is added after gelatinization of starch, the paste does not turn thin.

Fats   The presence of fat in starch-thickened pastes lowers the gelatinization and thickening temperature.

Milk proteins   Gelatinization temperature is lowered if milk is an added ingredient.

GELATION

Gelatinized starch mixtures may exhibit flow properties and remain a sol or may cool and set to form a gel. The amylose, which has leached out of the swollen starch granule, forms hydrogen bonds with other amylose molecules as the starch paste cools and loses energy. Amylose molecules move slowly forming bonds and a three-dimensional continuous network of amylose is formed in which swollen granules are trapped. This forms the continuous phase of the newly formed starch gel in which water is dispersed. The starch mixture is transformed into a gel and no longer exhibits flow properties.

Following are the factors affecting gelation:

1. Type of starch
2. Concentration of starch
3. Duration of heating
4. Stirring
5. Other ingredients
6. Aging of gel

Type of Starch

The proportion of amylose and amylopectin in the starch determines whether a gel will form and whether it will be permanent. The straight chains of amylose form bonds easily, while the branches of amylopectin come in the way and prevent the formation of a firm gel. Starches rich in amylose can form gels at low concentrations, while starches lacking amylose, e.g., waxy starches, can form soft gels at high concentrations.

Wheat and rice flours are good thickening agents but poor gelling agents. Arrowroot starch forms a soft gel, while potato and tapioca starches do not have a tendency to gel. Corn flour forms a stiff gel but retrogrades when frozen. Chemically modified starches form stable gels.

Concentration of Starch

Corn starch forms a firm gel at 10 per cent concentration, while waxy starches which lack amylose can form a soft gel at 30 per cent concentration. Starches containing large amounts of amylose will gel at low concentrations.

- 1 tbsp starch in 1 cup liquid—thin sauce
- 2 tbsps starch in 1 cup liquid—medium consistency
- 3 tbsps starch in 1 cup liquid—thick sauce

Browning of flour results in dextrinization with lessened thickening ability.

Duration of Heating

When starch is heated along with water, the hydrogen bonds in the starch granule break and amylose fraction of starch leaches into the surrounding water. A starch paste should be heated gradually for granules to swell and release sufficient amylose to form a gel. Prolonged heating results in fragmentation of amylose and formation of a weak gel with a pasty texture.

Stirring

Vigorous stirring during heating results in fragmentation of amylose. A firm gel forms when the paste is allowed to cool undisturbed. Amylose starts forming bonds as the mixture cools and starts gelling. Stirring disrupts the bonds and results in a weak gel. Essences and colour should be added to the starch mixture as soon as it is removed from the heat and not while the mixture is cooling.

Other Ingredients

Sugar, acids, etc., modify the behaviour of starch gels. The greater the amount of sugar in the product, the more delicate the gel formed, as sugar prevents water from binding to starch. Acids hydrolyse the amylose chains resulting in a more tender gel. This is seen when acids are added before gelatinization of starch. If acid is added after gelatinization of starch, the gel is soft because of extra liquid from lime juice or fruit juice. This can be corrected by calculating the liquid in the acidic substance and reducing that amount of liquid from the recipe.

Aging of a Gel

In a starch gel, water forms the dispersed phase and is trapped within the gel. Water is also bonded by hydrogen bonding to amylose molecules and starch granules which form the matrix of the gel. When a gel stales or its structure is disrupted by cutting the gel, water which is trapped in the gel is released and the gel collapses. This 'weeping' or loss of moisture from a gel is called syneresis.

RETROGRADATION

Starches rich in amylose form gels more readily but these gels are less stable. Amylose chains have a tendency to recoil and partially recrystallize. Some hydrogen bonds which hold the gel together break and amylose molecules move around forming new bonds. As the gel stales, amylose molecules rearrange themselves in an orderly manner in crystalline regions. This is accompanied by loss of solubility and release of water from the gel, causing food defects.

A starch gel which has retrograded loses its smooth texture and feels gritty when eaten. The rate and extent of retrogradation are influenced by temperature, size, shape, and concentration of starch. Starch retrogrades rapidly at 0°C.

Retrogradation occurs when a starch gel becomes stale or when it is frozen. Bread and starch-thickened puddings stored in the refrigerator develop undesirable textural changes because of retrogradation by formation of crystalline aggregates of amylose.

The texture defects caused by retrogradation in foods, which can be heated, are temporarily corrected by warming the food containing starch. Heat energy breaks the hydrogen bonds which hold amylose molecules together forming crystalline areas. Stale bread becomes soft when it is covered and reheated, but as it cools it develops an undesirable texture once again.

The problem of retrogradation is of concern in cold starch-based gels. This can be corrected by using starches which are stable to freezing and thawing. A number of modified starches are available in the market today.

DEXTRINIZATION

When starch is heated without any water, the temperature rises rapidly beyond 100°C. Water, which is naturally present in flour, and the high temperature brings about chemical degradation of flour splitting the starch molecule at one or more of the 1,4-α-glucosidic linkages. This reaction is called dextrinization, and the short chain starch molecules of varying lengths formed are called dextrins. Dextrinization is seen when flour in browned while making brown roux for gravies and sauces. Browned flour has lesser thickening ability because of formation of shorter chain dextrins.

TYPES OF FOOD STARCHES

Unmodified Starches

Starches from different plant sources differ in their size, shape, gelatinization temperature, gel forming ability, and texture. In the food industry, the behaviour of different starches as thickening agents and gelling or setting agents is an important consideration while selecting the starch. Starches can be extracted from grains, roots, tubers, and pith of trees in a comparatively pure form to be used in commercial food products.

Corn flour, rice flour, wheat flour, waxy corn, waxy sorghum, potato, tapioca, and *sago* are some of the common unmodified starches.

Modified Starches

Knowledge about the molecules of amylose and amylopectin in starch and the structure of different starch granules has enabled scientists to modify natural starches. Physical and chemical means have been used to develop a variety of special starches with unique characteristics to meet specific needs of the food industry.

Pre-gelatinized starch   These starches have been cooked till they are gelatinized and then they are roller dried after the starch granules are swollen. When water is added to the dehydrated starch, it swells to a desired thickness without heating. Instant pudding mixes, baby cereals, such as Farex and Nestum, are examples of convenience foods. In these products, a physical change modifies the characteristics of the native starch.

Acid modified or thin boiling starch   Starch is chemically modified by treating it with very dilute hydrochloric or nitric acid at temperatures below gelatinization. Starch is hydrolysed and gets fragmented. Its solubility increases and thickening ability decreases. When hot, thin boiling starches are very fluid and are used in making gum drops as they can be easily poured into moulds which form firm gels upon cooling and aging.

Oxidized starches   These are chemically modified thin boiling starches which have been treated with an alkali such as sodium hypo-chlorite. The starch granule is mildly oxidized and forms a soft gel.

Cross-linked starches   Cross-linked starches are formed when hydroxyl (OH) groups on two different molecules in the same granule are substituted by alkalis such as acetic anhydride or succinic anhydride. The greater the amount of cross-linking, the lesser the tendency to retrograde. Both acetate and succinate cross-linked starches are very useful as thickeners and stabilizers in salad dressings. Gels formed using cross-linked starches show minimal retrogradation during storage.

Unmodified waxy cereal starches and root starches produce undesirable stringiness in food products. They form clear pastes and do not gel. Cross-linking retains the good qualities, but controls the degree of thickening that causes long stringy pastes.

Starch phosphates　Starch is chemically esterified with sodium tripolyphosphate. The starch phosphates formed improve the texture of starch pastes and increases its stability. These pastes have excellent clarity and reduced syneresis or weeping. They have high freeze–thaw stability.

Modified cellulose is most widely used in the food industry as the sodium salt of carboxymethylcellulose also known as CMC or cellulose gum. It is used in ice creams to give a good body, texture, and to retard formation of large ice crystals on storage.

CEREALS AND CEREAL PRODUCTS

Cereals are a rich source of starch and are obtained mainly from cultivated grasses. The term cereals also include tapioca, arrowroot, potato, and *sago* as they are rich in starch and are widely used in the catering industry. They are used in some form or the other in all meals and form the staple diet of majority people across the world. Cereals are used mainly as flours. A wide variety of cereals is processed into breakfast foods and ready-to-eat snacks.

The basic structure of all cereal grains is similar with some variation in form. All grains have an outermost layer called the bran or *pericarp*, followed by an *aleurone* cell layer which surrounds the endosperm and is rich in nutrients. The endosperm is rich in starch and protein and forms the bulk of the grain. The embryo or germ is separated from the endosperm by the *scutellum* and is rich in protein, fat, and B complex vitamins. The endosperm makes up approximately 84 per cent of the grain, while the germ and bran constitute 14 per cent and 2 per cent of the grain, respectively. Refer Fig. 11.6 in Chapter 11 for the structure of a wheat grain.

Cereals used in the Catering Industry

The cereals used in the catering industry are as follows (see Table 4.3):

- Wheat
- Oats
- Rye
- *Bajra*
- *Sago*

- Rice
- *Ragi*
- *Triticale*
- Tapioca
- Potato

- Maize
- Barley
- *Jowar*
- Arrowroot

Malting of Cereals

Malt is prepared from *jowar*, barley, *ragi*, and wheat. The following steps are involved in malting of cereal grains.

1. *Selection of grains* Good quality grains which are of high germination rate and are free from infestation are selected. Grains are cleaned and graded to remove undersized grains.

2. *Steeping* Grains are washed and soaked in cold water for 36 to 72 hours. Water is changed twice or thrice. Time taken for steeping depends on the ambient temperature and is longer in cold climates.

3. *Sprouting* Water is drained and soaked grains are spread in a 2 to 3-inch thick layer on wire mesh trays supported on a stand. Sprouting or germination takes three days in the summer and up to six days in the winter. Grains should be mixed and water should be sprinkled on the grains once a day to prevent drying. During sprouting, the dormant grain becomes alive and enzymes amylase and protease are formed.

4. *Kilning* Kilning or controlled slow drying of the grains is the final stage of malting. During this stage the enzyme amylase acts on starch and hydrolyses it to *dextrins*, while protease acts on proteins breaking them down into proteoses and peptones. Temperature control is necessary to prevent the enzymes from getting inactivated. Enzymes are proteins in nature and get denatured at high temperatures. As drying proceeds, the fraction of water-soluble carbohydrates and proteins increases and the characteristic malt flavour develops. Grains are dried to approximately 13 per cent moisture.

5. *Removal of rootlets or sprouts* The rootlets which develop need to be removed from the grain. This is done by sieving through a wire mesh.

After removal of the rootlets, the malted grains are powdered and used for the preparation of malt extract, health foods, infant foods, and in the brewing industry.

Breakfast cereals The variety of ready-to-cook and ready-to-serve breakfast cereals available in the market today is unbelievable. Puffed, flaked, parched, shredded, granular, and extruded cereal grains are packaged in a wide assortment of combinations and shapes and have flooded the supermarkets. Dried and flaked fruits, nuts, and confections, such as marshmallows, are added to multigrain mixes to increase nutritive value and interest. They are served with milk and form a quick, convenient, and healthful alternative to breakfast items. For example, the popular brand of breakfast cereals, 'Kelloggs' has introduced Extra Muesli Nuts Delight, a ready-to-eat breakfast cereal which is a multigrain blend (containing wheat, corn grits, rolled barley, rolled oats, and rice) with dates, raisins, almonds, malt extract, and sugar. It is fortified with vitamins and minerals to meet 25 per cent of the RDA for most vitamins and minerals. Cereals and cereal products include a variety of bread, wheat, rice, and pastas (see Plate 1).

TABLE 4.3   Important cereals used in the catering industry

S. no.	Cereal	Products	Description	Uses
1	Wheat	Wholewheat flour (*atta*)	100 per cent of whole grain	Chapatti, brown bread
		Refined flour (*maida*)	Approximately 70 per cent to 85 per cent of the whole grain, mainly the endosperm	Bread, pasta, puff, and flaky pastry
		• Strong flour		
		• Soft flour		Cakes, biscuits, pastry except puff and flaky, batters, thickening and coating agent.
		Broken wheat (*dalia*)	Coarsely crushed whole wheat grain	Porridge
		Semolina (*rawa*)	Granulated hard flour prepared from central portion of the wheat grain	*Sooji halwa*, *upma*, *rawa dosa*, cous, and cous
2	Rice	Whole grain		
		• Long grain (basmati)	Narrow, pointed grains, stay firm separate.	*Pulao*, biryani, plain boiled rice
		• Medium grain	All purpose rice	All sweet and savoury rice dishes
		• Short grain	Small rounded grains with soft texture	Milk pudding
		Brown rice	Bran is retained	Boiled rice
		Ground rice	Coarsely ground grains	*Phirni*, idli
		Rice flour	Finely ground flour	Steamed *modak*, thickening agent
		Rice paper	Thin edible paper made from rice	Macaroon, nougat
		Wild rice	Seed of an aquatic plant of rice species, has nutty flavour, and different texture	Boiled rice
		Parboiled rice	Rice steamed with husk before milling to retain vitamins	Boiled rice, dosa, idli, and other south Indian preparations
		Parched rice (*poha*) or rice flakes	Paddy pressed through rollers and dried	Savoury snacks, breakfast cereal
		Puffed rice	Roasted rice grains	Savoury snacks
3	Millets, maize or corn	Corn on the cob	Entire corn with kernels	Roasted, boiled
		Sweet corn	Hybrid variety of corn	Used in soups, salads, and in a variety of preparations
		Maize flour	Ground grains	*Makki ki roti*, tortillas
		Corn flour	Crushed endosperm of the grain devoid of protein and fat	Custard, *blancmange*, cakes, and as a setting and thickening agent
		Cornflakes	Processed dried flakes	Breakfast cereal
		Corn grains	Dried to 13.5 per cent moisture	Popcorn

Contd

Table 4.3 Contd

S. no.	Cereal	Products	Description	Uses
4	Millets	*Jowar* or sorghum	Grains milled into flour	*Bhakri* from all millets
		Bajra	*Bajra* is parched like popcorn	Multigrain bread, biscuits, *thalipeeth*
		Ragi or finger millet	Used for preparation of malt	Malted grains are used commercially in infant foods
5	Oats	Oatmeal	Ground coarse, medium, or fine	Porridge, thickening agent, coating foods, enriched breads, cakes, cookies, haggis
		Oat flakes	Quick cooking as they are heat treated and rolled into flakes	Porridge
6	Barley	Whole grains or Scotch barley	Hard grains require soaking overnight	Barley water, soups, and stews
		Pearl barley	Grain polished after removing most of bran and germ	Breakfast cereals
		Malt	Grains malted and kiln -dried	Malt extract brewing vinegar
7	Rye	Rye flour • Light • Medium • Dark	Only flour apart from wheat which contains gluten but forms dough with sticky dense consistency	Rye bread
8	*Sago*	Round globules	Made from the pith of the *sago* palm	Milk pudding, *wadas*, *khichdi*, extruded snacks
9	Tapioca	Flake (rough) Seed (fine)	Obtained from the roots of the cassava plant	Milk puddings, soups, chips, wafers
10	Arrowroot	Flour	It is made from the roots of the *maranta* plant. Flour is easily digestible. Starch paste becomes transparent when boiled.	Cakes, puddings, foods for invalids and convalescents, and as a thickening agent in products requiring clarity
11	Potato	Potato flour • Floury • Firm • Waxy	Each variety of potato has specific cooking properties	Thickening agent in soups and sauces
		Sweet potatoes	Long tubers, yellowish flesh with sweet aromatic flavour	Sweet pudding
12	*Triticale*	*Triticale* flakes	Hybrid cereal from a cross between wheat (*Triticum*) and rye (*Secale*)	Breakfast cereal
		Triticale flour	Grain is hardier and higher in protein content (18 per cent) and in lysine compared to wheat (12 per cent protein)	Used in chapatti flour up to 50 per cent

SUGAR

The main sugar used in cookery is sucrose or common sugar. It is a disaccharide made up of glucose and fructose. It is extracted from sugar cane or sugar beet and is available in different stages of refinement and varying crystal sizes. Sugar is available as table sugar, as fine or granulated crystals, or as sugar cubes. Jaggery is the unrefined form, and brown sugar is the partially refined form of sugar. Molasses is a by-product of sugar used for making rum and industrial alcohol. Castor sugar or powdered sugar and icing sugar are other common forms of sugar.

Sugar solutions are used for different purposes in different concentrations. A thin syrup is sprinkled on fatless sponge while making pineapple pastries, syrups are used to soak *rasgullas* and *gulab jamuns*, while pulled sugar is made into baskets and fancy shapes. All these are made from sugar and require skill and precision.

Sugar Cookery

Three processes are of importance while making confections and preserves:

Inversion   When sugar is boiled in the presence of an acid, it is hydrolysed into glucose and fructose. This process is called inversion, and the mixture of equal parts of glucose and fructose is called invert sugar.

Invert sugar does not recrystallize.

$$\underset{\text{Sucrose}}{C_{12}H_{22}O_{11}} + \underset{\text{Water}}{H_2O} \xrightarrow[\text{Heat}]{\text{Acid}} \underset{\text{Glucose}}{C_6H_{12}O_6} + \underset{\text{Fructose}}{C_6H_{12}O_6}$$
$$\underbrace{\phantom{C_6H_{12}O_6 + C_6H_{12}O_6}}_{\text{Invert sugar}}$$

The acid used may be lime juice (citric acid) or cream of tartar. Confectionery glucose or liquid glucose contains readymade invert sugars. It is prepared by breaking down corn starch into dextrins and different types of sugars.

Crystallization   When a concentrated sugar solution is cooled gradually, large crystals are formed which impart an unpleasant gritty texture to foods.

Crystal formation can be avoided or the size of crystals can be reduced by:

Beating   While making fondants from sugar alone, the concentrated sugar solution is heated to 115°C to saturate it, then cooled to approximately 40°C, and beaten vigorously so that microcrystals are formed.

Inversion   Addition of cream of tartar before heating results in inversion of sugar and slow crystal formation, the fondant formed is mouldable.

Non-crystalline products are hard and glassy in appearance, e.g., *chikki*, pulled sugar, and spun sugar. They have a low moisture content and are boiled at high temperatures.

Caramelization   Caramel is formed when sugar is heated at high temperatures with minimum amount of water (refer the section on caramelization in Chapter 9).

Making Preserves

Jam, jellies, and marmalade are made by boiling sugar with fruit containing acid and pectic substances. The acid in the fruit inverts 25–40 per cent of the sugar and retards crystal formation during storage.

Honey

The flavour of honey depends upon the flowers from which nectar is collected. It is rich in fructose.

Artificial Sweeteners

They are also called non-nutritive sweeteners as they do not provide any calories or provide negligible calories as compared to sugar. (Sugar provides 4 kcal/g, i.e., 1 teaspoonful sugar provides 20 kcal.)

Low-calorie sweeteners are available as sugar substitutes in food and beverages. Low-calorie sweeteners, unlike carbohydrates, do not change blood sugar levels significantly.

Low-calorie sweeteners are of two types: bulk sweeteners and high-intensity sweeteners. Table 4.4 shows the relative sweetness of natural and artificial sweetners.

Bulk sweeteners are indigestible and include sugar alcohols, such as sorbitol mannitol, and xylitol. Some are found in natural foods, while others are manufactured. High intensity sweeteners include the artificial sweeteners and need to be added in very small amounts (see Table 4.4).

Table 4.4 Relative sweetness of natural and artificial sweeteners

Sugar	Relative sweetness
1. **Natural sugars**	(Sucrose 100)
Lactose	16
Maltose	32
Glucose	74
Sucrose	100
Invert sugar	130
Fructose	173
Sugar (stevia sugar)	100–300
Sorbitol	67
2. **Artificial sweeteners**	(No. of times as sweet as sucrose)
Cyclamate	30
Aspartame	160–200
Dulcin	250
Ace sulfame K	200
Saccharin	300–500
Sucralose	600

Sugar alcohols are used to sweeten chewing gum and other confectionery products. High intensity artificial sweeteners are a boon for diabetic and obese individuals. Use of saccharin is permitted in carbonated water, soft drink concentrates, *supari*, and *paan masala*. Artificial sweeteners, such as saccharin, aspartame, or ace sulfame, may be sold as tabletop sweeteners.

SOLUBLE FIBRES: PECTINS, GUMS, AND MUCILAGES

Pectin

It is a soluble polysaccharide present in the cellwalls of all plant tissues. It forms a viscous solution in water and is a gelling agent for jams, jellies, and marmalades. For a pectin gel to form, sugar and an acidic pH are necessary. Apples, oranges, and lemons are rich sources. Commercial pectin is available as a coarse or fine yellowish white powder which is added to fruit preserves which are low in natural pectin.

Agar

It is a polysaccharide complex extracted from algae. It forms a stiff gel at 1 per cent concentration. It is mainly used to prepare culture media and as a stabilizer in food gels.

Algin

Algin and alginates are extensively used in the food industry. Algin is sodium alginate, the sodium salt of alginic acid. It is extracted from giant brown seaweed or horsetail kelp. It is available as a cream-coloured powder soluble in water, which can form a viscous gel. Algin and alginates are used as stabilizers in the preparation of ice creams and other dairy products. They prevent the formation of ice crystals during freezing and give good whipping ability. They are used in cakes, fruit drinks, milkshakes, desserts, sugar confectionery, and wines.

Gums

A number of gums extracted from plants are used for a variety of purposes.

These polysaccharides are extracted from the seed, e.g., locust bean gum and guar gum, or as an exudate from several species of trees and shrubs, e.g., gum Arabic, gum tragacanth, gum karaya, and ghatti gum.

Gums are important for their thickening ability, stabilizing action in emulsions, retardation of crystals in sugar, etc.

USES OF CARBOHYDRATES IN FOOD PREPARATION

Starch from various sources in its natural form is used as a thickening and gelling agent in a wide range of products. It is the primary thickening agent in soups and roux-based mother sauces such as *béchamel*, *velouté*, and *espagnole* sauces. These sauces are used for casseroles and vegetable and meat-based preparations, salads, and pastas. It is used in custard sauce, puddings, pie fillings, and souffles.

Carboxymethyl cellulose (CMC), pectins, gums, and alginates have varied applications in their natural and modified forms (see Table 4.5).

Commercially, starch derivatives are used for an exhaustive range of products.

Sugars have a wide range of uses apart from sweetening and energy giving. Sugar cookery involves controlled formation of crystals which has a direct bearing on the texture of crystalline candies such as fondants and fudges.

Table 4.5 Some uses of carbohydrates

Carbohydrate	Use
Unmodified starch	
1. Refined flour	Thickening sauces and soups specially used in the form of a roux
2. Rice	Thickening soups and rice pudding (*phirni*)
3. Arrowroot	For clear sauces, e.g., lemon sauce and as a glaze for fruit flans
4. Tapioca	Used for pudding
5. Potato	Used to thicken soups which could curdle at high temperatures
6. High amylose starch	Edible films for wrapping candies
7. Waxy rice flour	White sauces and starch-thickened pudding which need to be stored frozen and thawed before cooking
8. Corn flour	Thickening soups, sauces, and gravies, anti-caking agent
Modified starch	
1. Starch phosphates	White sauces in cook–freeze operations
2. Oxidized starch	Products which need soft gels
3. Thin boiling starch	Gum drops
4. Pregelatinized starch	Instant pudding and soup mixes
5. Cross-linked starch	Thickeners and stabilizer in salad dressings
Other polysaccharides	
1. Cellulose	Powdered form used to provide bulk in weight-reducing foods
2. Cellulose compounds	Thickening and creaming agents
3. Dextrins	In coffee extracts
4. Pectin	Setting agent in jams, jellies, and marmalades
5. Gums	Thickening and gelling agent; stabilization of ice cream, cheese, and chocolate milk
6. Seaweed extracts (*algin* and *agar*)	Prevent ice crystal formation in ice cream, stabilize cream substitutes, modify crystal size in sugar confections, and are used in weight-reduction diets
Sugars	
1. Glucose	Used as a humectant in confectionery
2. Caramel	Used as a colouring and flavouring agent in christmas cake, soup mixes, instant puddings, etc.
3. Invert sugar	Prevents formation of sugar crystals in preserves and fondant

SUMMARY

Carbohydrates are one of the most important constituents of food. They are manufactured by green plants by a process known as photosynthesis. The glucose formed in this process is converted into starch and stored in various parts of the plant to be used as food. On the basis of saccharide or sugar units present, they are classified as mono-, di-, oligo-, and polysaccharides.

Starch is present in two forms: amylose and amylopectin. Amylose is a straight chain polysaccharide that is capable of forming a gel, apart from its thickening ability. The second and larger fraction is amylopectin which has a branched structure because of which it has thickening ability but no gelling power at normal concentrations. Both amylose and amylopectin are made up of glucose units linked to each other in long chains. Amylose and amylopectin are arranged in cell granules in an orderly arrangement and are tightly compacted.

When a mixture of starch and water is heated, the insoluble starch absorbs water and swells. On further heating, amylose gets leached into the water and the granule swells further, resulting in increase in viscosity.

The starch granule at this stage is gelatinized and as the starch paste cools, viscosity increases. If the percentage of amylose is adequate, the cooled paste sets into a firm gel. This step is called gelation. Many factors affect gelatinization and gelation of starch. As the gel ages or if the gel structure is disturbed, syneresis or weeping of a gel, and retrogradation or changes in texture of a gel are observed.

Cereals are a rich source of starch and include tapioca, arrowroot, potato, and *sago*. Cereals are processed to make breakfast foods and ready-to-eat snacks.

Sugars when cooked, show inversion, crystallization, and caramelization, all of which have a definite bearing on the quality of the product. A number of non-nutritive bulk and high intensity sweeteners are available in the market today. They are suitable for diabetics and calorie-conscious individuals. The unavailable or zero-calorie carbohydrates, such as cellulose derivatives, pectins, and gums, are used as thickening agents, stabilizers, setting agents, etc. The food industry depends on natural and modified carbohydrates for specific additive functions in many processed foods.

KEY TERMS

1,4-α-Glucosidic linkage   Linkage between Carbon 1 and 4 of first and second glucose units, respectively,

Amylase-rich food   These are germinated cereal flours rich in enzyme alpha-amylase, which can instantly reduce the viscosity of thick cereal pastes by splitting the long starch chains into shorter dextrins and provide infants with low viscosity, high energy weaning foods.

Amylopectin   Branched form of starch made up of chains of glucose units linked to each other by 1,4 linkages in the chain and 1,6 linkages at point of branching.

Amylose   Form of starch made up of long straight chains of glucose units linked together by 1,4 linkages.

Gelatinization   Swelling of starch granules on heating with water, resulting in thickening of starch pastes, and leaching out of amylose from the granule into water.

Golden rice   A term used for genetically modified rice with enhanced β-carotene, iron, and proteins (lysine) which has been specially developed to reduce the incidence of malnutrition worldwide.

Heteropolysaccharide   Also called heteroglycan, and is made up of more than one repeating unit of monosaccharide.

Homopolysaccharide Also called homoglycan, and is made up of one repeating unit of monosaccharide.

Implode Implode means to burst inwards.

Leucoplasts Colourless plastids in the cytoplasm of plant cell in which starch is stored.

Malted cereals These are grains, such as barley, *ragi*, *jowar*, which have been soaked in water, sprouted, and kiln-dried. They are used in making malted health drinks, infant foods, and in brewing and distilling alcoholic beverages.

Milling of paddy A process to remove the hull and coarse outer layers of bran and germ from the rice grain and polishing the rice grain to increase its acceptability.

Modified starches Starch, whose natural state has been changed by physical or chemical methods.

Molasses It is a sweetener produced as a by-product during refining of cane sugar. Local name *kakvi*.

Muesli Popular breakfast cereal based on whole grains, rolled oats, fruits and nuts, served with low-fat milk providing a hearty high-fibre breakfast.

This term was derived from the Swiss German word *mus* meaning mixture.

Parboiling An optional process prior to milling to enhance nutritive value of rice. Parboiling involves soaking paddy in water, steam heating, and drying before milling.

Photosynthesis The process by which green plants manufacture complex foods from carbon dioxide in the air, and water and minerals from the soil in the presence of sunlight.

Retrogradation Gradual increase of crystalline areas in starch gels during storage which affect texture and palatability of puddings.

Starch granule Formed in the leucoplast of the cell by deposition of amylose and amylopectin in layers.

Starch Complex polysaccharide made up of amylose and amylopectin.

Syneresis Separation of liquid from a gel caused by contraction of the solid phase thereby squeezing the liquid out or by cutting the gel.

Waxy starch Genetically modified starch containing only amylopectin.

REVIEW EXERCISES

1. Classify carbohydrates based on the number of saccharide units present.
2. Describe the process of photosynthesis and list parts of plant where starch is stored, giving suitable examples.
3. Define and explain the process of gelatinization and factors affecting the same.
4. Differentiate between the following:
   (a) Amylose and amylopectin
   (b) Gelation and gelatinization
   (c) Natural and modified starches
   (d) Nutritive and non-nutritive sweeteners
5. Explain the following:
   (a) Retrogradation
   (b) Dextrinization
   (c) Structure of a starch granule
6. List 10 recipes in which starch is used as a thickening agent.

ASSIGNMENT

Visit a local supermarket or grocery store and read the label for ingredients on any four of the following ready-to-cook/ready-to-serve convenience foods:

1. Breakfast cereals
2. Multigrain biscuits
3. Infant foods
4. Other foods

List the different cereals used in preparing the same and correlate the choice of cereal with nutrients present in them.

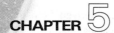

Proteins

LEARNING OBJECTIVES

After reading this chapter, you should be able to
- describe the chemical nature of proteins
- classify proteins on the basis of characteristics, structure, and functions
- understand the changes that take place when proteins are denatured
- understand the factors which affect gelation, emulsification, foam formation, and viscosity in commonly used protein-rich foods
- apply this knowledge in the kitchen and prevent undesirable changes in protein-based products
- describe the various pulses and the effect of steeping and cooking
- appreciate the importance of proteins in preparing high-quality products

INTRODUCTION

Proteins are complex organic molecules made up of carbon, hydrogen, oxygen, and nitrogen. Most proteins also contain sulphur and phosphorus, along with traces of other elements. Proteins are not only essential for life but also play an important role in food preparation. The final quality of many food products is influenced by how the proteins are treated while food is being prepared. An understanding of the structure and behaviour of protein in food products is necessary for every caterer.

BASIC STRUCTURE AND PROPERTIES

Proteins are made up of amino acids, which are organic acids with a carboxyl group (COOH) and amino group (NH_2) attached to a carbon atom. R is the functional group which differentiates one amino acid from another.

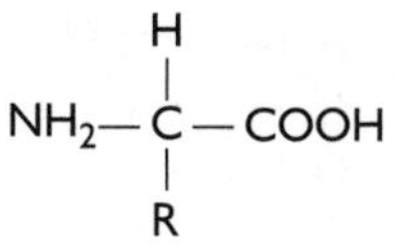

$$NH_2-\overset{\overset{\textstyle H}{|}}{\underset{\underset{\textstyle R}{|}}{C}}-COOH$$

Peptide Linkage

The carbon of the carboxyl group of one amino acid combines with the nitrogen group or amino group of another amino acid with the loss of one molecule of water. This bond, which unites the two amino acids, is called a peptide bond.

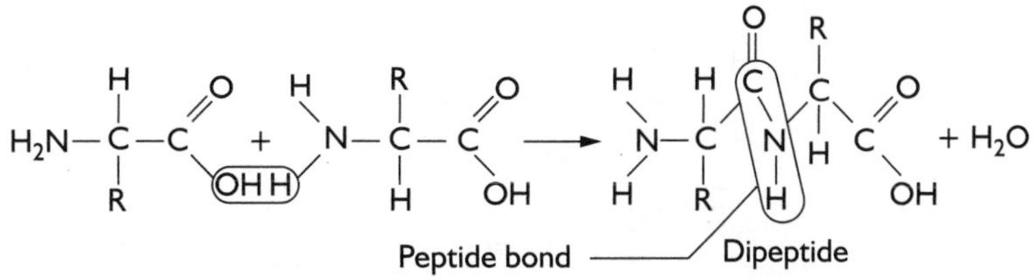

Peptide bond — Dipeptide

Protein molecules are polypeptides made up of repeating units of –C–C–N– group, which forms the backbone of the protein. Projecting alternately on either side of the main chain are the R groups (Fig. 5.1).

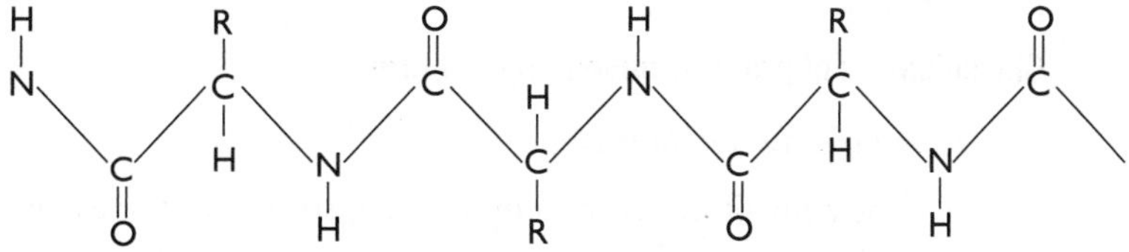

Fig. 5.1 Primary structure of protein

One protein molecule differs from another in the particular R group it contains (or the particular amino acids it contains) and in the order in which they are united in the long polypeptide chain.

The bonding angles between various atoms along the polypeptide backbone are arranged in a zigzag or spiral manner called the *helix*.

Holding the polypeptides in a helical configuration are the hydrogen bonds which are formed between the carboxyl (C=O) and imido group (N–H) along the polypeptide backbone. These hydrogen bonds are parallel to the major axis of the helix.

Some of the side chains (R group) contain carboxyl, amino, and imido groups which form *salt bridges*. These also hold the polypeptides in a helical manner. See Fig. 5.2 for the secondary structure of proteins.

(Salt bridges are formed between –COO⁻ group of an acidic amino acid radical and the –NH₃⁺ group of a basic amino acid radical, i.e., –NH₃⁺–COO⁻).

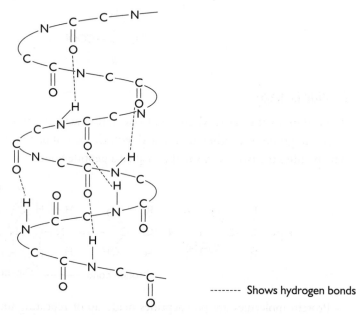

------- Shows hydrogen bonds

Fig. 5.2 Secondary structure of proteins

Classification of Protein

Classification of proteins based on structure

1. *Fibrillar or fibrous proteins*
   (a) The helix of the protein molecule is stretched. For example, in muscle myosin the helix is stretched but elastic.

   In collagen the helix is stretched to a great extent and is inelastic.
   (b) They are relatively insoluble in water and are resistant to acid, alkalis, and moderate heat.

2. *Globular proteins*
   (a) The helix is bent to give a compact shape, e.g., egg albumin, globin of haemoglobin, and globulin in meat and pulses.
   (b) These proteins are soluble in water and water solutions containing acids, alkalis, salt, and also in alcohols. They are easily affected by heat. This is due to the fact that the cross-links holding the helix are weak and hence slight increase in temperature or a change in pH disrupts these cross-links causing the chains to unfold, i.e., protein gets denatured.

Figure 5.3 depicts the tertiary structure of proteins.

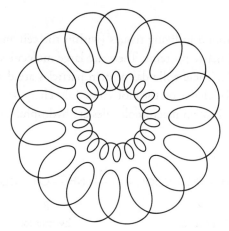

Fig. 5.3   Tertiary structure of proteins

Classification based on characterization

1. *Simple proteins*

   Those proteins which yield amino acids on hydrolysis, e.g., albumin in egg white, zein in maize, keratin in hair, and globin in haemoglobin.

2. *Compound or conjugated proteins*

   Those proteins which are combined with a non-protein molecule, e.g., haemoglobin (protein + haeme), casein (protein + phosphoric acid), mucin (protein + carbohydrate), and lipoprotein (protein + lipid).

3. *Derived proteins*

   Those proteins which are produced by the action of acids, alkalis, heat, or enzymes on native proteins.

   Proteins ⟶ Proteoses ⟶ Peptones ⟶ Polypeptides ⟶ Dipeptides

Classification based on function

1. *Complete proteins or first-class proteins*

   Complete proteins contain all the essential amino acids. They promote growth and maintain essential body processes as kinds and amounts of amino acids are proportional to body needs, e.g., animal proteins from milk, egg, fish, and meat.

2. *Partially complete or second-class proteins*

   These do not contain all the essential amino acids in required amounts. So they are capable of maintaining life but cannot promote growth, e.g., gliadin of wheat.

3. *Totally incomplete proteins*

   These are deficient in a lot of amino acids. They are incapable of meeting both major functions of growth and repair of proteins, e.g., zein in maize and gelatin.

NATIVE PROTEINS

Proteins found in living tissues (within the cell and in the fluids) of animals and plants are called native proteins. These are large molecules (macromolecule), which are sensitive and fragile. These colloidal protein particles are dispersed as a sol. All colloidal particles have similar charge on the molecules. Like charges repel each other and the particles remain dispersed. Protein macromolecules are hydrophilic colloids and are stabilized by a layer of water.

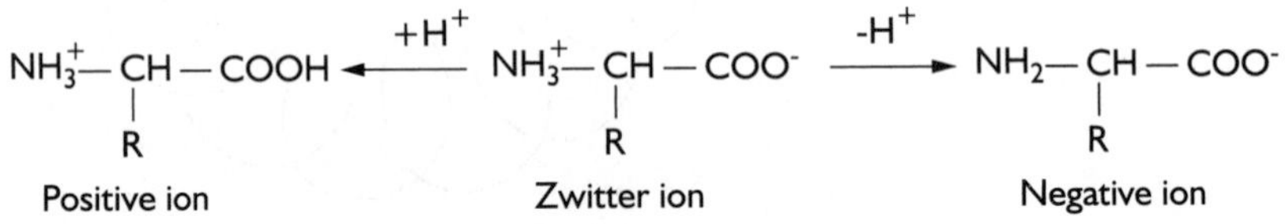

$$NH_3^+-CH-COOH \xleftarrow{+H^+} NH_3^+-CH-COO^- \xrightarrow{-H^+} NH_2-CH-COO^-$$

$$\underset{\text{Positive ion}}{\overset{|}{R}} \qquad \underset{\text{Zwitter ion}}{\overset{|}{R}} \qquad \underset{\text{Negative ion}}{\overset{|}{R}}$$

Fig. 5.4   Ionic character of an amino acid

This acts as an insulation and prevents bonding. Some amino acids with a ring structure (◯) and carbon chains (–C–C–C–C–) are hydrophobic, while the acidic group (COOH group) is hydrophilic. Figure 5.4 presents the ionic character of an amino acid.

The free amino and carboxyl groups in a protein molecule have an electric charge depending on the pH of the medium in which the protein is found. Proteins are said to be amphoteric, i.e., they can react with acids and bases. Hence, they act as buffers in food preparations.

In the presence of an acid, (the amino group neutralizes the acid) the protein molecules are drawn towards the cathode as a result of the net positive charge on them.

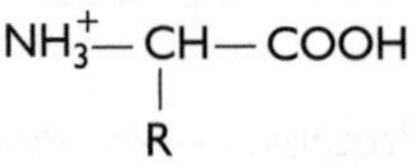

$$NH_3^+-CH-COOH$$
$$\overset{|}{R}$$

In the presence of an alkali, (the carboxyl group neutralizes the alkali) the protein molecule migrates towards the anode because of the net negative charge on them.

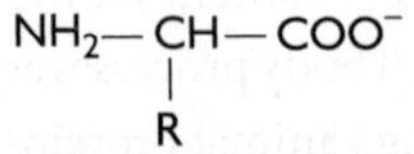

$$NH_2-CH-COO^-$$
$$\overset{|}{R}$$

This migration of proteins in an electric field at a definite pH is called electrophoresis. It depends on

1. Charge on the molecule
2. Size of the molecule
3. Shape of the molecule

Table 5.1	IEP for some proteins
Proteins	**pH**
Casein	4.6
Ovalbumin	4.6
Gelatin	4.9
Myosin	5.4
Gluten	7.0

At the isolectric point (IEP), the charge on the protein molecule is neutralized and they show no movement in an electric field. Proteins at the IEP are called zwitterions.

At this point, hydrophobic colloids, such as casein flocculate and hydrophilic colloids, show minimum hydration, e.g., gluten. The IEP for some proteins are given in Table 5.1.

When a fluid food containing protein is brought to its IEP, curdling is likely to occur (addition of acid while curdling milk) as there is no charge which keeps protein dispersed.

DENATURED PROTEINS

Denaturation is defined as any non-proteolytic modification in the original structure of the native proteins, giving rise to definite changes in physical, chemical, and biological properties. Denaturation is brought about by the following:

1. Denaturing agents such as acids, alkalis, salts
2. Increase in temperature
3. Extensive beating

Stages in Heat Denaturation

1. Unfolding of helix of the protein molecules as the cross-links holding the helix is disrupted.
2. R groups are exposed. Rebonding takes place between adjacent R groups of protein molecules leading to aggregation of the molecules, bringing about increased viscosity. This is the first change in denaturation which involves structural alteration (1st stage).

When sufficient proteins have united, the protein molecules are no longer dispersed as a sol. At this stage, the protein is said to have coagulated (second stage), i.e., water is held in the capillary spaces formed by united protein molecules and the coagulated proteins form a 'gel'.

If the liquid separates from the coagulated protein, the protein is said to be 'precipitated' or 'flocculated', i.e., 'curdling' takes place (third stage of denaturation). These stages can be observed while cooking scrambled eggs. If it is overcooked, liquid separates out.

Effects of Denaturation

Properties of denatured proteins are completely different from their native form.

1. Denatured proteins are easily attacked by proteolytic enzymes, e.g., cooked meat is more easily digested than raw meat.

2. They show decreased solubility, e.g., cooked egg white is not soluble in water.
3. They lose their biological activity as enzymes are destroyed, e.g., browning does not take place in boiled potato.
4. Denatured proteins lose their ability to crystallize.
5. There is an increase in viscosity of food.
6. Heat denaturation results in improved flavour and texture, e.g., cooking improves flavour in meat, and eggs give structure and improve texture of cakes.
7. Denaturation of food is irreversible unless it occurs under very mild conditions.

Factors Affecting Denaturation

pH Denaturation is brought about by controlling pH and occurs at the IEP when the protein is unstable.

1. Caseinogen is dispersed as a sol in milk. When milk turns sour (pH 4.6 ; IEP), it curdles (Third stage in denaturation).
2. Egg albumin is colloidally dispersed as a sol. It has a pH of 7.2–7.8. But when the pH is reduced to 4.6 (its IEP) by adding vinegar to water used for poaching eggs, the egg coagulates faster.

Heat When egg white is heated at 60°C the protein ovalbumin gets denatured. As temperature increases, coagulation takes place and egg white separates out as a solid.

If the temperature is below 100°C, e.g., poaching, then coagulation is slow and coagulated protein is soft and easily digested.

If temperature is above 100°C, e.g., boiling and roasting, coagulation is fast and coagulated protein is hard and more difficult to digest.
So 'a stew boiled is a stew spoiled'.

Surface denaturation This is brought about by mechanical means, e.g., beating egg white or milk to a foam. Surface denaturation of the protein takes place leading to pellicle or skin formation. This stabilizes the foam (pellicle is seen when foam has subsided).

If such a foam is heated, as in egg white foam, it becomes firm due to the coagulation of ovalbumin.

If pH of ovalbumin is at its IEP, then coagulation is faster. Hence, acidic substances (cream of tartar, lime juice, etc.) are added when whipping egg white.

Salts When present in a high concentration, it precipitates proteins out of solution and disperses them, e.g., cured ham baked in white sauce. The high salt concentration of the ham can cause the milk in white sauce to curdle.

Moisture Low moisture levels cause less denaturation than higher moisture levels at the same temperature.

FUNCTIONAL PROPERTIES OF SPECIFIC PROTEIN-RICH FOODS

Gelatin

Gelatin is a partially degraded protein prepared from collagen. Collagen is the intercellular cementing substance between cells. Skin, ligaments, and bones are hydrolysed by dilute acid or alkali, breaking collagen molecules into shorter fibrous molecules called gelatin. Gelatin contains a large proportion of amino acids which have a great affinity for water. The long thin fibres of gelatin help in forming firm gels at low temperatures.

Dry gelatin is soaked in cold water for preliminary hydration before adding some hot water. The mixture is stirred to form a sol. Alternatively, hydrated gelatin is heated in a double boiler for gelatin to dissolve. The concentrated gelatin sol is added to gel a liquid, stirring thoroughly to prevent gelatin from solidifying into rubbery strands or lump. Stirring also ensures even dispersion.

Gelation of a gelatin sol   Gelatin is a hydrophilic colloid. Polar groups on gelatin molecule bind water molecules in layers forming a shell around the molecule. Cooling of the gel increases its viscosity, and at chilling temperatures the fluid sol is converted into an elastic solid or gel. A three-dimensional network of gelatin molecules join to form a gel which entraps and immobilizes liquid in it. A gelatin gel is reversible. At 28°C it melts and forms a sol, which can reset and form a gel.

$$\text{Hydrated gelatin sol} \underset{\text{warming}}{\overset{\text{chilling}}{\rightleftarrows}} \text{Gelatin gel}$$

Once a gel is formed, rigidity increases with time and maximum gel strength is reached in 24 hours. As the gel ages, some of the liquid may escape from the network, a phenomenon studied earlier called syneresis.

The strength of a gelatin gel is affected by the following:

Concentration of gelatin   A concentration of 1–2 per cent gelatin can form a firm gel, which does not melt at normal serving temperature. Excess gelatin forms a stiff rubbery gel.

Sugar   Presence of sugar in excess increases the amount of gelatin needed for gelation.

Acid   Acid increases the clarity of the gel and lowers gel formation and melting temperature.

Fruits and vegetables   Uncooked pineapple and figs contain proteolytic enzymes, which hydrolyse gelatin and do not permit gelation.

Fruits and vegetables if added uncooked, float in jelly because of pockets of intercellular air. While making such jellies, blanch the fruits/vegetables and add them only when the gelatin sol is as viscous as thick raw egg white.

Whips, sponges, and creams These cold desserts are prepared by whipping the cold viscous gelatin sol. Whipping at this stage gives a foam double in volume of the original sol. After the foam is formed, the desserts are chilled for the gelatin to set. These desserts are a combination of a foam and a gel.

Pieces of baked fish skins, when cooled on the baking pan, stick to it because of conversion of collagen in the skin of fish to gelatin.

MILK

Milk is a solution of sugar lactose, and water-soluble vitamins and minerals. It is a colloidal dispersion of protein and an emulsion of fat in water. Water accounts for 87 per cent of milk.

Proteins in milk are of two types:

1. *Casein* Alpha, beta, and kappa caseins
2. *Serum or whey proteins* Albumin and globulins

They are of colloidal dimensions and make milk opaque. Casein is colloidally dispersed in milk as calcium phosphocaseinate. Casein molecules form micelles by aggregating with calcium and phosphorus.

Milk Cookery

Colloidal proteins remain dispersed in water as the molecules are hydrated. Molecules of water are bound to the polar groups of proteins. Besides the protective water layer, protein molecules are stabilized by the charge they carry as all molecules carry the same charge and like charges repel each other.

Effect of heat on milk proteins

1. Heat denatures and coagulates serum or whey proteins which settle to the bottom of the container.
2. When milk is heated in an uncovered vessel a skin forms on top. This is because of evaporation of water and concentration of casein, which blocks calcium salts and milk fats. The skin holds steam and makes milk boil over. A foam minimizes skin formation and this is the reason why hot coffee, cocoa, etc., are whipped to induce a foam or served with whipped cream. Casein is otherwise insensitive to heat.
3. The colour and flavour of condensed milk is because of browning caused by lactose and milk protein (refer Maillard browning in Chapter 9).

Effect of Acid on Casein

Fresh milk has a pH of 7.6 and casein micelles are dispersed as a colloidal sol. Acidity is increased when acid is added to milk, e.g., while making paneer, or acidity formed due to natural souring by lactic acid bacteria which ferment lactose to lactic acid, lowering the pH of milk. This reduces the stability of casein micelles and it coagulates, forming a gel. This is because addition of acid neutralizes the charge on protein.

$$\text{Calcium phosphocaseinate} \; + \; H^+ \; \longrightarrow \; \text{Neutral casein} + Ca^{++}$$
$$\text{(sol)} \qquad\qquad \text{(acid)} \qquad\qquad \text{(gel)}$$

If the gel formed is cut, stirred, or heated, liquid seeps out and the gel separates into two phases: the casein, rich solid called curd and the watery liquid called whey.

When milk or cream is added to acidic fruits, such as peaches and strawberries, the acid from the fruit lowers the pH of milk/cream causing it to thicken or even curdle.

While making curds or yoghurt, a starter culture of lactobacilli species is added to warm milk. The bacteria ferment milk sugar lactose to lactic acid and convert milk into curds.

$$\text{Milk} \; \xrightarrow[\text{bacteria}]{\text{lactic acid}} \; \text{Curds}$$
$$\text{(sol)} \qquad\qquad\qquad \text{(gel)}$$
$$\text{Warm temperature}$$

Yoghurt differs from curds because of the difference in species of lactobacilli used in the culture. The acid added to curdle milk for making paneer or cottage cheese is citric acid or, previously prepared whey water or lime juice.

EGGS

Eggs are used in a number of dishes because of the properties of egg white and yolk proteins.

Egg White

Nine proteins are dispersed as a sol in egg white. The two albumins, ovalbumin and conalbumin, which form 70 per cent of the proteins are fibrous proteins. Lysozyme is a globular protein and ovomucin gives thickness to the egg white. The protein avidin in raw egg white binds biotin, making it unavailable.

Egg Yolk

Proteins and lipids are the major constituents of dispersed phase in the yolk (Table 5.2). Many proteins are present as lipoproteins. Some lipoproteins contain lecithin, which is a natural emulsifying agent. Cholesterol is also present in the yolk.

TABLE 5.2 Composition of hen's egg

	Total Weight (%)	Water (%)	Protein (%)	Fat (%)
Whole egg	100	65	13	11
White	58	88	11	—
Yolk	31	48	18	33

Effect of Heat on Egg Proteins

Except for ovomucoid, all other egg white proteins are denatured by heat and get coagulated. The transparent viscous sol of egg white turns white and opaque, and forms a gel with water trapped inside.

The yolk, which is a thick liquid, becomes a solid with a mealy texture when denatured by heat. Egg white begins to coagulate at 60°C and is complete at 65°C, while the yolk starts to coagulate at 65°C and is coagulated at 70°C. Heating beyond this temperature shrinks and toughens the coagulated egg protein.

Egg Cookery

Cooking eggs in their shell   Eggs may be boiled in their shell to a soft or hard consistency. Sometimes a greenish grey layer forms on the surface of the yolk in a hard-boiled egg. This layer is ferrous sulfide formed by iron of the yolk reacting with hydrogen sulfide liberated by sulphur-containing proteins. This layer forms due to prolonged cooking. If hard-boiled eggs are immersed in cold water or cracked immediately after boiling, the H_2S formed is drawn away from the yolk.

Poached eggs   Eggs are cooked in hot water till the white is set and the yolk is semi-liquid. Vinegar added to poaching water hastens coagulation of egg proteins.

Fried eggs   The pan temperature should be above coagulation temperature. If the pan is too hot, the egg white toughens and develops a brown edge which is more flavoursome.

Scrambled eggs   The whole egg is blended with milk and heated to bring about coagulation of protein. Scrambled eggs should be moist, tender, and fluffy. Once the egg is coagulated, turn off the heat otherwise protein will get curdled, i.e., separate into curd and liquid.

Custards   An egg custard is prepared using one egg, a cup of milk, a tablespoon of sugar, and a pinch of salt. Milk is heated and added to beaten egg along with sugar and salt.

In egg custards, the egg protein ovalbumin gets denatured by heat and unites to form a network in which liquid milk is trapped to form a fragile gel. In a stirred custard, stirring breaks the gel as it forms and results in a smooth velvety texture. Heating should be done in a double boiler because the custard curdles at higher temperatures. Many factors affect the viscosity of the finished product such as the concentration of egg—more the egg, more viscous the custard. Sugar and salt help in gel formation by forming hydrogen bonds and salt increases viscosity. The quality of the egg and milk used for making the custard as well as the age of the custard affects its viscosity. Stale custards show syneresis. Beating egg to a foam before preparing custard gives desirable texture.

Egg Foams

Egg white is a viscous sol with proteins dispersed in it. It can be beaten into a foam. The proteins ovomucin, ovoglobulin, and conalbumin are necessary to form a fine foam with small air cells.

As air is incorporated into the liquid, protein molecules collect at the air-water interface. When more air is incorporated, the water layer gets thinner and protein molecules get stretched and unwind from their coiled structure. Surface denaturation takes place exposing the reactive 'R' groups along the protein molecules. These groups unite and give rigidity to the foam. Surface denaturation makes the foam rigid and when heat is applied, the proteins coagulate forming a permanent foam.

Stages of fresh egg white foam formation

1. *Foamy*
   (a) Bubbles form on surface, but all egg white is not broken up.
   (b) Foam is extremely unstable.
   (c) Air cells are generally large.
   (d) Mixture is still fluid.
   (e) Mixture starts to become opalescent. Acid, salt, and vanilla are added at this stage.

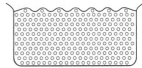

2. *Soft peaks*
   (a) Air cells are medium fine, all egg white exists as foam.
   (b) Foam is fairly stable, slight drainage occurs on short standing.
   (c) Mixture is shiny, flows easily in bowl, but is elastic
   (d) Soft peaks fall over to near the base of foam as beater is lifted from foam.
   (e) Sugar is added gradually at this stage.

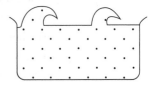

3. *Stiff peaks*
   (a) Air cells are fine, especially if acids are added at foamy stage. Mixture is white and opaque.
   (b) Foam quite stable, some drainage occurs on prolonged standing.
   (c) Mixture is shiny, flows slowly in bowl, but is still elastic.
   (d) Peaks are still quite soft, but the tip of the peak falls over as the beater is pulled from foam.
   (e) Egg whites for souffles and omelettes are beaten to this stage.
   (f) Egg white and sugar are beaten to this stage for angel cakes and pie meringues.

4. *Dry*
   (a) Air cells are very fine, mixture is extremely white.
   (b) Foam is not stable, drainage is rapid on long standing.

(c) Mixture is dull, has lost its ability to flow in the bowl.

(d) Mass is brittle and inelastic, peaks remain in rigid points.

(e) This stage is avoided for products of fresh egg white. Only reconstituted dehydrated egg whites must be beaten to this stage.

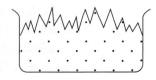

Once the beaten egg white has reached the desired stage, it should be used promptly otherwise it will stiffen upon standing without additional beating.

When egg white is beaten beyond the stiff peak stage a dry stiff foam, curdled in appearance, is obtained. Overbeating makes the surface a denatured film which is insoluble, so that liquid drains from the film and air bubbles coalesce. So, coagulation of protein can be due to overbeating as well as heating.

Egg yolks should be beaten extensively to form a fine, fairly stable foam. The foam is not denatured by beating unlike egg white.

Factors affecting egg white foam formation

1. Utensil should be large enough to allow for full increase in volume of foam. However, it should not be so large that the beater has no contact with egg white.

2. A rotary beater or wire whip should be used. Thinner the blade or finer the whip, the smaller are the air cells and finer is the foam.

3. Egg whites whip readily at room temperature than at refrigerated temperature. At colder temperatures, whites are too viscous to whip readily.

4. Presence of fat, even in traces, interferes with foaming and produces foam of less volume. So bowl and beater used should be perfectly dry and free of fat. Egg white should be separated completely from the yolk.

5. Salt and cream of tartar are used in egg white foams. Salt is used for flavour. Lemon juice or cream of tartar makes foam more stable. Both these ingredients delay foam formation, so should be added after the foamy stage is reached and not before you begin beating. Cream of tartar strengthens egg white protein and prevents foam from collapsing.

6. Addition of water up to 40 per cent of the volume of egg increases volume of foam. It also makes the product more tender, especially in omelettes and sponge cakes. However, water is incorporated towards the end.

7. Sugar acts as a dehydrating agent and excess beating is required to produce a foam. But once formed, the foam is stable and very fine but of less volume. Egg white foam is shiny as sugar prevents, in part, coagulation of protein that causes opaqueness. Excess sugar reduces extensibility of egg white foam.

Sugar added to foam prevents foam from being overbeaten inspite of longer beating time. Since sugar reduces coagulation with its accompanying loss of elasticity, a foam with sugar can be used for spreading without rupturing the air cells.

Meringues are egg white foams with sugar incorporated into it. There are two types of meringues: soft and hard.

1. Soft type are used for topping baked Alaska, cream, and chocolate pies. Equal amounts of sugar and egg white are used, i.e., 2 tablespoons sugar for every egg white which measures 2 tablespoons. Water in egg white is converted into a fairly concentrated syrup.

   Egg white is beaten to a foamy stage and then salt is added. Beating is continued till foam barely flows in the bowl. Sugar is added and foam is beaten till the soft peak with rounded top stage is reached. A meringue is more stable when sugar is beaten, rather than folded in.

   Soft meringues are spread on soft pie fillings and baked. Baking causes proteins in foam to coagulate and stabilize the foam without undue shrinkage. Two defects seen are as follows:

   (a) 'Weeping' or accumulation of liquid where the meringue and filling meet. This is due to under-coagulation of foam. This leakage can be overcome by placing the meringue on a hot filling (60–77°C or 140–170°F).
   (b) Appearance of amber-coloured droplets on the surface of the foam. This is due to overcoagulation of foam proteins due to the hot filling used. This beading can be overcome by baking meringue for a short time, i.e., hot oven 425°F for $4^1/_2$ minutes.

   A soft meringue is fluffy, slightly moist, and tender. The surface should be light brown with little contrast in colour between peaks and depressions. It should have a glossy sheen.

2. Hard meringues are used to make macaroons or as a base for pie fillings. It contains 1/4 cup sugar for every egg white used.

   Egg white is first beaten to soft peak stage, sugar is added, and then beaten again to form stiff peaks. Meringue mixture is spooned onto an oiled baking sheet. Hard meringues are baked at lower temperature (250°F) for 45–60 minutes. A good meringue should be dry, crisp, and tender. They should look puffy and be delicate brown.

   Omelettes For puffy omelettes, egg yolk with added liquid is beaten till thick and light lemon in colour. Egg white is beaten separately till stiff. The two foams are combined with gentle folding till a homogenous mixture is obtained. The mixture is poured into a preheated greased pan. When omelette sets along the edges, the pan may be covered and heat lowered to complete cooking. Air bubbles incorporated during foaming are poor conductors of heat.

A puffy omelette should be light and fluffy, uniformly cooked throughout, and should be well blended. It should be tender, slightly moist, and a delicate uniform brown.

Souffle and Fondue

Both contain milk, grated cheese, eggs, salt, and butter. Bread is used in fondue and flour in souffle. Fondue has double the amount of milk.

In fondue, milk is thickened with bread cubes. This hot milk–bread mixture is blended with egg yolk, then grated cheese, and finally beaten egg white is folded in.

In the case of souffle, a very thick white sauce is made. Egg yolk is blended in it followed by grated cheese. The white sauce should be hot enough to cause the fat in cheese to melt. The stiffly beaten egg white is then beaten in.

Both souffle and fondue are baked in a moderately hot oven at 350°F. The casserole, which contains the mix, is placed in a pan of hot water to protect the contents directly in contact with the baking utensil from overcoagulation.

As the product bakes, heat expands the air bubbles incorporated in the foam and the product rises. To prevent the product from falling as it cools, a high proportion of egg (which gives structure) should be used. A very thick white sauce base also helps. The souffle or fondue should be served immediately.

Cake

No baking powder is used in sponge and angel cakes as these are foam cakes. The proportion of egg, sugar, and water to cake flour is high. No fat is used.

The exception is chiffon cake in which salad oil is added at the last stage.

Functions of cake ingredients

Eggs

1. Incorporates air into the batter—leavening agent
2. Coagulated egg protein—structure
3. High water content of egg provides water which is essential for flour to form batter. Water converted to steam acts as a leavening agent.

Sugar

1. Castor sugar is a tenderizing agent which counterbalances the effect of egg and flour.

Acid

1. Cream of tartar or lemon juice changes the colour of egg white to a snowy white crumb.
2. Acid stabilizes protein film at air–water interface so that it lasts until heat penetrates batter and structure sets—the air cell walls are hence finer.
3. Lemon juice adds flavour to the product.

Flour

1. Flour provides structure. Good quality cake flour of fine granulation should be used so that it is evenly dispersed.

Flour should be folded in, not mixed. Excess manipulation should be avoided as flour will absorb liquid and foam will collapse and product will become tough.

In angel cake, only egg white is used. In sponge cake, the entire egg is used.

Baking is done at higher temperatures (400–425°F) for faster expansion of air cells and more rapid setting of batter and absorption of less water by starch of flour.

Role of Protein in Breadmaking

Bread is made from wheat, which is milled into flour. Wheat flour from hard wheat is higher in protein and is used for breadmaking, while soft wheat is low in proteins and yields a weak flour which is suitable for cakes and biscuits. The principal protein in bread is gluten, which is a protein complex made up of more or less equal amounts of glutenin and gliadin proteins. When flour and water are kneaded together, the gluten complex starts forming and an elastic dough is formed. This dough is extensible and when yeast produce carbon dioxide gas, gluten is stretched and forms air cells. On application of heat, the gluten coagulates and forms a fairly rigid cellular structure. The gluten matrix, thus, forms the foundation of the structure of all bakery products. Excessive mixing of the dough can weaken the gluten structure.

MEAT

Flesh food includes meat, poultry, and fish. The term meat is used for red meats from animal sources such as beef, veal, pork, lamb, or mutton.

Meat is composed of 15–20 per cent protein of high biological value, 5–40 per cent fat, B-complex vitamins, iron, and phosphorus. Lean meat is made up of one or more muscles. Each muscle is made up of many bundles of muscle fibres arranged in them. The simplest structure in meat protein is the protein molecules, myosin, and actin, which form myofilaments. Thick myofilaments are myosin and thin myofilaments are actin. Several myofilaments form myofibrils and bundles of myofibrils embedded in sarcoplasm are enclosed in a thin transparent membrane called the sarcolemma and form a muscle fibre.

Connective tissue consisting mainly of ground substance, collagen, and little elastin is found between each fibre. Connective tissue which surrounds each muscle fibre is called endomysium. Several muscle fibres are bundled together to form thicker fibrous bundles surrounded by connective tissue called perimysium. The outermost covering of the muscle which encloses many bundles of fibres is the epimysium. When meat is cooked, collagen is hydrolysed to gelatin. Figure 5.5 describes the structure of mutton muscle.

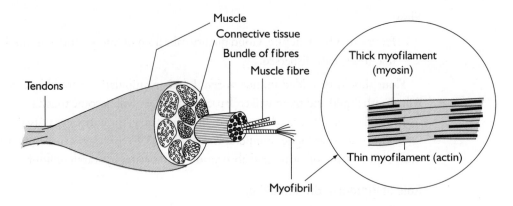

Fig. 5.5 Structure of mutton muscle

Fat is deposited in the connective tissue within the muscle and is called marbling. The amount of exercise, age, and feed of the animal influences the fat content of meat.

The colour of meat is due to pigment myoglobin and partly due to haemoglobin. In the living tissue, myoglobin which is purplish red exists in equilibrium with oxymyoglobin which is the bright red oxygenated form. After death of the animal, the colour changes to purplish red. On cutting the meat, due to oxidation, a bright red colour is formed. Further oxidation due to microorganisms and warm temperature change the colour to brownish red (see Fig. 5.6).

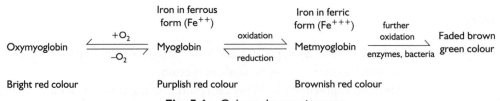

Fig. 5.6 Colour changes in meat

When meat is cooked, the proteins get denatured by continuous heating and denatured globin hemichrome is formed which is the denatured form of metmyoglobin that is greyish brown in colour (see Fig. 5.7).

Post-mortem Changes

When an animal is slaughtered, the skeletal muscles stiffen and remain stiff for about 24–48 hours after which they soften and become flexible once again. This condition is called rigor mortis. Many factors such as age, species of animal, and activity prior to slaughter affect rigor mortis. Meat cooked while in rigor mortis is much tougher.

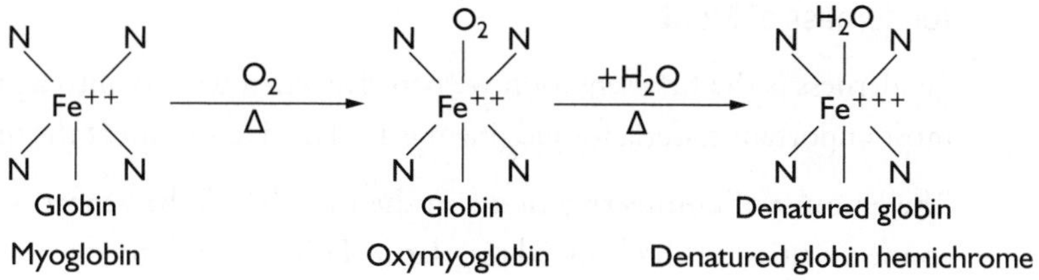

Fig. 5.7   Colour changes in cooked meat

After slaughter, glycogen store is broken down and lactic acid is formed lowering the pH to 5.6. Low pH in meat is desirable. It inhibits bacterial growth and is juicier. Animals prior to slaughter should be well rested, with a 1 per cent glycogen store so that maximum lactic acid is formed.

Ripening or Aging

After rigor mortis passes, meat gradually becomes more juicier and tender because of autolytic breakdown of cell proteins by enzymes. The flavour also increases. The time and temperature also influence the aging process. Planned aging is costly and is used for prime and choice grades of meat.

Changes in Meat during Cooking

The following changes are observed:

1. Cooking destroys microorganisms and their spores. If pork is infested with *Trichinella*, the cysts get destroyed at 77°C.
2. The jelly-like protein gel stiffens and toughens as proteins get denatured.
3. Hydrolysis of collagen, the main component of connective tissue surrounding meat fibres, takes place. Collagen gets hydrolysed to gelatin and the stock or gravy gels on cooling. As temperature increases, more collagen is lost.
4. Colour changes from red to purplish red to brown (Fig. 5.7). Pork should be cooked to the grey stage to ensure destruction of parasites.
5. When meat is cooked, liquid or drip separates out (drip formation), meat shrinks, and loses weight. Drip contains water-soluble compounds, protein, and fat.
6. Cooked meat has appetite-stimulating flavours. When meat is browned, amino acids are broken down forming volatile compounds which give a strong flavour to meat.
7. Cooking causes fat cells to rupture and fat to disperse in meat.
8. Overcooking toughens meat because of excessive loss of drip and loss of collagen and fat. Volatile flavour compounds are lost and mutton fibres become stringy.
9. There is a marked reduction in volume and increase in density caused by shrinkage of muscle fibres lengthwise.

Tenderness of Meat

Tenderness is the first sensation we perceive when we bite into a piece of meat. This is the most important criteria for judging meat. Many factors affect the tenderness of meat.

The amount of connective tissue in the muscle When meat is cooked, collagen in the connective tissue is hydrolysed to gelatin. This increases tenderness of meat.

The extent of hydration of proteins Aging results in greater hydration of proteins because of movement of ions into and out of the cells. Water is held by hydrogen bonds and this increases the tenderness of meat.

Marbling of meat Fat deposition in the connective tissue within the muscle is called marbling. In well marbled meat, fat lubricates the lean meat and makes it juicier.

Use of tenderizers Meat can be made more tender by using tenderizers. Tenderness can be increased by mechanical means, vinegar, enzymes, and salt.

Mechanical means When meat is subjected to mechanical treatment such as grinding, pounding, needling, scoring, or cubing, it becomes more tender. These methods cut or break the muscle fibres and connective tissues of meat.

Vinegar When the pH of mutton is lowered by adding vinegar, curds, or lime juice, there is increase in hydration of meat proteins and subsequent increase in tenderness.

Enzymes Proteolytic enzymes are often used to tenderize tough cuts of meat. Enzymes destroy the sarcolemma, and hydrolyse the proteins in the fibre and break down collagen and elastin. Cooking temperatures activate the enzymes and denature the connective tissue. Commercial papain extracted from the unripe papaya is applied to the surface of meat to be tenderized. The meat is pierced with a fork to allow the enzyme to penetrate the meat.

Other proteolytic enzymes are bromelin from pineapple, ficin from figs, and trypsin from fungal protease. Papain from unripe or green papaya is most common. Excessive use of enzyme results in an undesirable mushy texture.

Salt Salt used in moderation enhances the water retention and ultimately the juiciness. The bound water is held tightly and less juice is lost from meat during cooking.

Cured Meat

Cured and smoked meat develop a particular desirable flavour. Meat is cured using salt, sodium nitrite, sodium nitrate, sugar, and vinegar. These ingredients are used in the form of a rub, a pickle, or injected into the meat. Figure 5.8 shows a cross-section of mutton muscle.

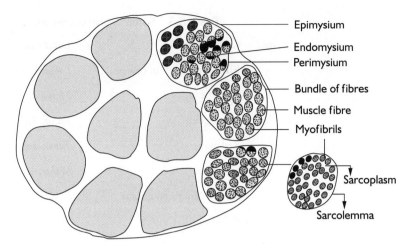

Fig. 5.8   Cross-section of mutton muscle

Salt acts as a preservative while nitrate reacts with myoglobin to form unstable nitric oxide myoglobin which is denatured by heat to nitrosomyoglobin giving a stable pink colour to cured ham, bacon, and beef.

Smoked meats are impregnated with constituents of smoke which have preservative action by destroying microorganisms. Smoking has a drying effect and imparts desirable organoleptic properties to meat. It brings out the colour inside the meat and gives a desirable gloss or finish to meat.

PULSES

Pulses or legumes are the dried seeds of pod-bearing plants. They belong to the *Leguminaceae* family. They are a good source of proteins, carbohydrates, and B-complex vitamins. With the exception of soya beans, they are deficient in fat. The plants of this family are not only an important source of proteins in vegetarian diets but also contribute towards soil fertility by their ability to fix atmospheric nitrogen, thereby increasing the nitrogen content of the soil. They are used in soups, stews, vegetable preparations, salads, and as an accompaniment to meat. In Indian diets, they are extensively used in combination with cereals in practically all meals. Table 5.3 shows some important pulses with their local names.

Pulses are available in five forms. These are

1. Whole grains, e.g., chickpea, kidney beans
2. Split and de-husked grains, *moong dal chilka*, yellow *moong* dal
3. Sprouted grains, e.g., *moong* sprouts
4. Pulse flour, e.g., *besan*
5. Parched pulses, e.g., roasted bengal gram

TABLE 5.3   Some important pulses

S. no.	Common name	Local name
1.	Black eyed beans or cow pea	*Lobia, chawli*
2.	Moth bean	*Matki*
3.	Horse gram	*Kulthi, kuleeth*
4.	Red gram	*Tuvar, arhar*
5.	Split peas	*Matar, vatana*
6.	Broad beans or fava beans	*Bakla*
7.	Field bean	*Sem*
8.	Lima beans	Butter bean
9.	Haricot beans or kidney beans	*Rajma*, French bean
10.	Chickpeas or Bengal gram	*Channa*
11.	Black gram	*Urad*
12.	Lentils	*Masoor*
13.	Green gram	*Moong*

Pulses contain about 18 to 25 per cent protein, 1.5 per cent lipids, and 55 to 60 per cent carbohydrates along with soluble sugars and unavailable carbohydrates. Oligosaccharides raffinose and stachyose are present in pulses and cannot be digested by humans because humans lack the necessary enzymes to digest them. They are broken down by microbial flora of the lower intestinal tract producing large amounts of gas, mainly carbon dioxide and hydrogen, along with small amounts of methane. Proteins in pulses have high molecular weight and compact molecules. Some proteins are complexed with carbohydrates and some with phytin. The protein in pulses have varying digestibility. The presence of trypsin inhibitors, polyphenolic compounds, such as tannin, fibre, and phytin, affect digestibility and availability of proteins and minerals.

In whole grains, the two cotyledons in the seed are tightly enveloped by a seed coat or husk. The husk can be removed and cotyledons split into dal by drying and controlling the moisture content in the grain. Pulses are milled to remove the husk. Milling improves digestibility and reduces fibre content which in turn increases nutrient availability. Anti-nutritional factors, such as polyphenols, which are mainly present in the seed coat, is removed during milling. However, during milling the germ may get removed along with skin, resulting in loss of thiamine.

Effect of Steeping

Most pulses have a hard outer covering and need to be soaked prior to cooking to reduce cooking time. Water enters the grain through the hilum and seeps into the grain causing the seed coat to wrinkle. After some time, the cotyledons swell and the wrinkles are removed. Steeping softens the hard seed coat, cells expand and intercellular adhesion caused by pectin is reduced. Whole pulses should be soaked in cold water overnight or in warm water for a few hours. Steeping pulses in water has many beneficial effects:

1. Cooking time is reduced
2. Oligosaccharides are reduced
3. Phytic acid content is reduced

However, when pulses are soaked in water, some water-soluble nutrients leach into the water and are lost if water is discarded. Losses are more in dals. To minimize such losses, water used for soaking can be used in cooking.

Effect of Cooking

Most pulses are cooked before they are served. Pulses need a longer cooking time as compared to cereals. Soaking or steeping pulses reduces cooking time drastically. Dals or dehulled split pulses cook faster than whole grains and are more acceptable in terms of taste, appearance, and texture. Overall protein quality is higher in pulses cooked by moist heat methods. Cooking by dry heat, e.g., by roasting and very high temperatures, reduce the essential amino acids lysine and methionine content.

Heat destroys anti-nutritional factors, and increases digestibility and availability of amino acids. Anti-nutritional factors, such as trypsin inhibitors, lathyrogens, haemagglutinins, and tannins, are removed or inactivated during cooking.

Trypsin inhibitors These are proteins that prevent the enzyme trypsin from digesting proteins in the diet. Proteins consumed are not fully utilized. They are present in soya bean and kidney bean. They are heat labile and are inactivated by autoclaving at 120°C for 15 to 30 minutes.

Lathyrogens Lathyrism is a disease of the spinal cord and nerves caused by excessive consumption of the pulse *Lathyrus sativus* or *kesari* dal. They can be removed by steeping *kesari* dal. When *kesari* dal is soaked in hot water for two hours, washed-and-sun dried, the neurotoxin β-N-Oxalyl-L-Alanine is removed. Parboiling *kesari* dal by soaking in cold water, steaming, soaking once again, and drying can help lower toxin levels to 10 to 20 per cent.

Haemagglutinins They are found in horse gram, double bean, and field beans and are heat labile. Also known as lectins, they are protein in nature and interact with digestive enzymes affecting the digestion and absorption of food.

Polyphenolic compounds   Tannins are polyphenolic compounds present in large amounts in the seed coat of most grains. They bind with iron and interfere with the digestion of carbohydrates and proteins, affecting their availability. Milling of grains reduces the tannin content.

In most dals, toxic constituents are inactivated in the normal cooking process. Therefore, pulses should be heat treated or at least steamed before consumption to denature the natural toxins present.

Addition of cooking soda or sodium bicarbonate reduces the cooking time of pulses by softening cellulose and tenderizing protein.

Addition of acidic foods in the form of tamarind, tomatoes, *kokum*, etc. to pulses before they are tender should be avoided as cooking time is increased.

Hard water contains salts of calcium and magnesium. When legumes are cooked with hard water, they take more time to cook. Calcium and magnesium chloride and sulphate react with pectic substances and phytates forming insoluble calcium and magnesium pectates in the cell walls, hardening the cellulose and delaying the cooking time.

Dehulling pulses or removal of seed coat reduces cooking time to one third and increases the digestibility of pulses.

Sprouting of Pulses

Dried whole grain pulses are dormant and germinate when they are steeped in water overnight, drained, and tied in a porous cotton cloth and kept in a warm place for 24 to 48 hours. Moisture and warmth are necessary for sprouts to form.

Sprouted grains have the following advantages.

- The nutritive value is enhanced. Dormant enzymes become active and begin the breakdown of starch into maltose, and proteins into essential amino acids. Pectinase enzyme is released which helps in the breakdown of cell walls and increase in the availability of nutrients. Minerals, such as calcium, iron, and zinc, are released from their bound form and phytic acid content is decreased thereby increasing availability of proteins and minerals. The content of B-complex vitamins, such as riboflavin, niacin, folic acid, choline, and biotin, increase. There is a significant increase in ascorbic acid or vitamin C content which is absent in the dormant grain and is synthesized during germination.
- Sprouts cook faster and can also be consumed uncooked or partially steamed in salads.
- Sprouting metabolizes oligosaccharides and prevents flatulence or gas formation.
- Sprouts are easier to digest.
- The thickening power of starch is reduced as starch is broken down into sugar. This property is made use of in preparation of infant foods.

Pulses play an important role in cookery not only because of their good nutritive value, but also because of their versatile use in food as a binding agent, as a thickening agent, for flavour and consistency, as an ingredient in seasonings, chutneys and chutney powders, and in stuffings and desserts. Their role in fermentation, along with cereals and the supplementary value of proteins, is discussed at length in this text.

COMMERCIAL USES OF PROTEINS

The major role of protein in food preparation includes the ability of proteins to

1. Form foams
2. Bind water and form viscous sols and gels
3. Get coagulated by heat
4. Exhibit emulsifying properties
5. Show enzymatic activity

No single protein exhibits all these properties and these complex reactions are influenced by other constituents present in food. Proteins are of major significance in determining the organoleptic characteristics and nutritional value of a food. Egg, milk, and gelatin are used for gels, foams, whips, souffles, meringues, custards, cakes, puddings, confections, soups, sauces, and gravies.

Proteins extracted from natural and novel sources are being extensively used in the manufacture of convenience foods for catering systems and for low-cost feeding programmes which rely on proteins to bridge the protein calorie gap.

Soya bean proteins, protein isolates from oilseed cakes, single cell protein, and milk proteins are being widely used today by the food processing industry. They are used in health drinks, weight-reduction foods, muscle-building foods, and many infant foods, and general convenience foods. Protein hydrocolloids have many uses in the food industry today.

Textured Vegetable Protein

Plant proteins can be used to produce textured protein products, also called protein analogs. They form an important substitute for expensive animal products. Textured vegetable protein (TVP) includes proteins manufactured from soya bean, groundnuts, and other oilseeds after oil has been expelled. Proteins can also be extracted from green leaves, grass, and certain species of microorganisms, such as yeast, mould, bacteria, and algae. Textured vegetable proteins are made by extracting the proteins from plants—mainly soya beans by treating it with alkali. The protein extracted is spun into fibres of nearly pure protein. The fibres are coloured, flavoured, and shaped into products that resembles and tastes like meat. They are often enriched with the essential amino acid methionine, B-complex vitamins, and iron to make it as nutritious as real meat.

These proteins are available in the market in the form of granules, nuggets, cubes, or slices. These products contain 50 per cent protein on dry weight basis. Table 5.4 discusses the percentage of protein in some novel sources of protein-rich food.

TABLE 5.4 Novel sources of protein

Source	Protein %
1. **Single cell protein**	
Bacteria	54
Yeast	65
Algae (blue green — *Spirulina*, green — *Chlorella*)	62
Fungi (*Fusarium*)	74
2. **Leaf protein (dry weight)**	50
Grass	
Foliage	
Harvested crops	
3. **Oilseed residues (pure protein isolated from seed cake)**	90
Groundnut	
Cotton	
Sesame	
4. **Textured vegetable protein (meat extenders)**	50
Soya beans	

The advantages of using TVP are as follows:

1. They can be used as a substitute for real meat in curries, biriyanis, etc.
2. Alternatively, they can be used along with real meat as a meat extender by mixing it with meat products as in cutlets, koftas, keema matar, etc.
3. They are equally nutritious as meat and cheaply priced, thereby cutting down on costs.
4. They are widely used in food processing industry.
5. They are acceptable to vegetarians and are used in nutrition feeding programmes.

Other Commercial Uses of Protein

1. Dehydrated egg whole, egg white	Cakes, omelettes, bakery products
2. Whey proteins	Health food, muscle building
3. Casein	Artificial whipped toppings, coffee whiteners
4. Gelatin	Gelling agent, whipping agent in foams, and clearing agent in wines and fruit juices Prevents ice crystal growth in ice cream
5. Synthetic amino acids	Lysine, methionine, and tryptophan
6. Protein hydrolysates	Beef and yeast extracts (flavour enhancers)
7. Milk solids	Health drinks, infant food

SUMMARY

Proteins are complex organic molecules containing nitrogen, which are not only essential for life but also play an important role in food preparation. They are made up of amino acids linked together into long chains by peptide linkages. These long chains or polypeptides form the backbone of the protein molecule.

Proteins differ from one another on the basis of amino acids present, and can be classified in various ways. Proteins found in living tissues are called native proteins and are present as macromolecules which are sensitive and fragile. They are hydrophilic colloids stabilized by charge on the molecules and a layer of water surrounding the molecules.

When proteins are heated, beaten, or subjected to acids, alkalis, etc., they show changes in physical, chemical, and biological properties. This is called denaturation. Many factors affect denaturation.

The proteins of specific importance to a caterer are milk, gelatin, egg, meat, and pulses. They are capable of forming gels, play a role in emulsification, used for various stages of foam formation, and increase the viscosity of many food products. Pulses play an important role in cookery, not only because of high nutritive value but also for multiple uses as binding and thickening agents. Apart from these properties, proteins in food have a wide variety of uses both in the kitchen as well as in the food processing industry. Proteins extracted from soya beans, oilseed cakes, foliage, and microorganisms are used extensively as food or in health foods to bridge the protein gap. Because of their properties, proteins have many commercial applications in the food and beverage industry.

KEY TERMS

Autolysis Breakdown of a cell by its own enzymes.

Coagulation Solidification of a liquid protein on heating.

Collagen Protein in bones, skin, and connective tissue which is completely hydrolysed to gelatin by heat during cooking. Collagen fibres predominate in meat.

Connective tissue Made up of four proteins, namely elastin, reticulin, ground substance, and collagen which is most important. It is present within and between muscles.

Denaturation Relaxation of the tertiary structure to the secondary structure, accompanied by decreased solubility of a protein.

Elastin Yellow connective tissue present in very small amounts in muscle and does not get gelatinized during cooking.

Epimysium Sheath of connective tissue which covers the muscle.

Ground substance Protein in meat in which collagen and elastin are held to form connective tissue.

Haemagglutinins Also known as lectins, they are protein in nature and interact with digestive enzymes affecting the digestion and absorption of food. They are found in horse gram, double bean, and field beans and are heat labile.

Micelles A colloidal ion composed of an oriented arrangement of molecules.

Myoglobin An oxygen carrying pigment found in mutton muscle and is oxidized to oxymyoglobin which is bright red in colour.

Nitrosomyoglobin Pinkish red coloured compound produced by action of curing salts on meat.

Organoleptic Qualities of a food which appeal to the sense of taste, smell, etc.

Perimysium Connective tissue binding groups of bundles of muscle fibres.

Primary structure   Covalently bonded backbone chain of a protein (–C–C–N–C–C–N–C–C–N–).

Rigor mortis   Stiffening of muscles immediately after animals have been slaughtered.

Secondary structure   The helical configuration of the backbone chain of a protein, held by secondary bonds.

Tertiary structure   Distorted convolutions of the helical configuration; the form in which many proteins occur in nature and which is held by secondary bonding forces.

Textured vegetable protein (TVP)   Prepared from soya bean and used as a meat extender and also in vegetarian dishes.

Trichinella spiralis   A nematode worm present in infected pork that causes trichinosis disease.

Trypsin inhibitors   Trypsin inhibitors are proteins that prevent the enzyme trypsin in the gastrointestinal tract from digesting proteins in the diet. Proteins consumed are not fully utilized because of such anti-nutritional factors. They are present in soya beans.

REVIEW EXERCISES

1. Classify proteins on the basis of their structure and on the basis of character.
2. Explain the ionic character of an amino acid and influence of acid and alkali on it.
3. Explain the term denaturation and list the factors which affect denaturation.
4. What points should be kept in mind while preparing a fresh fruit jelly?
5. Explain briefly:
   (a) Effect of acid on casein
   (b) Post-mortem changes in meat
   (c) Cured meat
   (d) Prevention of discolouration of boiled egg yolk
6. Explain the different stages in egg white foam formation. What products are prepared from egg foams?
7. With the help of a neat diagram explain the structure of meat and factors which affect tenderization.
8. Discuss the commercial uses of protein.
9. Give four reasons why pulses should be cooked before consumption.

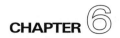
Fruits and Vegetables

LEARNING OBJECTIVES

After reading this chapter, you should be able to
• appreciate the importance of fruits and vegetables in our diet
• classify fruits and vegetables in different ways
• know the composition and tissue structure of fruits and vegetables
• understand the changes which take place in fruits and vegetables during ripening and storage
• select the appropriate procedures while cooking and processing fruits and vegetables
• suggest measures for retaining freshness, colour, and texture in fruits and vegetables
• understand the effect of cooking on plant pigments

INTRODUCTION

Fruits and vegetables are an important component of our daily diet. They not only add colour and a variety of textures to food but also provide significant amounts of vitamins, minerals, and carbohydrates including roughage. As discussed earlier in Chapter 4, fruits and vegetables are plant foods. Fruits are obtained from flowers. They are the ripened ovary or ovaries of a flowering plant together with the adjacent tissues. Most fruits are fleshy and pulpy or juicy and are pleasantly sweet and have a distinct appealing flavour when ripe. Except for rhubarb and cranberries, all fruits can be eaten uncooked. Vegetables are obtained from all parts of the plant, right from the root to the seed, depending on the specific plant. While some fruits of plants are classified as vegetables, most are called fruits depending on the amount of sugar and acid present in them.

CLASSIFICATION OF FRUITS AND VEGETABLES

Fruits can be classified on the basis of shape, cell structure, type of seed, or natural habitat. They may be grouped into soft fruits, segmented fruits, stone fruits, hard fruits, and tropical and other fruits.

TABLE 6.1   Classification of fruits

S. no.	Group	Examples
1	Berries or soft fruits	Strawberries, mulberries, cranberries, raspberries, gooseberries, blueberries
2	Citrus fruits or segmented fruits	Oranges, sweet lime, grapefruit, pomelos, kumquats, mandarin orange, tangerines
3	Drupes or stone fruits	Peaches, plums, apricots, cherries
4	Grapes	Green grapes, black grapes, seedless grapes
5	Melons	Watermelon, musk melon
6	Pomes or hard fruits	Apples, pears
7	Tropical and subtropical fruits	Bananas, guava, papaya, jackfruit, dragon fruit, custard apple, carambola or starfruit, kiwi fruit

Fruits may be further classified as berries, citrus fruits, drupes, grapes, melons, pomes, and tropical and subtropical fruits. A detailed classification with examples is given in Table 6.1. Each fruit has unique structural characteristics which is typical for the group. For example, berries have delicate cells with high water content, citrus fruits have segments while pomes have five encapsulated seeds in the core.

Vegetables are classified in different ways based on any one or more of the following criteria.

1. Nutritive value
2. Part of plant consumed
3. Pigments present
4. Season of the year

On the basis of nutritive value, they are grouped into four categories, namely

1. Beans and peas
2. Roots, tubers, and bulbs
3. Green leafy vegetables
4. Other vegetables

The botanical classification of vegetables is given in Table 6.2

TABLE 6.2   Botanical classification of vegetables

Roots	Tubers	Bulbs	Brassicas	Pods and seeds
Beetroot	Sweet potatoes	Spring onions	Cabbage	French beans
Carrots	Jerusalem artichokes	Garlic	Cauliflower	Butter beans
Horseradish	Potatoes	Onions	Broccoli	Runner beans
Radish	Yam	Leeks	Brussels sprouts	Cluster beans
Swedes	Colocasia	Shallots		Peas
Turnips				Sweet corn
				Okra

Contd

Table 6.2 Contd

Leafy	Fruiting	Stems and shoots	Algae and fungi	Seed sprouts
Fenugreek	Brinjal	Amaranth	Spirulina	Green gram
Lettuce	Plantain flowers	Asparagus	Oyster mushrooms	Moth beans
Spinach	Cucumber	Celery	Button mushrooms	Bengal gram
Watercress	All gourds	Kohlrabi	Shiitake mushrooms	
Mustard	Pumpkin	Globe artichokes		
Amaranth	Tomatoes	Ginger		
Coriander	Capsicum	Plantain stem		
Mint				

PLANT TISSUE SYSTEMS

Fruits and vegetables are made up of three types of tissue systems:

1. Dermal tissue
2. Vascular tissue
3. Ground tissue

The details of each system will vary from one fruit or vegetable to another.

Dermal Tissue System

Vegetables and fruits are covered with an outer protective coating called the skin or rind, which is called dermal tissue. This tissue encloses the vascular system and the ground system. Fluids, nutrients and waste products are transported through the vascular system, while the bulk of the edible portion of fruits and vegetables constitutes the ground system.

The dermal tissue comprises of the *epiderm*, which is a thin layer of epidermal cells that protect the surface. A layer of cutin and some waxes minimizes loss of moisture through evaporation. Vegetables that grow underground have a protective layer of cork-like cells called *periderm*.

Vascular Tissue System

The vascular system is composed of two parts, the xylem and the phloem. The xylem is made up of elongated tubular cells through which water moves, while the phloem tissue transports nutrients in solution.

Ground Tissue System

The ground system which forms the remaining edible portions of fruits and vegetables is mainly made up of parenchyma cells along with supporting cells and fibre.

Plant tissues are made up of cells which are of three types:

1. Parenchyma
2. Collenchyma
3. Sclerenchyma

Parenchyma cells

These cells are polyhedral with 11 to 20 faces and have intercellular air spaces in between, depending on how compactly the cells fit. Intercellular air spaces make up 1 to 25 per cent of the volume of fruits. The lesser the air spaces the more compact the texture. In apples, about 25 per cent of the volume is intercellular air space resulting in a slightly loose texture.

Supporting tissues may contain collenchyma and sclerenchyma cells, while most of the edible portion of plant foods is made up of parenchyma cells. The parenchyma cells (Fig. 6.1) consist of an outermost region called middle lamella, which is made up of pectic substances and cements the cells together. The primary cell wall is composed of several complex carbohydrates such as cellulose, hemicellulose, and pectic substances. There is a thin membrane between the cell wall and the interior of the cell called the plasmalemma which covers the protoplasm. The protoplasm contains several types of structures or organelles, namely

1. Plastids
2. Mitochondria
3. Nucleus

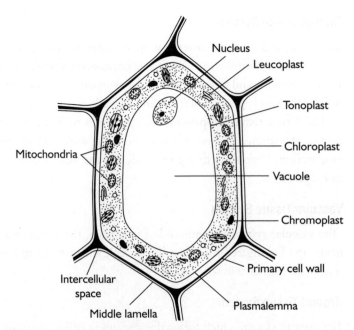

Fig. 6.1 Structure of a parenchyma cell

Plastids form and store two types of pigments and starch. They are of three types:

1. Chloroplasts which contain chlorophyll
2. Chromoplasts which contain carotenoids
3. Leucoplasts which form and store starch in the form of granules

The mitochondria are involved in plant respiration and have many enzymes which catalyze various biochemical reactions. The nucleus contains the hereditary material and plays an important role in cell division.

A thin membrane called tonoplast separates the protoplasm from the remaining interior of the cell. Each cell has a vacuole which gradually increases in size as the cell matures, while at the same time the proportion of the cell occupied by the protoplasm gradually reduces. The vacuole consists of a variety of flavouring compounds such as organic flavours, sugars, acids, and the flavonoid pigments. The vacuole occupies a large proportion of the cell at maturity and contains the following compounds.

1. Flavour components, such as organic flavours, which are distinct from one fruit or vegetable to another and also include sugars and acids
2. Flavonoid pigments, mainly anthocyanins and anthoxanthins
3. Cellular water which accounts for 90 per cent of water in the cell along with some nutrients and proteins

Collenchyma tissue

Collenchyma tissue or supporting tissue contributes to the overall structure of the edible portion of fruits and vegetables. Plant foods containing these cells are chewy and remain firm even after cooking. For example, elongated cells in the fibrous strands of celery are collenchyma cells.

Sclerenchyma cells

These are hard, wood-like cells that give a slightly gritty texture to fruits and vegetables. These cells have thick cell walls containing lignin, which is a wood-like compound. Fruits such as pears have sclereids, a type of sclerenchyma cells which give a unique gritty texture to pears, while fibers in green beans are also sclerenchyma cells which are supportive cells.

The structure and texture of fruits and vegetables also depends on the unavailable polysaccharides and lignin present. Cellulose, hemicelluloses, pectic substances, and lignin are present in varying amounts in fruits and vegetables (refer Chapter 4 on carbohydrates). Cellulose is a homogenous glucose polymer but differs from amylose because its glucose units are joined by 1,4-β-glucosidic linkages. These linkages render cellulose indigestible and are often responsible for the difference in texture. Hemicellulose is present in distinctly smaller quantities than cellulose and is a heterogeneous molecule containing both pentoses and hexoses, and uronic acids. Pectic substances are a group of galacturonic acid polymers present in the primary cell wall and middle lamella of fruits and vegetables. They include protopectin, pectin, pectinic acids, and pectic acids. Lignin is the structural component in some plant foods that needs to be removed to prevent toughness and rigidity in the texture of vegetables before they are cooked and served.

Fruits and vegetables differ from one another in their nutrient content and chemical composition. Apart from nutrients, they contain pigments, flavouring compounds, enzymes, and organic acids, all of which influence the taste and acceptability of the products.

Enzymes

Enzymes are protein in nature and are found in living cells. They act as catalysts in chemical reactions in the cell, e.g., browning reactions, tenderizing reactions, etc. They bring about ripening and spoilage of fruits and vegetables. They are inactivated by heat and addition of chemicals. Enzymatic activity can be stopped by mild heat treatment, as proteins get denatured by heat.

Organic Acids

Fruits and vegetables contain a number of organic acids such as citric, tartaric, succinic, acetic, malic, fumaric, and benzoic acid. Fruits contain a higher concentration of acids as compared to vegetables. The pH of potatoes and peas is near neutral while lime, unripe mango, and tamarind have acidic pH values. Other fruits and vegetables fall in between this range.

Pigments are discussed in detail at the end of this chapter, sugars are discussed in Chapter 4 on Carbohydrates, while flavouring compounds are discussed in detail in Chapter 8 on Flavour.

MATURATION AND RIPENING

As fruits and vegetables mature, the content of structural support tissue, namely cellulose, hemicelluloses, and lignin gradually increases. Vegetables lose their tenderness, e.g., French beans become stringy. Lignin content in vegetables increases giving them a tough, woody texture as seen in over-mature carrots. Vegetables should be harvested at the optimum stage of maturity to prevent toughening and loss of texture. Physical properties are modified as very long polymers of water insoluble protopectin are hydrolyzed and demethylated to form shorter, methylated water-soluble pectin which is capable of forming a gel with sugar and acid. As protopectin is converted to pectin, fruits gradually soften and develop flavour and aroma which were earlier not present in very hard green fruits.

Respiration rate is high in perishable vegetables, such as green leafy vegetables, as the uptake of oxygen and production of carbon dioxide is rapid. Respiration rate is affected by the following:

1. *Temperature* Respiration rate can be controlled by refrigeration
2. *Stage of maturity and ripening* Respiration rate is maximum just before the fruit is fully ripe
3. *Composition of surrounding atmosphere* Carbon dioxide is added to extend the shelf life of fruits and vegetables. This level varies from one produce to another. Ethylene gas is used to accelerate the ripening process.

In fruits, starch is converted to sugar during ripening whereas in vegetables, sugar is converted to starch.

POST-HARVEST CHANGES

Fruits and vegetables remain alive and continue to respire even after they are harvested. Most fruits and vegetables have a high percentage of moisture and retain optimum quality for few days only. Even after they are harvested the enzyme activity continues and they respire. This can be observed by keeping them in a polythene bag. Drops of moisture collect in the bag even on short storage. Loss of moisture results in limpness and wilting. To retain quality, it is essential that fruits and vegetables be harvested at optimum maturity and ripened under controlled conditions. Fruits and vegetables should be stored at the optimum temperature, humidity, and atmosphere to control the loss of moisture, retain freshness, prevent microbial spoilage, preserve the appearance, texture, flavour, and weight of products. During respiration, stored food is used up and the ultimate quality is affected. Flavour changes take place due to enzyme action and conversion of sugar to starch.

After fruits and vegetables are harvested, synthesis of virtually all organic compounds stop, but physiological changes continue during storage. Selection of proper storage area is of utmost importance and varies with the type of vegetable or fruit. Each type of vegetable or fruit has a temperature range over which it can be stored for at least a short time. Non-freezing very low temperatures may result in chilling injuries.

Climacteric fruits

Fruits which are harvested when they are horticulturally mature but not ripe and have the ability to continue to ripen after they are harvested, are termed climacteric fruits. Their respiratory rate is maximum just prior to full ripening.

Non-climacteric fruits

For fruits such as pineapple, citrus fruits, and grapes, the respiration rate does not accelerate after harvesting. Such fruits are of best quality if they are harvested when ripe.

Bulbs, roots, tubers, and seeds become relatively dormant during optimum storage, while fleshy fruits and vegetables undergo ripening after maturation and then lose palatability.

Changes are seen with reference to

1. Weight
2. Texture
3. Flavour
4. Taste

Biochemical changes seen in fruits and vegetables are

1. Respiration
2. Changes in certain constituents in cell walls
3. Conversion of sugar to starch in vegetables and starch to sugar in fruits

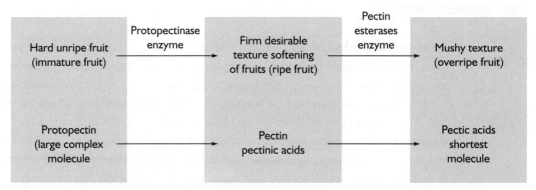

Fig. 6.2 Changes in pectic substances in fruits during maturation and ripening

Fruits undergo a number of chemical changes after they are harvested. Pectic substances in the cell wall are degraded by the action of enzymes during storage, converting pectin to pectic acid which is more soluble. The sweetness in fruits increases. Some complex polysaccharides, such as cellulose and hemicelluloses, are broken down resulting in release of sugars and increase in sweetness. Starch is converted to sugar by the enzyme amylase and sucrose is broken down in green leafy vegetables and fruits by the enzyme invertase.

The shelf life of perishable and semi-perishable fruits and vegetables can be extended by altering the relative proportions of atmospheric gases that surround the food. This technique, called modified atmosphere packaging (MAP), is commonly used nowadays (refer Chapter 13 on New Trends in Foods). In this technique, the normal composition of air of 78 per cent nitrogen, 21 per cent oxygen, and 0.03 per cent carbon dioxide is modified to match the respiration rate of fruits and vegetables and varies from one product to another. New packaging techniques are being developed to retain freshness in fruits and vegetables. The proportion of oxygen inside the package should be lower and the proportion of carbon dioxide should be higher than the normal composition of air. This reduces the rate of respiration and retards microbial growth, thereby preventing rot and decay during post-harvest storage.

NATURAL COLOURING PIGMENTS

Fruits and vegetables are appealing because of their bright and variable colours. These colours are present due to pigments present in the cell, mainly in the plastids, i.e., in the chloroplasts and chromoplasts and to some extent in fat or water droplets in the protoplasm of vacuoles.

Pigments are classified into three major groups, namely

1. Chlorophylls   2. Carotenoids   3. Flavonoids

Flavonoids and carotenoids present in strawberries, black grapes, melons, and pineapples add colour to our meals (see Plate 1).

To retain the attractiveness of fruits and vegetables and preserve their bright appealing colours, it is necessary to understand the effect of different cooking processes and medium of cooking on the pigments.

Chlorophylls

Chlorophyll is the bright green-coloured pigment present in chloroplasts which play an important role in photosynthesis, a process in which carbohydrates are synthesized from carbon dioxide and water. Chlorophyll is a fat-soluble pigment with a complex structure. It is present in two basic forms, namely chlorophyll *a* and chlorophyll *b*. Chlorophyll is a very large complex tetrapyrrole structure containing a magnesium ion, a phytyl group making it hydrophobic in nature, and a functional group that differs in chlorophyll *a* and chlorophyll *b*.

Note: In chlorophyll *a*, R = CH_3; in chlorophyll *b*, R = C (CHO)

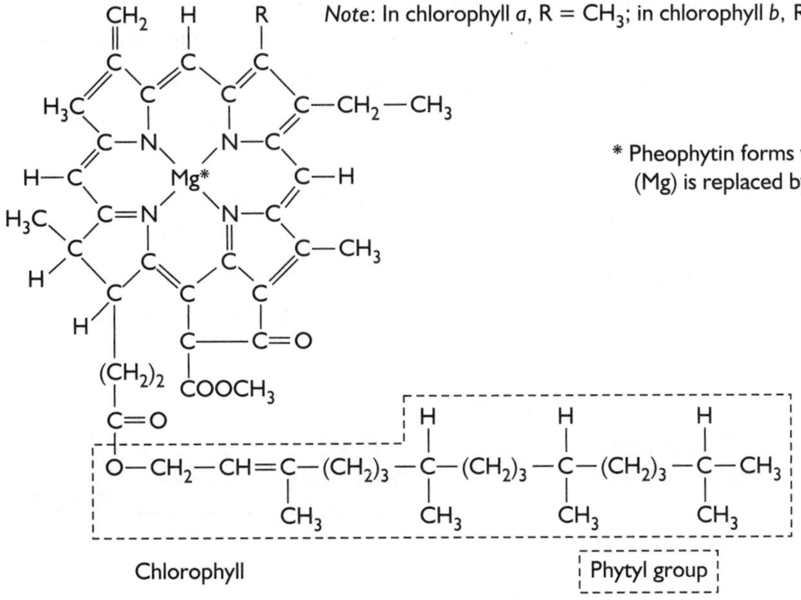

* Pheophytin forms when magnesium (Mg) is replaced by hydrogen (H)

Fig. 6.3   Structure of chlorophyll *a* and *b*

Chlorophyll *a* differs from chlorophyll *b* in that chlorophyll *a* has a methyl group at R position, while chlorophyll *b* has an aldehyde group (see Fig. 6.3). Chlorophyll *a* occurs in abundance in nature and is a bluish green pigment, whereas chlorophyll *b* is yellowish green in colour. The range of green hues present naturally in vegetables is possibly because of the varying ratios of chlorophyll *a* to chlorophyll *b* and also because of the presence of other pigments along with chlorophyll. Chlorophyll is present in unripe fruits and masks the colour of the other pigments present. These pigments become visible as the fruit ripens and chlorophyll content diminishes.

Effect of cooking on chlorophyll

When green vegetables are cooked in water, the cooking water turns slightly green. This is because of the action of chlorophyllase enzyme present in some vegetables, which removes the phytyl group from the chlorophyll molecule rendering it water soluble and changing it to chlorophyllide.

When green vegetables are heated, a gradual change in colour is observed. Air is expelled from intercellular spaces and the colour turns intense and brighter green. On further cooking, the bright green colour changes gradually to an unappetizing olive green colour. This is because the magnesium ion in the molecule is replaced by hydrogen and chlorophyll is converted to pheophytin *a* or *b* respectively. The conversion occurs when green leafy vegetables are cooked for at least 5 to 7 minutes. Some dilute acids are released into the cooking liquor and these acids facilitate the conversion of chlorophyll to pheophytin. If vegetables are cooked uncovered, some of the volatile acids are released along with vapour and the green colour is partly retained.

The green colour of vegetables can be preserved by the following practices.

1. Add vegetables to boiling hot water to reduce cooking time.
2. Cook vegetables uncovered for the first few minutes to allow volatile acids to evaporate.
3. Cook in sufficient water to dilute the effect of acids.
4. Blanch vegetables to enhance green colour by expelling air .

Addition of baking soda to neutralize the acidity of the medium helps in preserving the bright green colour of chlorophyll. However, an alkaline medium destroys vital vitamins,

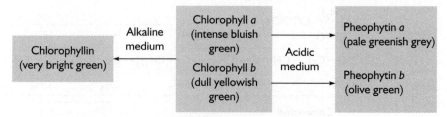

Fig. 6.4   Effect of pH on chlorophyll pigment

results in a mushy texture and an unnatural bright green colour as chlorophyll is converted to chlorophyllin (see Fig. 6.4).

Carotenoids

Carotenoids are a large group of yellow, orange, red pigments present in fruits and vegetables. In unripe fruits and vegetables, these pigments are masked by chlorophyll. The carotenoids are large molecules comprising of at least 40 carbon atoms with a high degree of unsaturation. They are broadly divided into two main groups, namely carotenes and xanthophylls.

Classification of carotenoid pigments

The β-carotenes (Fig. 6.5) have vitamin A activity. However, the intensity of colour is not necessarily an indicator of vitamin A content as all carotenoid pigments cannot be converted to vitamin A.

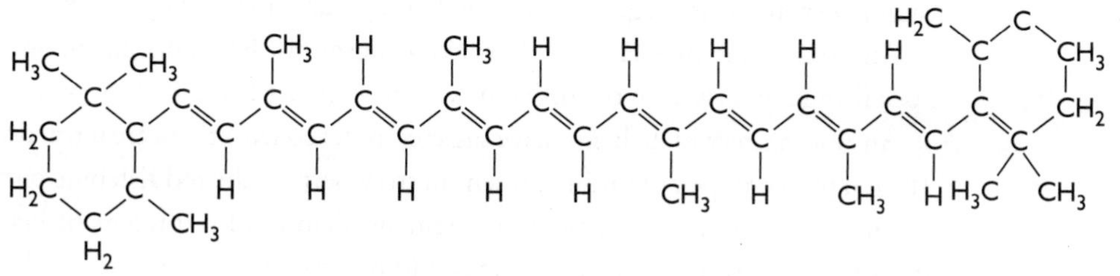

Figure 6.5 Structure of β-carotene

Effect of cooking on carotenoid pigments

As carotenoids are fat-soluble pigments, normal cooking procedures have little effect on the colour or vitamin A content. They are stable pigments. The colour of the pigment is very slightly affected by acids, alkalis, and volume of cooking liquor.

However, being highly unsaturated they are susceptible to oxidation and carotene is lost during drying of fruits and vegetables rich in carotene. Colour loss is also due to a shift from *trans* form to *cis* form as carotenoids with a *cis* configuration have a lighter hue.

When carotene-rich foods are cooked in fat, significant amounts of carotenoids get dissolved in fat.

Carotenoids can be preserved by

1. Cooking in a covered pan or for shorter periods
2. Blanching prior to dehydration to destroy enzyme activity
3. Low cooking temperatures
4. Reducing amount of surface area exposed to oxidation by cutting vegetables and fruits into larger pieces

Flavonoids

Flavonoids are water-soluble pigments which are dispersed in the vacuole in plant cells. The flavonoids are a group of closely related chemical compounds which are made up of two phenyl rings connected by a five or six-membered ring and have a basic structure.

They are divided into two main groups on the basis of the charge present on the oxygen atom in the central ring, namely

1. Anthocyanins
2. Anthoxanthins

In anthocyanins, the central ring is positively charged whereas in anthoxanthins, there is no charge. Anthocyanins are red to purple to blue in colour and are present in strawberries, black grapes, cherries, *kokum*, pomegranates, and in the leaves of red cabbage. They are also present in the peel of apples, table radish, sweet potato, and brinjal. Anthoxanthins are colourless, white, cream to yellow in colour depending on the pH and are present in practically all plants along with other pigments. They are present in onions, potatoes, cauliflower, and leafy vegetables where their colour is masked by chlorophyll.

Anthoxanthins may also be classified as flavanols, flavonols, flavonones, and flavones. Specific pigments within the different subdivisions are listed in Table 6.3.

Anthocyanins which do not have sugar complexed with them are termed anthocyanidins. The red pigment, pelargonidin, present in strawberries; the reddish blue pigment, cyanidin, present in raspberries; and the blue pigment, delphinidin, present in black currants, are examples of anthocyanidins. Anthocyanidins can form complexes with sugars to form anthocyanins which give food a reddish hue in an acidic medium and a violet colour in an alkaline medium.

TABLE 6.3 Classification of flavonoid pigment anthoxanthin

Flavanols		Flavones	Flavonones	Flavonols
Catechins	Leucoanthocyanins			
Gallocatechin	Leucocyanidin	Rutinol	Hesperidin	Kaempferol
Catechin			Naringin	Myricetin
				Quercetin

Betalains

Betalains are a group of pigments that are closely related to the anthocyanins but contain nitrogen in their structure. Beetroots contain betalains. There are two groups of betalains:

1. *Betacyanin* This group includes water-soluble pigments—betanidin and betanin—which give beetroots their crimson maroon colour.
2. *Betaxanthin* These pigments are yellowish in colour.

The betacyanin pigment is held tightly within the cells and diffuses rapidly into the cooking water when a raw beetroot is cut and boiled, resulting in the loss of colour in the boiled vegetable.

Effect of cooking on flavonoid pigments

The flavonoid pigments are water soluble and will easily leech out into cooking liquor. Anthoxanthins are colourless to creamy white in colour and a change in the colour of vegetable as well as cooking liquor is seen when the pH of the medium changes. In light-coloured vegetables, such as cauliflower, an acidic pH has a bleaching effect making the vegetable whiter. In an alkaline medium or on addition of cooking soda, cauliflower turns yellow. Similar changes in colour are also observed in the cooking water. Anthoxanthins can form complexes with metal ions causing discolouration. When yellow onions and green leafy vegetables are cooked in aluminium pans, the flavones present scavenge aluminium and form a flavone-aluminium chelate which gives a yellowish discolouration to cooking water. Cast iron pans and tin cans bring about similar discolouration and unappetizing darkening of vegetables. Some anthoxanthins are easily oxidized. They undergo browning or blackening when fruits and vegetables containing these polyphenolic compounds are exposed to oxygen from the air or from intercellular spaces. When fruits and vegetables are cut or bruised, enzymes present in them act on the polyphenolic substrate and cause enzymatic browning. The enzyme polyphenoloxidase act on flavonoid (polyphenolic) compounds to cause discolouration of cut surfaces. Refer Chapter 9 on Browning Reactions for more on this topic.

Anthocyanins show striking changes in colour when fruits and vegetables containing these pigments are blended with other ingredients while preparing and serving food. If tap water is alkaline, colour changes to an unattractive bluish grey. In an acidic medium, the colour brightens. At pH 3, the oxygen atom in anthocyanin is positively charged and colour is red. At neutral pH, red colour changes to violet purple and turns bluish grey as alkalinity increases. At pH 14, the colour changes to bright green probably because anthoxanthin, which is widely present in all plants along with other pigments, turns yellow and the mixture of the two pigments yellow and blue appears green.

To preserve the colour of red cabbage and prevent it from turning to an unpalatable blue shade, it is necessary to keep the pH of the medium acidic. This can be done by adding an acidic fruit like apple while cooking the cabbage.

Metals have a marked effect on anthocyanin pigment. While canning anthocyanin rich foods, special enamel-coated cans need to be used to prevent reactions between tin and pigment. Copper, iron, aluminium, and tin react with anthocyanins changing the reddish pigment to shades of blue grey and green. Iron causes black discolouration of red pigments.

Dramatic colour changes result from a change in pH, oxidation, high temperature, prolonged storage, or contact with metals. This point needs to be kept in mind while processing fruits and vegetables if attractive colours have to be retained. Table 6.4 highlights the effect of pH, oxidation, metals, and cooking processes on plant pigments.

Flavonoid pigments can be preserved by the following practices.

1. Do not boil vegetables containing flavonoids in aluminium or cast iron pans.
2. Use stainless steel knives and containers to cut and process fruits and vegetables.
3. Keep flavonoid rich fruits and vegetables in specially enameled cans.
4. To prevent leaching losses in cooked beetroot, cook whole keeping skin intact.
5. Understand the effect of pH on pigments while blending juices.

TABLE 6.4 Effect of cooking on colour of plant pigments

Pigment	Solubility in water	Oxidation	Acidic medium	Alkaline medium	Metals
Chlorophyll (green)	Almost insoluble	No change	Olive green/grey	Intense green	Copper and weak acid enhance colour
Carotenoids (yellow/orange/red)	Insoluble	Loss of colour	No significant change	No significant change	No significant change
Anthoxanthin (colourless/white/creamish yellow)	Soluble	No change	Bleaching effect, whiter vegetable	Distinct yellow	Aluminium, iron pans, and tin cause yellow discolouration
Anthocyanin (red/purple/blue)	Soluble	No change	Red pigment turns deep crimson red	Red pigment turns blue grey, sometimes green	Copper, iron, aluminium, and tin cause red pigment to change to shades of blue, grey, and green
Betalains (deep crimson red/maroon)	Highly soluble	No significant change	Bright reddish colour	Brownish blue colour	No significant change

SUMMARY

Fruits and vegetables not only add colour and texture to food but are also a source of essential nutrients. Most fruits can be eaten uncooked while most vegetables, except for salad vegetables, need some form of cooking. They can be classified in different ways based on nutritive value, part of plant, pigments present, and natural habitat. The tissue system comprises of dermal tissue, vascular tissue, and ground tissue. The ground tissue which is made up of parenchyma cells forms the main edible portion of fruits and vegetables. The attractive appearance is due to several pigments which are stored in the cell. The structure and texture of fruits and vegetables also depends on unavailable polysaccharides and lignin present. Fruits and vegetables differ from one another in their nutrient content and chemical composition. Apart from nutrients, they contain pigments, flavouring compounds, enzymes, organic acids, and sugars, all of which influence the taste and acceptability of the fruit or vegetable. Fruits and vegetables remain alive even after they are harvested. To retain quality, it is necessary that they are harvested at optimum maturity and stored under controlled conditions to preserve freshness, texture, flavour, and weight of products. Storage conditions vary from one fruit or vegetable to another. The main groups of pigments in plants are the chlorophylls, carotenoids, and flavonoids. It is necessary to understand the effect of acids, alkali, metals, and oxidation while cooking food to preserve the original attractiveness and appeal of fruits and vegetables.

KEY TERMS

Anthocyanidin It is anthocyanin type of pigment that is devoid of a sugar molecule in its structure.

Betalains This is a group of two pigments, betacyanins and betaxanthins, which are closely related to anthocyanin, containing nitrogen in their structure, responsible for the colour of beetroot.

Carotenoid A large group of stable, fat-soluble pigments present in plastids in the cell, which impart yellow orange red colour to fruits and vegetables. Some pigments have vitamin A activity.

Chlorophyll This is the dominant fat-soluble green pigment in plants present in plastids in the cell, which play an important role in photosynthesis and change colour during cooking and processing.

Chlorophyllin This is an unnatural bright green colour pigment formed in an alkaline medium when methyl and phytyl groups are removed from chlorophyll.

Climacteric It is the period of highest respiratory rate seen in many fleshy fruits just before they are fully ripened.

Flavonoid It is a group of chemically related pigments which are water soluble, unstable, and are present in the vacuole in the cell, with a wide range of colours from colourless-white-creamish-yellow to highly pigmented red-purple-blue. Some flavonoid pigments are capable of changing colours dramatically during cooking and processing.

Fruits Fruits are the ripened ovary or ovaries of a flowering plant together with the adjacent tissues.

Pheophytin It is an unappetizing dull olive green colour formed in an acidic medium when magnesium is removed from chlorophyll and is replaced by hydrogen.

Vegetables Vegetables are the edible portion of plants and are obtained from all parts of the plant, right from the root to the seed, depending on the specific plant.

REVIEW EXERCISES

1. Classify vegetables based on part of plant consumed, giving one suitable example for each.
2. Discuss the main functions of the three tissue systems in fruits and vegetables.
3. With the help of a neat labelled diagram, explain the structure of a parenchyma cell.
4. Briefly explain the various chemical constituents in fruits and vegetables.
5. Which points should be kept in mind while storing green leafy vegetables?
6. Discuss the changes observed in pectic substances present in fruits during maturation and storage.
7. How can the respiration rate in fruits and vegetables be controlled?
8. Discuss major pigments present in fruits and vegetables.
9. What measures will you take to preserve the green colour of *palak paneer*?

CHAPTER 7

Fats and Oils

LEARNING OBJECTIVES

After reading this chapter, you should be able to
- appreciate the importance of the different types of fats and oils available in the market
- understand the properties of various fats and oils
- know the factors which contribute towards flavour changes in fats and oils and their control
- classify fats and oils on the basis of origin and degree of saturation
- describe the steps in extraction, refining, and winterizing fats and oils
- distinguish between rancidity and reversion of fats and oils
- know the role of shortenings and apply the same in the bakery
- understand the importance of nuts and oilseeds in our diet
- state the commercial applications of fats and oils

INTRODUCTION

The basic use of fats and oils in cookery is to add richness and flavour to food and as a cooking medium to fry or cook food. They improve the texture of various preparations such as cakes, pastries, and biscuits.

Fats and oils are found in plant, animal, and marine foods. The properties of fats and oils depend on their source as well as a number of other factors. The quality of the food product depends largely on the fat or oil which is used while preparing it. The storage conditions of fat as well as preparation temperatures and time influence the quality of the final product. Figure 7.1 classifies lipids on the basis of origin and the degree of saturation.

Fats and oils are organic compounds composed of carbon, hydrogen, and oxygen. They are collectively known as lipids. Unlike carbohydrates, lipids contain a smaller proportion of oxygen and a larger proportion of hydrogen and carbon. This is why lipids provide more energy per gram than carbohydrates.

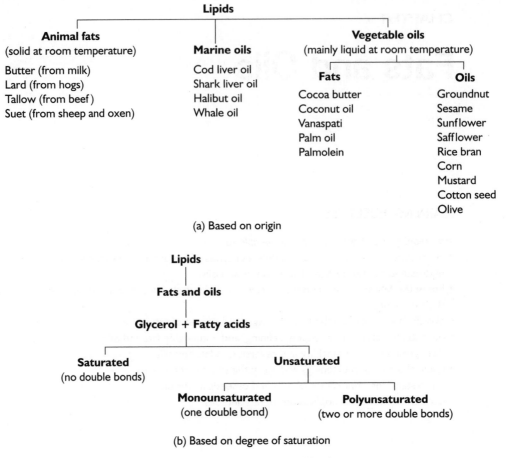

Lipids

Animal fats
(solid at room temperature)

Butter (from milk)
Lard (from hogs)
Tallow (from beef)
Suet (from sheep and oxen)

Marine oils

Cod liver oil
Shark liver oil
Halibut oil
Whale oil

Vegetable oils
(mainly liquid at room temperature)

Fats

Cocoa butter
Coconut oil
Vanaspati
Palm oil
Palmolein

Oils

Groundnut
Sesame
Sunflower
Safflower
Rice bran
Corn
Mustard
Cotton seed
Olive

(a) Based on origin

Lipids

Fats and oils

Glycerol + Fatty acids

Saturated
(no double bonds)

Unsaturated

Monounsaturated
(one double bond)

Polyunsaturated
(two or more double bonds)

(b) Based on degree of saturation

Fig. 7.1   Classification of lipids

STRUCTURE

Simple fats and oils are of great importance in food preparation. They are composed of glycerol and fatty acids linked together to form an ester. One, two, or three fatty acids may be esterified with glycerol to form monoglycerides, diglycerides, or triglycerides, respectively.

The most common form of food fats are triglycerides. Triglycerides are made up of three fatty acids esterified to the glycerol molecule. This is the maximum number of fatty acids that can be attached.

In Fig. 7.2, R is the symbol for the fatty acid half of any chain length. The fatty acid chain is generally of 16 to 18 carbon atoms. The most common fatty acids found in fats are palmitic, stearic, oleic, and linoleic. In a simple triglyceride, the three fatty acids that combined with glycerol are similar. In a mixed triglyceride, more than one kind of fatty acid is present.

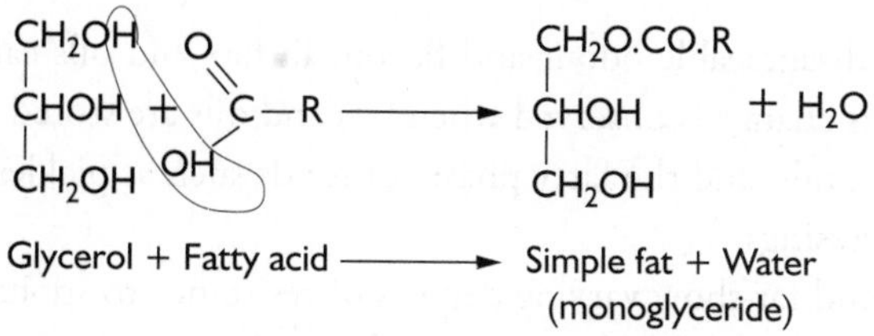

Fig. 7.2   Formation of a monoglyceride

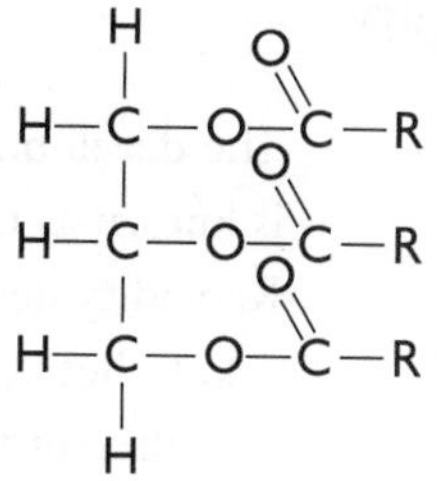

Fig. 7.3   A triglyceride

The fatty acids present in fats may be saturated, unsaturated, or polyunsaturated. The flavour and hardness of a fat depend on the kinds and amounts of fatty acids present. Fats found in foods are a mixture of saturated, unsaturated, and polyunsaturated fatty acids. The fat is classified on the basis of the amount and type of fatty acids present. A food fat is called saturated if it contains more saturated than unsaturated fatty acids. Such fats are solid and are generally found in animal food. When polyunsaturated fatty acids (PUFA) are more in a fat than saturated fatty acids, the fat is generally liquid and found in vegetable oils. The exception to this rule is fish liver oil which is liquid, and cocoa butter, palmolein, and coconut oils, which are solid inspite of their vegetable origin.

In a saturated fatty acid, each carbon atom in the fatty acid carries all the hydrogen atoms possible. In unsaturated fatty acids, the full complement of hydrogen atoms is not received. This leads to the formation of double bonds between the atoms, e.g., oleic, linoleic, linolenic, and arachidonic acid with 1, 2, 3, and 4 double bonds respectively. Figure 7.3 shows the structure of a triglyceride.

Properties

1. Fats are insoluble in water and soluble in a fat solvent such as ether and acetone.
2. They are greasy to touch.
3. They have a specific gravity less than one.
4. At room temperature, fats are solid due to the high percentage of saturated fatty acids. Oils are liquid because of the higher percentage of unsaturated fatty acids.
5. Fats do not melt sharply but soften over a range of temperature. This is because fats are generally mixed triglycerides, each one having its own melting point.
6. The spreading quality of a fat is due to its plastic nature. Solid fats which spread are composed of a mass of tiny crystals in a matrix of liquid fat. The crystals slide over one another as they are not trapped in the liquid oil and permit the fat to be deformed.
7. When fat or oil is heated, the temperature at which a thin bluish smoke is given off is called the smoke point. Fats used for deep fat frying should have a high smoke point.
8. When fats and oils are heated to high temperatures, the fat is decomposed into glycerol and free fatty acids. Glycerol is further broken down by high temperature and acrolein is formed. Acrolein has a sharp odour and irritates the nose, throat, and eyes.
9. Iodine value is a measure of the extent of unsaturated fatty acids present in fats and oils.

RANCIDITY

The development of any disagreeable odour and flavour in fats and oils causing spoilage is known as rancidity. This change is observed when fats and oils are stored for sometime. Rancidity develops in fats, oils, and the fatty phases of foods such as pickles, fried snacks, cakes, cheese, and salad dressings.

Different types of oil and fat show varying degrees of resistance to spoilage, thus most vegetable oils deteriorate very slowly whereas animal fats deteriorate more rapidly, and marine (fish) oils which contain a relatively high proportion of highly unsaturated fatty acids deteriorate most rapidly.

Vegetable oils resist oxidation because of the presence of antioxidants, which occur naturally in the tissues and which are present in oil when it is pressed, e.g., vitamin E or tocopherols. The antioxidants get readily oxidized themselves and protect the oil from oxidation.

Types of Rancidity

Two types of rancidity is commonly observed in food, namely

1. Hydrolytic rancidity
2. Oxidative rancidity

Hydrolytic rancidity is brought about by hydrolysis of triglyceride molecule to glycerol and free fatty acids by the presence of moisture in oils. The rate of hydrolysis is hastened by

1. The presence of enzymes, e.g., lipases present in oils which have not been subjected to heat treatment
2. Microorganisms, such as molds, yeasts, and bacteria, present in oils or contaminants during processing

The nature of the unpleasant flavours and odours produced by hydrolysis depends upon the fatty acid composition of the triglyceride. If the triglyceride contains low molecular weight fatty acids (4 to 14 carbon atoms), hydrolysis yields free radicals having characteristic unpleasant taste and odour. For example, hydrolysis of butter yields the rancid-smelling butyric acid. Oils containing fattyacids with more than 14 carbon atoms yield free acids which are odourless and flavourless.

Auto-oxidation   The spontaneous uptake of oxygen by the unsaturated oils exposed to air is known as oxidative rancidity (Fig. 7.4). It is the most common and important type of rancidity which results in the production of rancid or tallowy flavours. It is caused by the reaction of unsaturated oils with oxygen. Moisture and impurities do not have any effect on oxidative rancidity. Pure and refined oils can turn rancid on exposure to oxygen. Oxidative rancidity is a complex process in the form of a chain reaction. Once the reaction begins, it is a continuous process.

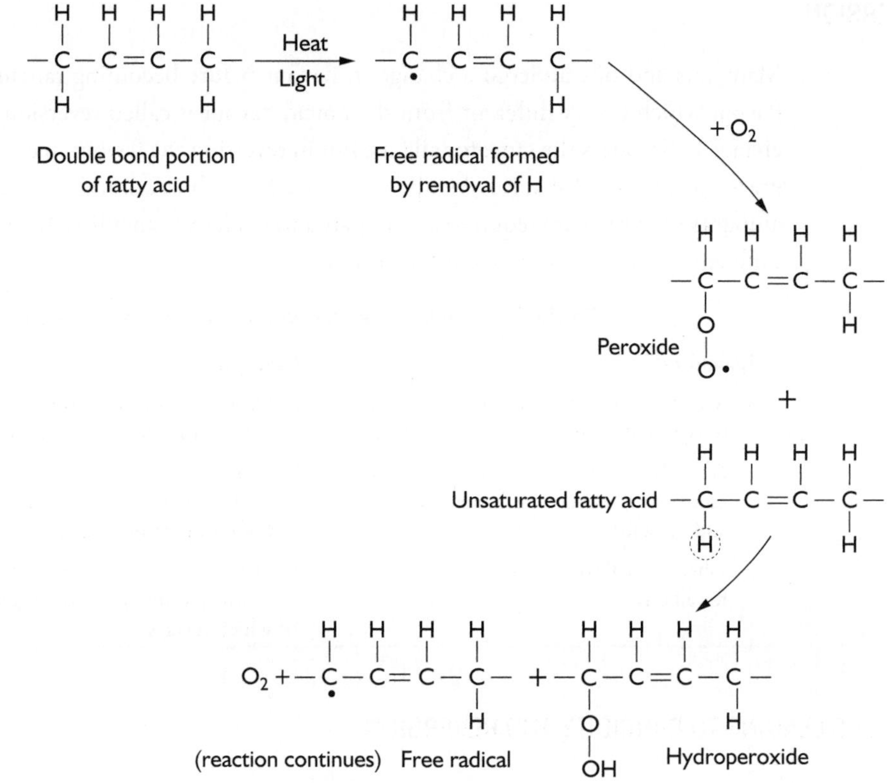

Fig. 7.4   Auto-oxidation

The reaction occurs in two stages:

1. Induction period in which the fat or oil gradually takes up oxygen from the air. Heat, light, and traces of metal help in the formation of free radicals. The free radical is formed by the removal of a hydrogen atom from the carbon adjacent to the carbon involved in the double bond. The free radical combines with two oxygen atoms, forming a peroxide. The peroxide formed combines with another hydrogen atom from another fatty acid to form a hydroperoxide and a new free radical. This new free radical again takes up two oxygen atoms and the chain reaction continues till all unsaturated fatty acids are used up or all oxygen gets exhausted.

   The products of oxidation are auto-catalytic so that the uptake of atmospheric oxygen is accelerated as rancidity progresses and new free radicals continue to be formed. Rancidity is detected at this stage.

2. In the second stage the peroxides and hydroperoxides formed rapidly break down into aldehydes, ketones, and alcohols which contribute to the undesirable flavours and odours in rancid fat.

REVERSION

Many fats and oils undergo a change in flavour before becoming rancid. This change in flavour which is very different from the rancid flavour is called reversion. In rancidity the change in flavour is the same for all fats. But in reversion the flavour may be buttery, beany, grassy, painty, and fishy. Reversion is seen in fish oils, linseed, and soya been oil. Very small amounts of oxygen are required as compared to oxidative rancidity. Table 7.1 discusses the differences between rancidity and reversion.

Table 7.1   Differences between rancidity and reversion

Rancidity	Reversion
1. May be hydrolytic or oxidative leading to typical flavour changes of rancid oil	1. Flavour change develops before onset of rancidity with very little oxidation
2. All oils can turn rancid, e.g., maize, groundnut, sesame, sunflower, safflower, and mustard	2. Only some oils revert, e.g., soya bean oil, rapeseed, fish oils, and linseed oil, i.e., oils with high proportion of unsaturated fatty acids
3. Change in flavour is typical and same for all oils	3. Flavour developed may be fishy, buttery, beany, painty, or grassy depending on the oil which reverts

FACTORS LEADING TO RANCIDITY AND REVERSION

Temperature

High storage temperatures accelerate the development of off-flavours and odours in fats and oils.

Moisture

Low moisture content in cereals, specially breakfast cereals, to keep them crisp, accelerates their deterioration due to rancidity.

Presence of moisture in butter and oils brings about hydrolytic rancidity. In butter, the enzyme lipase hydrolyses butter fat to butyric acid, which gives stale butter a rancid smell. When butter is heated to prepare clarified butter or pure ghee, the enzyme lipase is inactivated and moisture from butter is removed by heat. Clarified butter can be stored at room temperature and does not turn rancid.

Air

The amount of air in contact with the fat or oil is an important factor in determining its shelf life. Auto-oxidation or oxidative rancidity occurs when fats are exposed to oxygen. Reversion occurs with very minor amounts of oxygen. Potato chips and salted nuts, because of their large surface area, turn rancid at a faster rate.

Light

Light accelerates the development of both rancidity and reversion.

Metals

The presence of metals in traces accelerates the development of both rancidity and reversion as they are active pro-oxidants. Metal contamination can occur from equipment used for extraction and refining of oils. Rust from steel equipment, traces of copper, lead, zinc, and tin can accelerate the onset of rancidity.

Degree of Unsaturation

This is an important criteria for oxidative rancidity and reversion.

Oils containing high proportions of unsaturated fatty acids and shortenings made from such oils show flavour reversion. Oils with high proportions of linolenic and linoleic acids revert. Oils with unsaturated fatty acids turn rancid.

Absence of Antioxidants

The natural presence or addition of antioxidants to oils prevents rancidity. Vitamin E or tocopherol is naturally present in vegetable oils and acts as an antioxidant preventing auto-oxidation of oil. The antioxidant takes up oxygen and gets oxidized, thereby preventing rancidity.

PREVENTION OF RANCIDITY

Disagreeable odours and flavour in fat can be prevented by the following ways.

1. Store fat at low temperatures in a cool, dark place.
2. Use airtight containers. Keep minimum headspace.
3. Do not keep strong smelling foods in the vicinity of fats and oils as they absorb foreign odours and get tainted.
4. Copper containers and rusted iron accelerate rancidity. Only steel or aluminium should be used.
5. Avoid undue exposure to light and air. Expose minimum surface area.
6. If antioxidants are added to fats rich in unsaturated fatty acids, oxidative rancidity can be significantly delayed. Tocopherol (vitamin E) and lecithin are antioxidants naturally present in some oils. Synthetic antioxidants, such as butylated hydroxy toluene (BHT), butylated hydroxy anisole (BHA), and tertiary butyl hydroquinone (TBHQ), are added to oil in which snacks are fried. Ethylenediamine tetraacetic acid (EDTA), citric acid, or ascorbic acid may be added to fats to prevent rancidity. These substances act as scavengers and bind copper and other metals present which cause oxidative rancidity. Tocopherols and ascorbic acid are excellent antioxidants.

7. If fats and oils have to be stored for sometime, they should be hydrogenated and stored. Hydrogenation increases the shelf life of fats and prevents rancidity.

EFFECT OF HEAT ON FATS AND OILS

During cooking or prolonged heating of fats and oils certain changes are seen:

1. There is an increase in the free fatty acid content
2. Smoke point is lowered
3. Iodine number decreases
4. Melting point falls
5. Fat turns darker in colour
6. Fat gets polymerized
7. Refractive index increases.

All these changes influence the overall quality of food. These changes are faster when the cooking temperature is increased.

POLYMERIZATION

This takes place because of the intense heat which the fat is subjected to during frying. Lipolysis or lipid breakdown takes place and free fatty acids are released. These free fatty acids undergo further changes and form polymers. Polymerization is generally seen in fatty acids with one double bond. The larger polymers increase the viscosity of the hot fat. The colour darkens and the quality deteriorates. Gum may be formed at the edge of the vessel.

It is of utmost importance to avoid unnecessary heating of fats and oils and controlling frying temperature and time. If the fat is not hot enough, excess fat is absorbed by the food. If the fat is too hot, the surface browns but the food is not cooked. The moisture should be removed before frying a food. Fat used for frying should have a high smoke point.

CARE OF FATS AND OILS

Fats and oils are used in many preparations and as a method of cooking food. If care is not taken while heating and storing fats, it may result in wastage of food as well as the fat used in preparing it. The following points should always be kept in mind while handling fats and oils in the kitchen.

1. Do not overheat fats, as they decompose at high temperature.
2. Follow a time and temperature chart for frying foods.
3. Cover fats when left in the deep fat fryer and ensure that the temperature does not exceed 200°F.

4. Strain fat after use and used fat should be stored in closed containers in the refrigerator.
5. When fat has to be reused for frying, replace with equal quantity of fresh fat.
6. Do not use fats with a low smoke point for frying.
7. To prevent fat from going rancid, it should be stored in an airtight container away from light.
8. Fat should be stored in tall containers to keep minimum surface area exposed.
9. Always remember that fats and the fatty phases of foods take up flavours and odours of other foods stored nearby.
10. Copper or rusted containers should not be used for storing fats.

EXTRACTION OF FATS AND OILS

There are three methods for extraction of fats and oils from animal or vegetable tissues.
1. Rendering
2. Pressing
3. Solvent extraction

Rendering

This method is mainly used for extracting animal fat from fatty tissues. The tissue from which fat is to be extracted is carefully removed from the carcass and chopped or minced. Rendering is of two types: wet rendering and dry rendering.

Wet rendering   It is carried out in the presence of water. The chopped tissue is treated with very hot water or steam. Fat melts and forms a layer on top, which is skimmed off. Fat obtained by this method has a bland flavour and complete extraction is not obtained. Antioxidants are added to prevent rancidity.

Dry rendering   The chopped tissues are heated without addition of water. Lipids escape from the cells and melted fat is removed by draining and squeezing the fat out of the residue.

Pressing

In this method, oil is extracted by the application of high pressure to oilseeds or fruit rich in oil. The oil obtained is filtered to remove all extraneous matter. Oil obtained from the first pressing is called virgin oil and is particularly bland in flavour.

In hot pressing, the oil bearing tissue is rolled, crushed, or ground into flakes, and then heated by steam to 70°C. The hot tissues are pressed to extract oil. Along with oil, gums and free fatty acids are also extracted.

Solvent Extraction

The crushed or flaked tissue is agitated along with a solvent to extract the oil. This method is used to extract the fat remaining in the seedcake after pressing. The solvent is separated from the mixture by evaporation.

REFINING

The oil extracted by rendering, pressing, or solvent extraction is called crude oil. It may contain undesirable constituents such as gums, free fatty acids, pigments, cellular material, and odourous compounds such as aldehydes, ketones, and essential oils.

Crude oil needs several types of treatment to extend its shelf life and make it suitable and pure for use.

Steps in refining oil are as follows:

1. *Settling*   The cell debris is allowed to settle down and is removed by filtration.
2. *Degumming and neutralization*   The gum and free fatty acids present are removed by steam distillation. Steam is passed through hot oil under pressure. Water-soluble low-molecular-weight fatty acids which are volatile are removed.

    Hot oil is treated with sodium hydroxide or sodium carbonate. The free fatty acids saponify and soap is separated out. This step is called alkali refining.
3. *Bleaching*   This step removes undesirable colouring and flavouring contaminants. Pigments are removed by filtering the oil through activated charcoal till it is light in colour.
4. *Steam deodourization*   Steam is injected into the hot fat under pressure. Low molecular weight aldehydes, ketones, peroxides, and free fatty acids are removed. The oil is cooled rapidly.

WINTERIZATION

After steam deodourization, the oils are chilled rapidly without stirring so that large filterable crystals are formed. These crystals are composed of high molecular weight triglycerides which have a high melting point. They are separated out by filtration and the cold viscous oil obtained is said to be winterized.

Winterized oil does not turn cloudy or solidify in the refrigerator. It is suitable to be used in foods which require refrigeration, e.g., salad dressings and mayonnaise which can be poured even when chilled. It is an important step in refining oil. Olive oil is not winterized or deodourized as desirable flavour is lost in these processes.

HYDROGENATION OF OILS

Liquid oils can be converted to solid fats by a process known as hydrogenation. In this process, hydrogen is added to unsaturated fatty acids. Some unsaturated fatty acids become saturated and the melting point of the fat increases.

The hot oil and finely divided nickel catalyst is stirred together under an atmosphere of hydrogen. Hydrogen is introduced under pressure so that maximum is dissolved in oil. The oil and catalyst are heated under vacuum. The reaction is continued till the desired consistency of fat is obtained. The oil is cooled, filtered to remove the catalyst, and chilled rapidly. By chilling, small crystals are formed and the fat gets a grainy texture.

$$-\overset{\displaystyle|}{\underset{\displaystyle|}{C}} = \overset{\displaystyle|}{\underset{\displaystyle|}{C}} - \quad \xrightarrow[\;+H_2\;]{\text{Nickel}} \quad -\overset{\displaystyle H}{\underset{\displaystyle H}{C}} - \overset{\displaystyle H}{\underset{\displaystyle H}{C}} -$$

Unsaturated	Saturated
(double bond)	(no double bond)

Hydrogenation is utilized in the manufacture of a wide variety of fats such as *vanaspati* and margarine. These can replace costly animal fats such as butter and clarified butter. The hardness of a fat depends on the degree of hydrogenation. Sometimes additives, such as antioxidants, monoglyceride, and vitamin A and vitamin D, are added to the fat. Air may be whipped in to impart a snow white colour.

Palm oil, palmolein, rice bran, cotton seed, sunflower, maize, soya bean, groundnut, and sesame oils are generally hydrogenated.

SHORTENINGS

Shortening Power of Fats and Oils

All baked goods use fat as a shortening, the amount varying from 5–10 per cent in biscuits and cookies, 10–20 per cent in cakes, and 15–30 per cent in pound cakes.

Fats impart flavour, texture, and tenderness to the product.

In *pound cake*, air is incorporated by creaming of fat. Each little air bubble is surrounded by the gluten of flour which stretches and sets to a rigid structure when the cake is baked. The extent of creaming the fat affects the texture. The tenderness of the product is also due to fat. Fat lubricates the tough and hard gluten and starch so that they slide over one another and the walls crumble (tenderness) when the cake is bitten.

In *butter cake*, leavening depends on air and steam as well as on carbon dioxide (CO_2) produced from baking powder. The air bubble serves as the nucleus for CO_2 gas.

In *pastry*, the fat is flattened into sheets between layers of flour and water (stiff dough) and causes their separation. This produces flakiness. The fat gets squeezed between the gluten strands so that a continuous tough matrix is not formed, but pastry is brittle or short.

Fats have different shortening abilities. The *shortening ability* of a fat is determined by a shortometer, which measures the load required to break a wafer or a pastry. If a small force is required to break a wafer, then the wafer is said to be very short.

The fat that covers the greatest surface area of the flour particles in a particular baked product is said to have the *greatest shortening power*.

The following factors affect the shortening power of fats.

The nature of the fat   Fats with the greatest unsaturation (3 or more double bonds) have the greatest shortening power. Greatest shortening power means greatest surface area of flour covered in a particular product. Polar groups are strongly attracted to each other. Water is polar. Fats contain both polar groups (COOH group and double bonds and phosphorus) as well as non-polar groups (hydrocarbon chain). When a small amount of oil is placed on a large clean surface of water, it spreads rapidly until a definite area is covered and then shows little tendency to spread further. This is because of the attraction of polar groups of fat for water. Fats with more polar groups will spread more.

Concentration   As the concentration of fat increases, its shortening power is also increased, e.g., butter has less shortening as compared to hydrogenated fats.

Temperature   Fats are less plastic and oils are more viscous at low temperatures. Therefore, they spread less readily and area covered is smaller with the same amounts of mixing than at higher temperatures.

Other ingredients   Presence of other ingredients may modify the shortening power of fat. When oil or melted fat is used in a batter with egg yolk, the fat is emulsified as an oil in water (O/W) emulsion and has less shortening power.

Manipulation of fat   It includes creaming or stirring the fat to soften it, thoroughly mixing fat with flour, way of rolling and handling and this affects shortening power.

For example, pastry making—relaxation of dough in a cool place between rolling is important in pastry making because if fat melts, then layers are not formed.

Shortenings available in the market are mixtures of high melting animal fats, low melting animal fats, and low melting hydrogenated fats or oils. They are called compound shortenings and are mixtures of oleostearin, edible tallow with hydrogenated cotton seed or groundnut oil. The oils are carefully blended and hydrogenated to obtain longest possible keeping period, plasticity, and consistency for incorporation in batters and doughs. A balance should be maintained between oleic, linoleic, and linolenic acid as excess linoleic/linolenic acid shows signs of reversion and excess oleic acid hardens the fat and reduces its plasticity. Shortenings available in our country are mainly of vegetable origin.

Diet Margarines

They contain half as much fat as other margarines and twice as much water.

Whipped Butter and Margarine

Butter and margarine are whipped mechanically into fat foam which is lighter, more airy textured, and have fewer calories per gram.

Soft (Tub) Margarines

They are made with higher content of PUFA and low melting point fats.

Peanut Butter

It contains oil, protein, and other components of groundnuts, which are finely blended into a smooth paste.

Stick Margarine

Stick margarine spreads are made by hydrogenating plant oils and made to resemble butter by adding colour, flavour, milk solids, and water. Cheese spread, garlic spread, tofu spread, and many other flavours are available in the market.

POPULAR FATS AND OILS AVAILABLE

A wide varity of fats and oils are available in the market today.

Oils

Oils from different oil seeds are available refined or unrefined as a single type of oil or as a blend of two or more oils. Single oils are preferable for deep fat frying as each oil has a different smoke point.

Butter

It is available salted or unsalted.

Spreads

These are emulsions of oil in water as compared to butter and margarine which are emulsions of water in oil (W/O).

The consumer can choose from a large number of spreads which unlike butter/margarine are easy to spread even when removed from the refrigerator. Spreads may be blends of hydrogenated plant oils, water, milk solids, flavouring, and colouring.

They may be whipped into a foam to increase volume. They have a light texture and provide lesser calories per teaspoon as the water and air content is more. They are marketed as diet spreads or low-calorie spreads. They contain half the fat and twice the water of ordinary margarine.

Vanaspati

It is prepared by hydrogenation of oil to varying degrees to give a soft grainy fat or a hard fat. They are usually prepared from a blend of different oils.

Margarine

It is a synthetic emulsion containing at least 80 per cent or more fats and oils. Margarine used for spreads is more plastic, while cakes and pastries need harder margarine. The fats and oils used may be from plant, animal, or vegetable sources. Margarine is a saturated fat.

In India, it is made from a blend of different oils. Since it is a substitute for butter, it is fortified with vitamin A, 25 IU, and vitamin D, 2 IU, per gram. After the fats and oils are refined and hydrogenated, it is ripened with pasteurized milk inoculated with Streptococci for 12–24 hours to develop butter flavour. The fat–milk emulsion is further treated and kneaded to obtain a hard fat which has no crystals.

Compound Fats

These are special blends of hydrogenated fats that are available to the bakery industry for specific use (refer the section on commercial uses of fats and oils).

Suet

It is the solid fat deposits around the kidneys of various animals. It is used for making suet puddings.

Dripping

When meat is roasted, especially beef, the drippings are clarified and fat which rises to the top is separated and used for shallow frying.

Olive Oil

Virgin olive oil extracted by cold pressing is of premium quality and is used for salad dressings such as mayonnaise and vinaigrette dressing.

Canola Oil

Canola oil is extracted from the seeds of the canola plant grown in the cold regions of Canada. It is a hybrid variety of the rapeseed plant *Brassica napus* or *Brassica campestris*, in which the levels of toxic erucic acid have been lowered as compared to traditional rapeseed oil.

It is a versatile cooking oil which can withstand high temperatures of baking and deep fat frying, ensuring crispiness, colour, and flavour of the product. Because of its neutral flavour, it is popular in dressings, salads, and bakery products. Its main benefits are its high stability and healthy fatty acid profile.

Fresh Cream

Cream is obtained by skimming whole milk and contains 18–55 per cent fat. It is available as single cream, double cream, sour cream, whipping cream, and clotted cream. *Synthetic cream* which is dairy free is available in the market and is a convenient substitute to fresh cream because of its enhanced properties. It is made from oils and does not contain cholesterol. It is 100 per cent vegetarian and does not curdle, but blends well with other ingredients.

It is available in two forms: for whipping and for cooking.

Both are purchased in the frozen form and at −18°C have a shelf life of one year.

They are prepared using vegetable oils, water, sugar or cornsyrup, soyprotein concentrates, emulsifiers, stabilizers, and added flavours.

NUTS AND OILSEEDS

Nuts and oilseeds are an important group of foodstuff in our daily diet. Nuts are the reproductive seeds of the fruits of the plant or tree from which they are obtained. They consist of an edible kernel rich in fat covered with a hard or brittle shell. They are very nutritious because they are rich in proteins, fat, B-complex vitamins, and minerals and are of special importance in vegetarian diets, if consumed in moderate amounts.

Oilseeds are grown mainly for oil extraction. As they are rich in oils, they are perishable as oil may get rancid or the nuts may get infested with insects. They contain small amounts of moisture and are a concentrated source of energy. They should be consumed in moderation as they may be difficult to digest. Soaking nuts and proper mastication improves their digestibility. Oilseeds need to be stored in airtight containers in a cool, dry, and well-ventilated store. Oilseeds may be consumed as such or may be used for extraction of oil. The oilseed cake or meal which remains after oil is extracted, is an excellent source of protein. Earlier, this residue was used as cattle feed. With developments in science and technology, the percentage of oil which is extracted is higher, and if oilseeds are carefully selected and handled, the residue which remains can be recycled as a rich source of proteins. The de-oiled cake is used in developing nutritious products, for feeding programmes, and also to isolate proteins from the oilseed cake. These protein isolates are of importance in supplementary feeding programmes and in the pharmacological industry. Like pulses, nuts and oilseeds are rich in amino acid lysine and deficient in amino acid methionine. Compared to other oilseeds, *gingelly* or sesame seeds are richer in essential amino acid methionine. The protein from oilseed meal is combined with cereals to improve the protein quality of food, especially infant foods, e.g., it is used in multi-purpose food (MPF). Flaxseeds are rich in omega-3 fatty acids.

Oilseeds are subjected to fungal contamination if they are not dried and stored properly. The fungus *Aspergillus flavus* grows on groundnuts and produces the toxin aflatoxin which causes liver damage and is carcinogenic.

The nutritive value of some nuts and oilseeds is given in Table 7.2 and local names for some nuts and oilseeds are given in Table 7.3.

TABLE 7.2   Nutritive value of some nuts and oilseeds

Name	Protein (g)	Fat (g)	Energy (kcalories)	Calcium (mg)	Iron (mg)	Niacin (mg)
Almond	21	59	655	230	5	4.4
Cashew nut	21	47	596	50	6	1.2
Coconut dry	7	62	662	400	8	3.0
Garden cress seeds	25	25	454	377	100	14.3
Gingelly seeds/sesame	18	43	563	1,450	9	4.4
Ground nut/peanut	25	40	567	90	2.5	19.0
Linseed/flaxseed	20	37	530	170	2.7	1.0
Niger seeds	24	39	515	300	57	8.4
Walnut	15	65	687	100	2.6	1.0

Note: Values per 100 g edible portion

Role of Nuts and Oilseeds in Cookery

Nuts and oilseeds are available in many forms: whole inside the shell, shelled, halved, flaked, nibbed, ground, or desiccated. They are consumed fresh, boiled, roasted, or fried.

Uses

1. Nuts are used as a salted snack. For example, almonds, groundnuts, pistachio, macadamia nuts, cashew nuts.
2. Nuts and oilseeds, such as coconut, *gingelly*, groundnut, linseed, and niger seeds, are used in wet and dry roasted chutneys.
3. Coconut, poppy seeds, *gingelly*, and cashew nuts are used as thickening agents to add richness to gravies.
4. Nuts are used in sweetmeats and confections such as *pista burfi*, *kaju katli*, and groundnut *chikki*/peanut brittle.
5. Nuts are used in cakes and confectionaries such as marzipan, praline, ice creams, sorbets and puddings.
6. Nuts are used in savoury snacks, gravies, curries, sauces, pastas, and as a stuffing.
7. They are used as a garnish on many foods.
8. They are used as a spread, e.g., peanut butter is a nut spread for toast.
9. They are used as beverages, e.g., coconut milk, groundnut milk, and *thandai*.

TABLE 7.3 Local names for some nuts and oilseeds

Name	Local name	Name	Local name
Almond	*Badam*	Niger seeds	*Karale*
Cashew nut	*Kaju*	Piyal seeds	*Charoli*
Coconut	*Nariyal*	Pine nuts	*Chilgoza*
Garden cress seeds	*Ahliva*	Pistachios	*Pista*
Gingelly seeds	*Til*	Safflower seeds	*Kardai*
Linseed/Flaxseed	*Jawas*	Sunflower seeds	*Suryamukhi*
Groundnut/Peanut	*Moongfali*	Walnut	*Akhrot*
Mustard seed	*Sarso*		

COMMERCIAL USES OF FATS AND OILS

Fats and oils are used in the food industry because of their ability to

1. Increase tenderness and make the product short
2. Form emulsions
3. Spread and be plastic
4. Fry or cook food
5. Get creamed and form foams
6. Impart flavour, aroma, and colour to food.

Fats available in the market are specially manufactured for a variety of applications. Separate hydrogenated fats are available for each of the following:

1. Crispness of biscuits
2. Puff pastry and *kharis* for excellent layer separation, i.e., highly plastic variety available as vanaspati or as margarine
3. Soft and tender cakes with high volume
4. Softer bread with easy dough handling
5. Cream filling for cakes and biscuits
6. Crunchy cookies and biscuits
7. Easy release of baked products from the baking pan.

Shortening Power

Superglycerinated or high ratio shortenings are specially manufactured to achieve a desired consistency by hydrogenation of oil. Mono- and diglycerides are added to improve the emulsification ability of the shortening in batters and doughs. The amount of water and sugar used in a recipe can be increased and these are used to produce high ratio cakes of sufficient strength. The usual sugar:flour ratio is 1:1, but with high ratio shortenings it is possible to prepare cake with a 1.4:1 ratio. Antioxidants are generally added to prevent the development of rancidity.

These shortenings are not suitable for deep fat frying as they have a lower smoke point.

Mono- and diglycerides added are glyceryl monostearate (GMS) and glyceryl mono-oleate (GMO) which help in softening the crumb, reduce spattering in margarine when it is heated, and are good emulsifying and stabilizing agents.

SUMMARY

Fats and oils are unimportant components of our daily diet. Most of the fat which we consume is simple fat made up of one molecule of glycerol and three molecules of fatty acids. Fatty acids may be saturated, mono-unsaturated, or polyunsaturated. Fats and oils are mixed triglycerides containing different fatty acids and hence have different properties. The hardness of fats depends on the fatty acids present in the fat. Saturated fats have higher melting points and liquid oils can be converted to solid fat by a process known as hydrogenation.

Undesirable odours and flavour changes develop in fats and oils due to hydrolytic rancidity, oxidative rancidity, and reversion. Hence, fats and oils have to be stored in cool dry places in containers.

When fats are heated during cooking and frying, certain changes are seen. Hence, care should be taken when fat is used as a cooking medium. Fats should be stored properly to prevent uptake of flavours or turn rancid.

Fats and oils have to undergo several steps in processing before they are fit for the table. These include extraction, refining which means degumming, neutralizing, deodourizing, bleaching, winterizing, and hydrogenation. Depending on the degree of hydrogenation, various shortenings specific for certain food products have been manufactured for the bakery industry.

Nuts and oilseeds are rich in nutrients and can contribute significantly to the nutritional value of vegetarian diets as they are versatile and can be used in a wide variety of preparations.

Fats have many uses in food processing such as tenderizing, emulsifying, medium for cooking, creaming and foam formation, preparation of low-calorie diet spreads, and to impart flavour, aroma, colour, and texture to food. Fats are available as *vanaspatis* of varying degree of hardness to be used over an extensive range of products.

KEY TERMS

Acrolein   A highly irritating volatile substance formed when glycerol is heated till it is broken down.

Antioxidant   A compound that is oxidized very readily. Thus, preventing unsaturated fatty acids from getting oxidized quickly.

Auto-oxidation   Oxidation reaction which is auto-catalytic and continues easily once it begins with little added energy.

Bleaching   A step in refining oil in which oil is filtered through charcoal to remove colouring and flavouring matter.

Cholesterol   Lipid widely distributed in animal tissues only, not in plant tissues. It is synthesized by the body.

Cold pressing   Mechanical pressing of ripe olives to extract oil without using heat, producing excellent quality pure virgin oil.

Degumming   A step in refining in which natural gums are removed from oil.

Deodourizing   A step in refining to remove low molecular weight aldehydes, ketones, peroxides, etc., which could affect flavour and aroma of fats and oils.

Free radicals   Groups containing an unpaired electron.

Hydrogenation   Addition of hydrogen to an unsaturated fatty acid in the presence of a catalyst to increase saturation and melting point.

Lipolysis   Reaction of a molecule of water with a fat molecule to release a free fatty acid in the presence of lipase or heat.

Neutralization   A step in refining to remove free fatty acids from oils.

Plasticity   The property of solid fats to spread and get deformed when pressure is applied.

Polyunsaturated fatty acids   Fatty acids containing two or more double bonds between the carbon atoms in the carbon chain.

Rancidity   Development of off-flavours and odours in fats because of oxygen, lipases, heat, etc.

Rendering   Process by which fat is extracted from animal tissues using dry or moist heat.

Superglycerinated fats   They are not triglycerides but are mono- or diglycerides, e.g., glyceryl monostearate (GMS) used as an emulsifier and stabilizer and as a plasticizer in bakery products.

Triglyceride   Esters of glycerol with three fatty acids to form a simple fat.

Unsaturated fatty acid   Fatty acid having one or more double bonds in the carbon chain.

Winterization   Removal of high molecular weight triglycerides with high melting points by chilling the oil, so that oil remains clear and pourable at refrigeration temperatures.

REVIEW EXERCISES

1. Differentiate between:
   (a) Fat and oil
   (b) Saturated fatty acid and unsaturated fatty acid
   (c) Rancidity and reversion
   (d) Butter and margarine
   (e) Smoke point and melting point
2. Classify fats on the basis of saturation giving two examples for each.
3. What is hydrogenation? What are its advantages and disadvantages?
4. How can you prevent fats and fatty phases of food from going rancid?
5. Briefly explain the various stages in refining of oil.
6. What is the role of shortenings in the bakery industry?
7. Explain the commercial significance of fats and oils.
8. Explain the following terms:
   (a) Polymerization
   (b) Superglycerinated fats
   (c) Spreads
   (d) Rendering
   (e) Virgin olive oil
9. Discuss the uses of nuts and oilseeds in cookery.

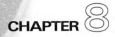

Flavour

LEARNING OBJECTIVES

After reading this chapter, you should be able to
- understand the significance of flavour in the food industry
- classify different flavours present in food
- know various flavouring agents and flavour enhancers permitted in food
- differentiate between the terms herbs, spices, condiments, and seasonings
- know the different herbs and spices popularly used in cookery
- explain and control the effect of cooking and processing on flavour retention and development

INTRODUCTION

The enjoyment and acceptance of a meal depends to a large extent on the blend of different flavours present in food. Flavour is the most important attribute of food. It is detected by our senses of taste and odour. It is produced by aromatic chemicals that stimulate the senses of odour and taste. These stimulating components are synthesized in plants and animals. They may be further modified by cooking and processing. The intrinsic flavour of food represents the complex effect of these aromatic substances on our senses of odour and taste.

There are four basic tastes: sweet, bitter, salty, and sour. All other tastes are permutations and combinations of these four taste sensations. Taste is detected by the 10,000 taste buds located mainly on the tongue while odour is detected by extremely sensitive 10 million cells situated in the upper portion of the nasal cavity. Sweetness and saltiness are detected by taste buds on the tip of the tongue, sourness on the sides of the tongue, and bitterness at the back of the tongue (Fig. 8.1).

The level at which a taste can be identified is called the threshold level. This level may vary from one individual to another. Even at sub-threshold levels, one taste can modify another taste, e.g., a pinch of salt added to a glass of lime juice increases the apparent sweetness of sugar.

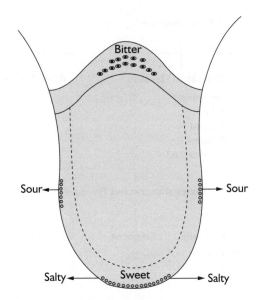

Fig. 8.1   Site of taste detectors on the tongue

Definitions

Flavouring   It is a substance which can impart flavour and is generally used to impart taste or odour or both to a food.

Aroma   It refers to a pleasant, often spicy odour, fragrance, or smell.

Flavour   It is a blend of taste and odour perceptions experienced when food is in the mouth.

Aftertaste   It is the flavour that lingers in the mouth after food has been swallowed.

Flavour intensifier   It is a compound that enhances the flavour of other foods without contributing any flavour of its own.

The flavour of any food depends upon minute quantities of 100 or more chemicals that are present in food. These flavouring components are present in concentrations ranging from a few ppm to 0.1 per cent. Food flavours are broadly classified as natural food flavours, processed flavours, and added flavours which may be natural extracted flavours or synthetic flavours (Fig. 8.2).

NATURAL FLAVOURS

These are usually extremely complex mixtures of many different substances. Sometimes, the flavour of a natural flavouring agent may depend upon a single substance, e.g., the flavour of clove oil is because of the chemical eugenol that constitutes 85 per cent of clove oil or it may be present in extremely small amounts, such as citral in oil of lemon which constitutes

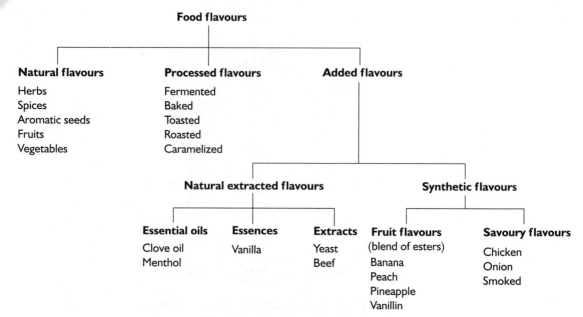

Fig. 8.2 Classification of flavours

5 per cent of the oil. Natural flavouring agents are composed mainly of aromatic organic compounds present as volatile essential oils or as non-volatile constituents such as resins and oleoresins. They are formed in the plant during normal plant metabolism and remain as such when the plant is harvested.

Some Flavoursome Plant Products

Herbs Basil, parsley, celery, thyme, mint, etc.

Fruits Orange, lemon, apple, banana, strawberry, pineapple, etc.

Spices Cardamon, clove, turmeric, peppercorns, etc.

Vegetables Mushrooms, corn, peas, onion, garlic, cabbage, turnips, etc.

Aromatic seeds Aniseed, cumin, fennel, dill, caraway, etc.

The aroma of onion, garlic, cabbage, etc. is mainly due to sulphur-containing compounds. These vegetables should not be overcooked. Other flavouring components in vegetables are methanol, acetone, propanal, etc.

Fruits such as apple owe their distinct flavour to 131 chemical components, while fresh strawberries contain over 100 volatile components. The flavour and aroma of fruits and vegetables is because of the presence of volatile organic chemicals such as esters, aldehydes, acids, alcohols, ketones, and ether present as essential oils in natural foods.

PROCESSED FLAVOURS

These flavours develop during processing by decomposition, combination with other compounds, or formation of a new compound. The following flavours form during processing of various foods.

1. Flavour resulting from enzyme action: When vegetable tissues are cut or damaged, e.g., onion and garlic, the crushed garlic odour is because of the formation of diallyl disulfide.
2. Flavour produced by microbiological action during fermentation of sugar to alcohol by yeast and fermentation of milk to curd and cheese by bacteria.
3. Flavours formed during cooking and other heat processing, e.g., cooked meat flavour and aroma of freshly baked bread or roasted coffee beans (refer the section on Maillard reaction in Chapter 9).
4. Undesirable flavours caused by oxidation, e.g., oils turning rancid in pickles and fried snacks such as *chiwda* and *chakli* (refer the section on rancidity in fats in Chapter 7).

ADDED FLAVOURS

Natural flavours or synthetic flavours are often added to food to increase its acceptability. With advanced techniques used in the food industry and development of new food products such as bakery and confectionery items, ready-to-cook, ready-to-eat foods, beverages, and fast food items, the role of added flavours has gained importance. Although some flavours develop during processing of some foods, natural flavours are often lost during cooking and processing. These flavours can be replaced by either of the methods discussed here.

1. Adding natural flavourings and extracts, e.g., natural essences from fruits, essential oils extracted from spices, beef extract, yeast extract, etc. Vanilla essence is prepared by extracting the essential oil from vanilla pod with ethanol.
2. Adding imitation or synthetic flavours that consist of a blend of chemicals which smells like the original substance, e.g., saffron flavour instead of pure saffron, vanillin is the synthetic flavour instead of vanilla.

Synthetic flavours are easy to prepare when the natural flavour is composed of a single chemical. With the advent of modern analytical techniques, the food technician can understand and develop flavours to closely match natural flavours. Perfect matching of the flavour profile is possible, but is a costly process. The electronic nose is a gadget which can measure the quality of odour very quickly and objectively. Synthetic chemicals are blended to match a natural flavour, but there is generally a detectable difference between the natural and synthetic flavours.

The number of flavours used today is so large that flavours form the largest group of food additives.

Commercial flavour is usually a mixture of essential oils, aroma chemicals, gums, resins, emulsifiers, etc. in which the actual flavour ingredient is approximately 1 per cent.

Other substances which contribute towards the flavour of food are sweeteners and flavour enhancers.

Sweeteners   The basic taste of a food, especially the acid:sweetness ratio also affects the effectiveness of flavours used. Sweeteners used in food may be natural or artificial. Natural sweeteners or carbohydrate sweeteners are also called nutritive sweeteners. Artificial sweeteners or synthetic sweeteners are also called non-nutritive sweeteners as they provide no calories (refer Chapter 4 on carbohydrates).

Sugar is added to savoury dishes in minute amounts to improve the flavour of the dish.

Flavour enhancers   They are chemicals which by themselves have little or no odour or taste. When they are added to food, even in small quantities, they are able to bring out the existing flavour of the food. In other words, they are capable of enhancing, modifying, or intensifying the original flavour.

The following chemicals are used as flavour enhancers.

1. Monosodium glutamate (MSG) is also called *aji-no-moto* or Chinese salt. It is the sodium salt of glutamic acid, an amino acid. Glutamate is present naturally in many foods such as meat, fish, poultry, milk and many vegetables such as peas, mushrooms, and tomatoes. Although glutamic acid is present in many foods, its content decreases during harvesting to processing, causing a natural loss of flavour. This can be partly restored by adding MSG to food. It draws out the hidden flavour of food and reduces the less-desirable flavours. Monosodium glutamate increases salivation and its excessive consumption leads to a condition known as 'Chinese restaurant syndrome' in which people suffer from various symptoms such as a burning sensation, migraine-like symptoms, and chest pain.

   Monosodium glutamate is used worldwide as a flavour intensifier in soups, sauces, gravies, taste makers and flavourings, canned and frozen vegetables, meat, poultry, and combination dishes. A level of 0.05–0.8 per cent by weight in foods gives best flavour enhancement and excessive use decreases the palatability of food. Under the Prevention of Food Adulteration (PFA) Act, MSG has been banned in foods meant for infants below 12 months of age, and should not exceed 1 per cent by weight in foods meant for adults.

2. Nucleotides are flavour enhancers widely present in plant and animal cells. Like MSG, nucleotides bring out the flavour of foods. They are 50 to 100 times stronger than MSG and cover more flavours than MSG, which is basically a 'meaty' flavour enhancer. The two are ideally used together in the ratio of 1:50, i.e., 1g of nucleotides is used with 50g of MSG, with a flavour enhancing effect equal to 100 g of MSG used alone.

It is used in processed foods such as potato chips, peanuts, dry and canned soups, sauces, ketchups, sausages, canned vegetables, and meat. The quantity of nucleotide added is very low.

Professor Kikunae Ikeda was the first to isolate glutamic acid in 1908 from a bouillon as the ingredient which gave the taste to soups.

3. Maltol is used as a flavour enhancer for sweet flavours. It is found in several plants and is formed when cocoa, coffee, and malt are roasted and in bread, when it is baked. It is synthesized from soya bean protein fermentation and is used as a fragrant, caramel-like flavour for addition to fruit-based products, ice creams, chocolates, and candies. It imparts a 'freshly baked' flavour to breads and cakes.

   It is also used in cookies, beverages, instant pudding mix, and soup mixes at levels ranging between 50–300 ppm.

4. Salt is used in food for its flavour, as a preservative, and as a dietary constituent. The main role of salt in food is for salty taste, flavour intensification, and as a digestive stimulant. It is used at 2 per cent level.

   Salt also blends with and enhances other flavours present. It is capable of reducing the sourness of acids and increasing the sweetness of sugar. If small quantities of salt are added to soft drinks, the amount of sugar required may be reduced by 5 per cent.

5. Sodium-restricted flavouring: When salt is restricted on health grounds because of hypertension, oedema, kidney disorders, etc., the flavour of food can be improved by using herbs and spices such as pepper, dry mustard, paprika, lime juice, mint, celery, onion, ginger, garlic, and bay leaf. If small quantities of sugar are added to vegetables while cooking, the natural flavour of food is brought out.

   Salt substitutes are salts which do not contain sodium but contain potassium or ammonium instead, such as potassium chloride and ammonium chloride. To improve the palatability of the diet, salt mixtures are available which contain potassium and ammonium chloride, citrates, formates, phosphates, and glutamates along with herbs and spices.

SPICES AND HERBS

Spices and herbs contribute natural flavours to foods in which they are used or added to. They are used to enhance the flavour of foods. The flavour is due to essential oils and other flavour components present in plants. Herbs and spices are used in small amounts to flavour foods and increase its palatability and acceptability. Herbs are the leaves of fresh or dried plants, while spices may be the aromatic part of plants, usually the dried buds, fruits, berries, roots, or bark. They both have nutritive and medicinal properties and are used in cuisines all over the world. Spices have stronger flavours than herbs. Since they are more concentrated in flavour, they should be used sparingly. They contain oils which help in digestion by stimulating the flow of saliva and gastric juice. Other natural and processed flavouring agents are condiments and seasonings. The terms herbs and spices and seasonings and condiments are often used interchangeably. A condiment was originally defined as any item added to a dish to give flavour such as herbs, spices, and vinegar. The term condiment now also includes cooked or prepared flavourings or accompaniments such as relishes, prepared mustards, ketchup, proprietary sauces, and pickles.

A seasoning is traditionally defined as any item added to enhance the natural flavours of a food item without changing its flavour dramatically. Salt is the most common seasoning, although all herbs and spices are often referred to as seasonings. Table 8.1 describes popular herbs and spices.

TABLE 8.1 Popular herbs and spices

Herbs	Description	Spices	Description
Basil	Small leaves with pungent flavour	Ajwain	Small round seeds with sharp pungent taste
Bay leaf	Dried aromatic leaf of the laurel tree	Allspice	Berries with flavour of cloves, nutmeg, and cinnamon
		Aniseed	Seeds look like cumin and has delicately sweet liquorice aroma
		Star anise	Pretty star-shaped fruit with aniseed flavour
Chervil	Looks like parsley with delicate stem and soft, almost wilting leaves; has faint flavour	Asafoetida	Strong-flavoured dried resin with strong smell
Chive	Tender green shoots with mild onion and scallion flavour	Cardamom	Black large pods and green small pods with pleasing warm aroma
Coriander/ cilantro	Looks like parsley; piquant taste and intense flavour with a fresh pungency	Chillies	Numerous varieties of dried ripened green chillies with varying degrees of pungency
Curry leaves	Long slender shiny dark green leaflets; strong warm spicy aroma curry flavour	Cinnamon	Delicate inner sweet and fragrant bark of small evergreen laurel-like trees
Dill	Fine feathery green strands with sweet aromatic flavour of caraway and lemon	Cloves	Dried unopened flower buds with a sweet pungent flavour and aroma
Fennel	Fine wispy leaves with mild aniseed and dill flavour	Coriander seeds	Yellowish brown round light seeds with pleasant flavour
Horseradish	Long tapering root with powerful smell and fiery taste	Cumin and caraway seeds	Caraway seeds are smaller new moon-shaped seeds resembling cumin; pungent, sharp, and astringent tasting seed
Kaffir lime leaf	Looks like bay leaf but fresh, green, and smaller with aromatic lime flavour		
Lemon grass	Pale green long sturdy leaves with distinct lemony flavour	Fennel seeds	Sweet aniseed-like flavour
Marjoram	Similar to oregano but slightly sweeter flavour and a sweet, almost perfumed aroma	Fenugreek seeds	Small aromatic curry flavoured hard beige-coloured seeds

Contd

Table 8.1 Contd

Herbs	Description	Spices	Description
Mint	Leaves of spearmint plant containing peppermint oil	Galangal	Galangal is similar to ginger
Oregano	Wild variety of marjoram with a stronger flavour; warm aroma and pleasant slightly musty flavour	Garlic	Bulb with characteristic flavour of diallyl disulphide and high medicinal value
		Kokum	Dried sour fruit rich in anthocyanin
Parsley	Refreshing flavour with grassy undertones	Ginger	Rhizome or root with sharp burning sensory stimulation, used fresh or dried.
		Mace and nutmeg	Mace is the outermost covering of the nutmeg fruit while nutmeg is the fruit; both have aromatic sweet and warm flavour
Rosemary	Narrow spiky leaves with a fragrant evergreen smell	Mango powder	Substitute for tamarind and lime
Sage	Pale green leaves with earthy flavour	Mustard seeds	Hot pungent taste, small round black, brown and yellow seeds
Tarragon	Slender leaves with intense sweet aniseed/ vanilla flavour	Pepper	Dried pungent small round berries, black, red, green and white in colour; also classified as condiment
Thyme	Tiny greenish grey petals with pungent earthy flavour	Pomegranate seeds	Dried seeds of fruit with sharp sour taste used for sourness
Wasabi	Root with delicate apple-green flesh; flavour milder than horseradish	Saffron	Stigmas of a crocus which are dried and used for distinctive flavour and bright yellow colour; very expensive spice.
		Tamarind	Sour, fruity flavour, brown bean-like seed pod
		Turmeric	Rhizome with bright yellow colour used in curry powder

Bouquet garni is a combination of herbs (parsley stalks, sprig of thyme, a bay leaf along with celery or rosemary or fennel) tied together and used to flavour soups and stews. They are removed before the dish is served.

Herbs are available in three forms: fresh, dried, and frozen. Delicate herbs, such as basil, chives, tarragon, chervil, coriander, dill, and parsley, can be preserved by freezing. All herbs cannot be preserved by drying as they lose their aroma. Although frozen herbs lose their fresh appearance and texture, they can be used successfully in cooked items and have a shelf life of three months if stored at proper temperatures. Herbs to be frozen should be washed well. They can be frozen in plastic containers or in freezer bags, either as sprigs or finely chopped. Air should be expelled from the freezer bag in which sprigs are to be frozen. Finely chopped herbs are preserved as ice cubes. They are half-filled in ice cube trays, topped with water and frozen. The frozen ice cubes can be stored in freezer bags and used in hot soups, stews, etc.

Dried herbs are a convenient alternative for fresh herbs. They should be used carefully as they have a more concentrated flavour than fresh herbs and should be given sufficient time to rehydrate and soften. They should be stored carefully in sealed, airtight jars in a cool and dark place to prevent spoilage and loss of flavour by exposure to light.

USE OF FLAVOURS IN FOOD PREPARATION

Retaining the natural flavours while processing food is an art. An understanding of volatile and non-volatile flavours is necessary for any chef. Flavours are often lost when food becomes stale, and off-flavours may develop. Processing of food results in both development of flavour and loss of flavour. Different processes and ingredients used give different flavours to food. These flavours can be altered, modified, or intensified by the use of flavouring agents.

Flavouring agents are widely used in the food industry to

1. Enhance a food flavour, e.g., addition of chocolate essence to chocolate cake.
2. Replace flavours lost while processing food.
3. Give a particular flavour to a food.
4. Mask some undesirable flavours in order to increase the acceptability of a food, e.g., adding essence to egg nog to mask the eggy flavour.

Table 8.2 presents some flavours in food and Table 8.3 shows taste components in fruits and vegetables.

TABLE 8.2   Some flavours in food

Natural flavours	
Foodstuff	*Principal flavouring agent*
Mint	Menthol
Thyme	Thymol
Cloves	Eugenol
Pepper	Piperidine
Butter	Diacetal
Orange	Limonene
Lemon	Citral
Garlic	Diallyl disulfide
Turmeric	Curcumin
Synthetic fruit flavours	
Flavour	*Chemical (mixtures of esters and alcohols)*
Banana	Ethyl butyrate + amyl acetate
Peach	Benzaldehyde, benzyl alcohol
Apple	Ethyl acetate
Pineapple	Pentyl acctate
Strawberries	Methyl and ethyl acetates propionates and butyrates
Flavour enhancers	
Foodstuff	*Flavouring compound*
Chicken soup	Monosodium glutamate
Mushrooms	Nucleotides, i.e., GMP Disodium-5-guanylate

TABLE 8.3 Taste components in fruits and vegetables

Taste	Substance
Sweet	Glucose, galactose, fructose, ribose, arabinose, and xylose
Bitter	Quinone-like compounds
Sour	Organic acids such as citric, tartaric, oxalic, malic, isocitric, succinic acid, etc.
Salty	Small amount of salt

SUMMARY

Flavour is an important attribute of food which contributes to its palatability and acceptance. It is produced by aromatic chemicals that stimulate our senses of odour and taste. Flavouring agents may be naturally present in food as volatile essential oils or non-volatile chemicals. Flavours may be complex, consisting of 100 or more chemicals present in varying proportions.

Flavours are classified as natural flavours, processed flavours, and added flavours which may be natural extracts or essential oils in an alcoholic base or they may be synthetic chemicals which are blended to match a natural flavour as closely as possible.

Sweeteners and flavour enhancers also contribute towards the flavour of foods. Sweeteners may be nutritive sweeteners such as sugar and jaggery, or non-nutritive sweeteners such as saccharin or aspartame. Flavour enhancers include monosodium glutamate, nucleotides, maltol, sodium chloride, and sodium-restricted flavourings.

They are widely used in the food industry to enhance flavours, replace flavours, add flavours, or mask undesirable flavours. Processing of food needs to be carefully controlled to develop the desired flavour in a food.

KEY TERMS

Bouquet garni Parsley stalks, a sprig of thyme and a bay leaf along with a stick of celery (for poultry), rosemary (for red meat), fennel (for fish), bundled together and tied with a string or wrapped in muslin and added to soup, stew, etc. for flavour and removed before the dish is served.

Condiment Originally defined as any item added to a dish to give flavour, such as herbs, spices, vinegar, now also includes cooked or prepared flavourings or accompaniments such as relishes, prepared mustards, ketchup, proprietary sauces, and pickles.

Electronic nose An instrument with multisensors and pattern recognition techniques which can measure the quality of odour very quickly and accurately.

Essential oils Volatile, natural flavouring agents present in plants which are oily but chemically not related to fats and oils.

Flavour intensifiers These substances enhance the flavours of other substances without itself imparting any characteristic flavour of its own, e.g., monosodium glutamate, small quantities of sugar, salt, and vinegar.

Herbs   Any of a large group of annual and perennial plants whose leaves, stems, or flowers are used as a flavouring; usually available fresh and dried.

Nucleotides   Compounds made up of five carbon sugar ribose, phosphoric acid, and an organic base such as guanine. They are present in animal tissues and give a characteristic meaty taste to food.

ppm   Parts per million

Seasoning   Traditionally, an item added to enhance the natural flavours of a food without changing its flavour dramatically. Salt is the most common seasoning, although all herbs and spices are often referred to as seasonings.

Spices   Any of a large group of aromatic plants whose bark, roots, seeds, buds, or berries

are used as a flavouring; usually available dried either whole, ground, or finely powdered. Also available as spice oils and oleoresins.

Synthetic flavours   Mostly mixtures of esters which give an imitation flavour when added to food, e.g., banana flavour is a mixture of ethyl butyrate and amyl acetate.

Taste threshold   It is that critical concentration value at which the presence of a taste can be just detected.

Vanilla   It is the extract of the vanilla bean. The beans are allowed to ferment till they become dark brown in colour. Flavour is extracted by crushing the beans and adding alcohol. Synthetic vanillin is $3\frac{1}{2}$ times as strong as the natural vanilla extracted from beans.

REVIEW EXERCISES

1. How are food flavours classified?
2. What are flavour intensifiers? Which flavour intensifier will you use in
   (a) Hypertensive diets
   (b) Cookies
   (c) Cream of mushroom
   (d) Tomato ketchup
   (e) Lime juice
3. Explain the following:
   (a) Types of sweeteners
   (b) Detection of taste
   (c) Commercial flavours.
4. Why is flavour an important characteristic of food?
5. Define the terms herbs, spices, seasoning, and condiment giving five suitable examples for each.
6. Explain how the following herbs can be preserved to ensure non-seasonal availability:
   (a) Mint leaves   (c) Basil
   (b) Fenugreek leaves   (d) Parsley
7. Classify the following into herbs/ spices/ seasonings/ condiments:
   (a) Balsamic vinegar   (g) Pepper
   (b) Fennel seeds   (h) Bay leaves
   (c) Mustard paste   (i) Soya sauce
   (d) Thai red curry paste (j) Salt
   (e) Onion   (k) Garlic
   (f) Nutmeg

CHAPTER 9

Browning Reactions

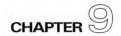

LEARNING OBJECTIVES

After reading this chapter, you should be able to
- understand the different types of browning reactions seen in food
- appreciate the need for controlling the extent of these reactions in different food products
- gain insight into factors which accelerate and retard these reactions
- gain knowledge as to how these reactions take place
- understand other changes which accompany these reactions and their effect on nutritive value
- identify desirable and undesirable browning reactions

INTRODUCTION

Browning is a common colour change seen in food during pre-preparation, processing, or storage of food. It occurs in varying degrees in some food material. The colours produced range from cream or pale yellow to dark brown or black, depending on the food item and the extent of the reaction.

Browning reactions may be desirable or they may be undesirable. In some foods, the brown colour and flavour developed during browning is highly desirable and is associated with a delicious, highly acceptable, and quality product. Browning reactions contribute to the aroma, flavour, and colour of the product such as the brown crust of bread and all baked goods, potato chips, roasted nuts, roasted coffee beans, caramel, peanut brittle, and many other processed foods.

The undesirable effects of browning reactions is seen in dehydrated food, such as milk, eggs, dry fruits, in cut fruit and citrus fruit juices and juice concentrates, in canned milk, and in coconut. The colour varies from light cream to black while coconut develops a saffron colour. The off-colour and off-odour developed in foods depend on the extent to which the browning reaction has progressed. Off-flavours may vary from mild flavour changes to stale and very bitter.

Controlled browning is necessary even in foods where browning is desired because excessive browning can produce an undesirable product. Changes in odour and flavour, which may also develop along with browning, may be characteristic of a food and desirable or may be bitter, making the food unpalatable.

TYPES OF BROWNING REACTIONS

Browning reactions observed in food may be classified as *enzymatic browning* and *non-enzymatic browning*.

Non-enzymatic browning may be further classified as shown in Fig. 9.1.

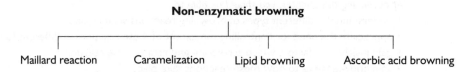

Fig. 9.1 Classification of non-enzymatic browning reactions

Enzymatic Browning

Some light-coloured fresh fruits and vegetables darken when exposed to air as a result of the presence of oxidative enzymes. Enzymatic browning occurs in these fruit and vegetable tissues when cellular organization is disrupted by cutting, bruising, or other injury to the tissues. This is due to the action of oxidative enzymes on the phenolic substances present in the fruit or vegetable tissues. Apples, bananas, pears, brinjals, and potatoes undergo enzymatic browning. The cell contents come in contact with each other resulting in browning of uncooked fruits and vegetables which are cut or bruised.

Enzymatic browning takes place only in fruits and vegetables which contain phenolic compounds. These phenolic compounds act as the substrate, and in the presence of oxygen and by the action of enzymes, the following oxidative reaction is observed (Fig. 9.2).

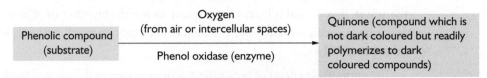

Fig. 9.2 Enzymatic browning reaction

The formation of O-quinone is the first step in brown colour formation. Quinones are polymerized to form complex compounds which darken in colour.

The details of chemical changes which take place in conversion of colourless substrate in the intact fruit to the brown-coloured reaction product in the damaged tissues are not known. First quinols are formed, which change to quinones. Polymerized quinones are oxidized non-enzymatically and are responsible for brown colour formation.

Phenol oxidase enzymes are specific for certain substrates and are present in many fruits and vegetables such as apples, bananas, pears, peaches, potatoes, and brinjals.

Phenolic compounds present, such as tannins, and related phenolic substances, such as leucoanthocyanin, contribute towards the astringency of food.

Prevention of enzymatic browning

Enzymatic browning can be prevented by the following methods.

By inactivating enzymes   Enzymes can be inactivated by any of the following measures.

Application of heat   Blanching or cooking fruits and vegetables which are prone to browning prevents discolouration. Enzymes are protein in nature and heat denatures proteins there by inactivating the enzymes.

Addition of salt   Vegetables may be immersed in a solution of sodium chloride to retard enzymatic browning. The chloride ion in NaCl inhibits enzyme activity. However, this is a temporary measure to retard browning, as the amount of salt required to prevent browning temporarily would make the food unpalatable.

Lowering the pH   Enzymatic browning is prevented by lowering the pH to 2.5–2.7 by addition of acid. Acids used to prevent browning are ascorbic acid, malic acid, citric acid, and lime juice. Ascorbic acid or vitamin C acts as an antioxidant and retards enzymatic browning. The quinones formed by the action of enzymes are reduced to their dihy droxyl state by vitamin C and in turn vitamin C is oxidized to dehydroascorbic acid.

Chilling a food below temperatures optimum for enzyme activity   Optimum temperature for enzymes to act is 43°C (109°F). In cold storage, the browning reaction slows down, but even fruits stored in frozen storage brown unless they are treated.

By avoiding contact with oxygen   Oxygen should not come in contact with the substrate. This can be achieved by any of the following measures.

Coating fruit with sugar   Coating fruit with sugar or covering it with syrup keeps atmospheric oxygen away from the surface. Intercellular oxygen is present in fruits, but sugar reduces the concentration of oxygen dissolved in the syrup and at the same time suppresses enzyme activity.

Immersing vegetables in water   Contact with atmospheric oxygen can be avoided by immersing cut vegetables in water. Since water contains dissolved oxygen, it is more effective if it is first boiled to remove dissolved air.

Vacuum packing   Protecting food from contact with oxygen as in vacuum packing prevents enzymatic browning since it is an oxidation reaction.

By elimination of substrate   This method of prevention is not practical. A variety of peach called 'sunbeam' is an exception because it is deficient in substrate.

Sulphuring of fruits prior to dehydration   Sulphur prevents oxidative browning due to enzyme activity. Fruit is treated to sulphur fumes prior to drying. Treatment with sulphur dioxide (SO_2) gas or sulphurous acid solution (H_2SO_3) or 0.25 per cent sodium sulphite for 45 seconds is adequate to prevent browning. Bisulphites and metabisulphites are also used. Sulphurous acid is a strong reducing agent and prevents discolouration.

Non-enzymatic Browning

Maillard reaction

Maillard was the first to describe the development of a brown colour in mixtures containing amino acids and reducing sugars. The reaction between certain free groups of amino acids, such as the NH_2 group and a carbohydrate, affects the product in many ways in addition to the colour change. The aroma and flavour of the ready product is also affected. The reaction is also known as car bonylamine reaction or protein sugar reaction. Figure 9.3 shows Maillard reaction.

The brown pigment formed contributes to the aroma, flavour, and colour of many ready-to-eat cereals, toffees, malted barley, and bakery products such as bread, cakes, and biscuits. If the dough contains less reducing sugar then the colour of the crust is light. The more the percentage of reducing sugar, the darker the crust in bakery products such as dinner rolls.

Condensation of amino group of protein

+

Carbonyl group of sugar

various reactions such
as rearrangement,
fragmentation, and
polymerization

Brown pigment

Fig. 9.3   Maillard reaction

The characteristic flavour developed differs in different products because of the amino acid involved in the reaction. For example,

- Food product   –   Amino acid involved
- Beer   –   Glycine
- Fresh bread   –   Leucine
- Maple syrup   –   Aminobutyric acid

Conditions which favour Maillard reaction

High temperature   The rate of browning increases rapidly with a rise in temperature.

Moisture   Certain amount of moisture, approximately 13 per cent will favour the reaction. Very high or very low water levels will decrease the rate of the reaction.

pH value   Browning is accelerated by an increase in alkalinity, i.e., a pH above 7.8. Presence of phosphate, citrate, and acetate buffer salts acelerate the rate of browning.

Concentration and type of amino acid and sugar present   Maximum browning effect is observed with amino acid lysine and sugar glucose.

Presence of catalyst   Browning reaction is generally catalyzed by the presence of metals such as copper and iron.

Desirable changes   Many favourable changes in colour, flavour, and aroma are seen during roasting of coffee beans and nuts and improvement in quality of bread during baking.

This reaction is also partly responsible for the flavour of meat extracts, breakfast cereals, and all bakery items.

Undesirable changes   Maillard reaction is also responsible for certain undesirable effects seen in dried foods such as

- Off-odour
- Off-flavour—mild, stale, or bitter
- Off-colour—ranging form mild cream to nearly black.

Dried milk powder and condensed milk darken on storage for a long time. Coconut turns saffron in colour. Undesirable Maillard browning can be prevented by low pH and low temperatures during processing and storage.

There is some loss of nutritive value because of the presence of nutrients involved in the reaction. Several essential amino acids, especially lysine and methionine, undergo this reaction and the substances formed cannot be hydrolyzed by digestive enzymes. Losses of amino acids lysine and methionine in toasted and flaked breakfast cereals are quite significant because amino acids involved in the reaction are unavailable to the body.

Bread loses 10–15 per cent lysine during baking, 5 per cent during staling, and 5–10 per cent during toasting. Lysine is also lost when meat is roasted.

Caramelization

Sugars are caramelized at 163 to 170°C or 325 to 338°F because of action of heat. Darkening of syrups, brown colour of candies such as caramels, taffy, and brittle are because of caramelization reaction. Caramelization or sugar browning reaction occurs with sugar alone. Sugar is broken down into a number of compounds because of intense heat.

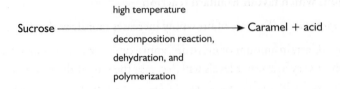

Sucrose →(high temperature) Caramel + acid
decomposition reaction,
dehydration, and
polymerization

Stages of sugar cookery   When sugar is boiled, it passes through regular stages till it gets caramelized at 163°C.

The various stages of sugar cookery are listed in Table 9.1.

The rate and extent of browning in carbohydrate solutions are influenced by the following factors.

Heat   For caramelization to take place, high temperature is necessary. Temperature can be lowered by the presence of a catalyst.

Effect of pH   Both acids and alkali increases browning, but alkalis are more effective.

Type of sugar   Fructose shows the greatest degree of browning, followed by sucrose. Glucose shows least browning.

TABLE 9.1   Stages of sugar cookery

Stage	Temperature (°C)
1. Small thread	102
2. Large thread	103
3. Pearl	106
4. Soft ball	114
5. Hard ball	120
6. Soft crack	143
7. Hard crack	156
8. Caramel	163 to 177

Presence of catalysts   Metals such as iron and copper aeclerate the rate of reaction.

Caramel is used to flavour and colour alcoholic beverages, soups, gravies, sauces, soup cubes, cake mixes, coffee products, canned meat products, etc.

Ascorbic acid browning

Kokum and strawberry preserves undergo a change in colour during storage. The original bright red/crimson of the anthocyanin pigment in the fresh fruit becomes dull and develops a rusty brown colour. A similar change in colour is also seen in citrus fruit juices and squashes.

The ascorbic acid present in these fruits undergoes oxidation with the formation of a compound which produces a brown pigment and causes discolouration. The oxidized ascorbic acid hastens the degradation of the red pigment of anthocyanin giving the product a dull brownish colour. Factors which hasten this reaction are

1. Presence of oxygen
2. Reducing sugars present
3. High pH
4. Warm storage temperatures

Lime juice cordial loses its lemon colour to become darker and brown. This type of browning is seen in preserves. To prevent this discolouration, strawberries are kept as frozen stock and made into preserves only as and when required. Low storage temperatures and addition of bisulphites retard the reaction.

Lipid browning

This type of browning is seen in fats and fatty phases of food. The amino groups of phospholipids and lipoproteins can react with aldehydes and reducing sugars resulting in browning.

This type of browning is quite uncommon and may be observed in fats stored for long periods. It is an undesirable reaction.

ROLE OF BROWNING IN FOOD PREPARATION

Browning reactions may be desirable or undesirable affecting the appearance, flavour, and aroma of food. All browning reactions can be controlled and hence it is essential that the caterer is aware of all factors which influence these reactions.

Enzymatic browning is considered unsightly and undesirable, especially while preparing salads and fruit salads. Natural browning is usually undesirable but normal cooking processes, such as roasting, grilling, or baking, bring about brown colouration. This is expected and desirable and contributes to the acceptance and palatability of food. Cooking brings about chemical breakdown which along with colour, adds flavour to food. The aroma of freshly baked bread and roasted coffee beans is due to desirable Maillard reaction.

Food components interact chemically and give rise to a brown colour accompanied by modifications in flavour, aroma, and taste. Because food components are involved in the formation of the brown colour, there is some loss of nutritive value.

DETRIMENTAL EFFECTS OF BROWNING

Enzymatic browning   Enzymatic browning of apples and bananas makes fruit salads unappetizing and cannot be served to customers.

Maillard reaction   In baked and toasted products and in milk, some lysine and methionine are lost.

Ascorbic acid browning   Some ascorbic acid is lost from citrus juices and strawberries because of auto-oxidation of vitamin C.

In desirable browning reactions, it is necessary to control cooking temperatures to prevent blackening or burning of the product.

Enzymatic activity can be retarded by blanching vegetables and fruit to inactivate the enzymes. Cooked food is not discoloured by enzymes.

Browning plays an important role in the aesthetic value of food. A baked product, e.g., cake or bread, would lose its acceptability if the golden brown crust and the accompanying aroma is absent. The kitchen staff should understand the various factors which can prevent undesirable browning and control them.

SUMMARY

Browning reactions occur very widely in food products and bring about changes in colour ranging from cream or pale yellow to dark brown or black.

These reactions may be desirable as in the brown crust of bakery items and caramelized sugar in peanut brittle. It may be undesirable in some fresh fruits and vegetables, such as bananas and apples, when they are cut or bruised or the darkening of milk powder and strawberry preserves.

Browning reactions need to be controlled as excessive browning may make the product unpalatable. Changes in odour and flavour may also accompany the reaction.

They are broadly classified as enzymatic browning and non-enzymatic browning. Enzymatic browning is seen in fresh, uncooked fruits and vegetables which contain phenolic compounds. In the presence of oxygen, specific enzymes bring about discolouration of phenolic substrate. This type of browning can be controlled by inactivating the enzymes.

Non-enzymatic browning is accelerated by temperature and is further classified as
1. Maillard reaction
2. Caramelization
3. Ascorbic acid browning
4. Lipid browning

While most Maillard reactions and caramelization are desirable reactions, ascorbic acid browning and lipid browning are undesirable. Since food components are involved, the nutritive value is reduced to a small extent in some reactions.

Browning plays an important role in food preparation and it needs to be controlled to ensure high acceptability of the product. The development of colour in baked goods along with enhanced flavour and aroma increases the acceptability and quality of food.

KEY TERMS

Carbonyl group   Free group of reducing sugars.

Enzyme   Catalyst made up of protein and responsible for most reactions in living tissues. Destroyed by heat as protein gets coagulated.

Maillard reaction   A reaction between proteins or amino acids and sugars resulting in a brown colour, often accompanied by aroma and flavour when food is cooked.

Oxidation   A reaction in which oxygen is gained or hydrogen is lost or loss of electrons.

Phenol oxidases   Enzymes that oxidize phenolic compounds to quinones causing browning in some fruits, vegetables, and mushrooms in which they are present.

Phenolic compounds   Group of aromatic compounds (with a ring structure) that undergo oxidative enzymatic browning, e.g., tyrosine,

catechins which are colourless pigments in plants.

Reducing sugars   Sugars that contain the aldehydic or ketonic reducing group, e.g., glucose, fructose, lactose, and pentoses (five carbon sugars).

 REVIEW EXERCISES

1. Classify the different types of browning reactions seen in food.
2. You have been asked to prepare fresh fruit salad. What precautions would you take to prevent enzymatic browning.
3. Explain briefly:
   (a) Uses of caramel
   (b) Factors affecting Maillard reaction
   (c) Measures to retain red colour in strawberry preserves.
4. List any five examples of desirable browning and the five examples of undesirable browning, mentioning type of browning reaction.

CHAPTER 10

Food Microbiology

LEARNING OBJECTIVES

After reading this chapter, you should be able to
- understand the significance of food microbiology in the food industry
- define important terms related to food sanitation
- identify different microorganisms found in food and understand where they are found and how they multiply
- classify microorganisms on the basis of their morphology
- know the factors which influence microbial growth
- describe sources of contamination and cross-contamination
- appreciate the economic importance of microorganisms
- understand how pathogenic microorganisms are transmitted
- understand causes of food spoilage and control measures
- distinguish between food poisoning and food infection
- apply this knowledge to prevent foodborne illnesses

INTRODUCTION

Having understood the chemistry of food, the food handler needs to understand the various interactions that take place between microorganisms and foods. This chapter introduces the reader to the different types of microorganisms present in food which may be useful or harmful to humans, what factors affect their growth, and how their growth can be controlled to prevent the spread of foodborne illnesses.

Some microorganisms cause food spoilage and foodborne illness, but others are beneficial in food processing and preparation. The composition of food dictates which microorganisms will be present in it, while steps in handling food determine which microorganisms can contaminate food. Hygienic food handling based on sanitary principles is essential if wholesome food is to be served. The term hygiene is derived from the Greek word *Hygieia* (the goddess of health) and means using sanitary principles to maintain health. Sanitation, in the food industry, means creating and maintaining hygienic and healthful conditions. The word 'sanitation' comes from the Latin word *sanus* which means 'sound and healthy' or 'clean and whole'.

Sanitation can reduce the growth of microorganisms on equipment and surfaces, the spread of foodborne illnesses and spoilage and wastage of food. Sanitation is more than just visible cleanliness. Food or equipment may be free of visible dirt but may harbour invisible microorganisms which can cause spoilage or disease. A hygienic environment can be created in the food industry by food handlers who use scientific principles to produce wholesome food. Knowledge of factors affecting growth of microorganisms and how their growth can be controlled is essential for all those who handle food if foodborne illnesses are to be prevented.

Microbiology is the study of microorganisms. A microorganism is a microscopic form of life which like any living creature uses nutrients, eliminates waste products, grows, and reproduces. We cannot see them with the unaided eye, but they are responsible for food spoilage and foodborne illnesses. They can be seen under a microscope after they are magnified. A compound microscope magnifies a microbe up to 1,500 times while an electron microscope is required to study viruses and has a magnifying power up to 5,00,000 times. Microorganisms are ubiquitous, i.e., they are present everywhere. They are found in the air, soil, water, all surfaces, food, and in and on the bodies of all living beings. There are five groups of microorganisms that are important in food microbiology. They are

1. Viruses
2. Bacteria
3. Fungi—yeasts and molds
4. Algae
5. Parasites

IMPORTANT MICROORGANISMS IN FOOD MICROBIOLOGY

Viruses

Viruses, the smallest form of microorganisms, can only grow and reproduce inside living cells, i.e., they are strictly parasitic. They feed on living cells of plants and animals and are pathogenic. They are very minute in size, approximately one-tenth to one-hundredth the size of bacteria and can only be seen under an electron microscope. They vary in shape and size from 0.015 micrometres to 0.2 micrometres. A micrometre or a micron is a unit of length equal to one-thousandth of a millimetre, the smallest marking on a foot ruler.

Viruses attach themselves to plant, animal, or bacterial cells and the nuclear material present in the virus is released in the cell. At the expense of the cell, the virus multiplies inside the cell. When sufficient numbers of particles are formed, the cell bursts and the released viruses attack other cells. Some viruses cause foodborne infections such as hepatitis. Other common viral diseases are poliomyelitis, influenza, common cold, mumps, measles, and chicken pox.

Bacteria

Bacteria are microscopic, unicellular organisms of different shapes, sizes, and activity. Their size varies from 0.2 μm to 10 μms and is one micrometre on an average. They are identified on the basis of their morphology, i.e., their shape, size, cell arrangement (Fig. 10.1), and special structures (Fig. 10.2), if present like flagella for locomotion, capsule or slime layer, and endospores. Four shapes are observed: rod shaped, spherical, spiral, and comma shaped.

1. Rod-shaped bacteria may have flagella, while some species are capable of forming a resistant structure called endospores when conditions are unfavourable for growth. Some coliform bacteria (so called because they are present in the large intestine or colon) which form part of the normal intestinal flora, are also rod shaped. Their presence in food or water indicates faecal contamination. Enteric pathogens which cause typhoid, dysentery, and Clostridium food poisoning are rod shaped.
2. Spherical or round bacteria are also called cocci. They exhibit the following arrangements:
   (a) pairs of cocci called diplococcic;
   (b) chains of cocci called streptococci, e.g., bacteria causing sore-throat;
   (c) irregular clusters of cocci called staphylococci, e.g., bacteria causing Staph food poisoning;
   (d) tetrads or cubes of four to eight cocci causing spoilage of food.
3. Spiral-shaped bacteria, also called spirilla, cause diseases such as syphilis.
4. Comma-shaped bacteria, also called vibrios, cause diseases such as cholera.

When conditions are suitable, bacteria reproduce asexually by binary fission (see Fig. 10.3), a process in which the full grown cell divides into two new cells every 20 to 30 minutes. A single cell can produce approximately two million cells in 7 hours under optimum conditions for growth. When the food supply is exhausted or waste products accumulate, the environment becomes unfavourable for growth. In these conditions, spore-forming bacteria form a single resistant endospore, while non-spore forming bacteria die.

This large group of microorganisms is of greatest concern because it is capable of flourishing and multiplying to enormous numbers at room temperature. Most food poisonings and food infections are of bacterial origin. Bacteria are also responsible for spoilage of food.

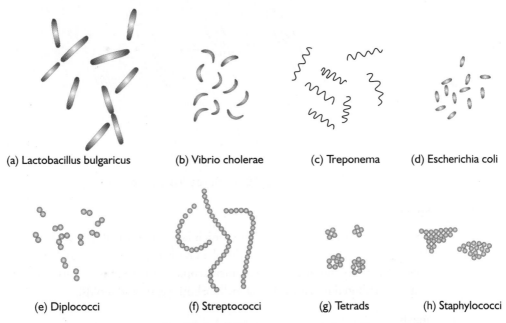

(a) Lactobacillus bulgaricus   (b) Vibrio cholerae   (c) Treponema   (d) Escherichia coli

(e) Diplococci   (f) Streptococci   (g) Tetrads   (h) Staphylococci

Fig. 10.1   Cell arrangements in bacteria

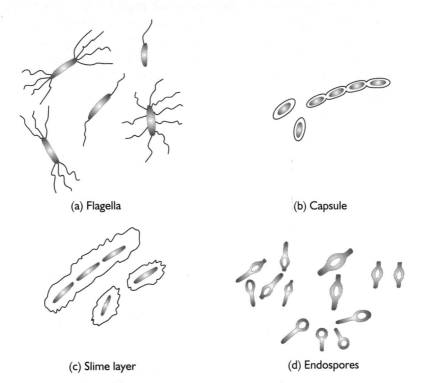

(a) Flagella   (b) Capsule

(c) Slime layer   (d) Endospores

Fig. 10.2   Special structures in bacteria

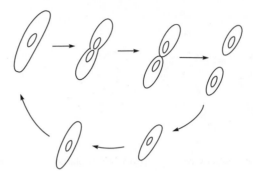

Fig. 10.3   Binary fission in bacteria

Fungi

This group includes the lower plants which lack chlorophyll and are mainly saprophytic. They are usually multi-cellular, but the plant body is not differentiated into root, stem, and leaves. They vary in size from small microscopic yeasts to mushrooms in the fields and are widely distributed in nature. Fungi include both yeasts and molds.

Yeasts

Yeasts are single-celled organisms which require food, particularly carbohydrates and moisture for growth. They are found naturally in soil and dust. They are much larger in size than bacterial cells, approximately 5 to 10 micrometres, and are oval, lemon shaped, or elongated. They mainly reproduce asexually by polar budding (see Fig. 10.4). During budding, a small protuberance or bud grows on the mother cell. This bud or daughter cell grows in size, breaks off, and eventually grows into an identical cell.

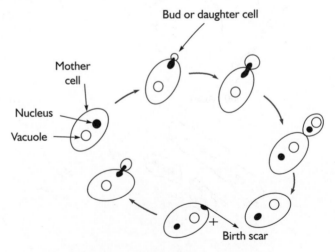

Fig. 10.4   Yeast cells showing budding

Yeasts can grow at refrigeration temperatures as well as at room temperatures. They are capable of fermenting sugars anaerobically to alcohol and carbon dioxide. The yeast *Saccharomyces cerevisiae* is of industrial importance in bakeries and breweries. Yeasts can grow on the surface of high acid and salt containing pickles and chutneys and spoil them. Some are osmophilic and can grow well in high concentrations of sugars and salt. Yeast contaminations can be identified by a slimy or powdery film, cloudy sediments in liquids, or by the presence of gas bubbles often accompanied by an alcoholic or fermented smell. Yeasts, most often, grow on fruits and preserves such as jams, jellies, syrups, dried fruits, cottage cheese, and curds. They require a moisture level above 20 per cent to survive and multiply.

Molds

Molds are multi-cellular microorganisms which are often seen as fuzzy, velvety, or powdery patches on the surface of foods with low moisture content. Their bodies are thread-like or filamentous with spore heads of varying shapes and sizes when observed under the microscope. The filaments are called hyphae and the entire plant body is called mycelium. Hyphae may be submerged, i.e., growing within the food or aerial, i.e., growing into the air above the food. They reproduce asexually by spores borne in hundreds on the aerial spore heads. The spores are liberated once the spore head matures. The spores are very light and are dispersed into the atmosphere. When they settle on a suitable substrate, the spores germinate into a new mycelium. They are 2 to 10 micrometres in diameter and several millimetres in length. They can exist at almost any storage temperature under almost any conditions. Figure 10.5 shows the various molds of economic importance.

Foods most susceptible to mold growth are bread, meat, fruits, jam, and cheese. Some molds produce harmful toxins, e.g., the mold *Aspergillus flavus* produces a toxin called aflatoxin when it grows on inadequately dried peanuts or grains.

Algae

Algae include both unicellular and multi-cellular organisms found naturally in water. They contain chlorophyll and are photosynthetic. They vary in shape and size from one micrometre to many feet. They are generally non-pathogenic, although some may have an unpleasant odour or slimy texture. Unicellular algae are of importance in water purification and sewage treatment plants. They are also important as primary producers of food for the aquatic environment. A pathogenic algae *Gonyaulax catenella* is found in seaweed planktons. Molluscs which feed on this plankton become poisonous. Multicellular algae is of importance as a source of agar for preparation of culture media.

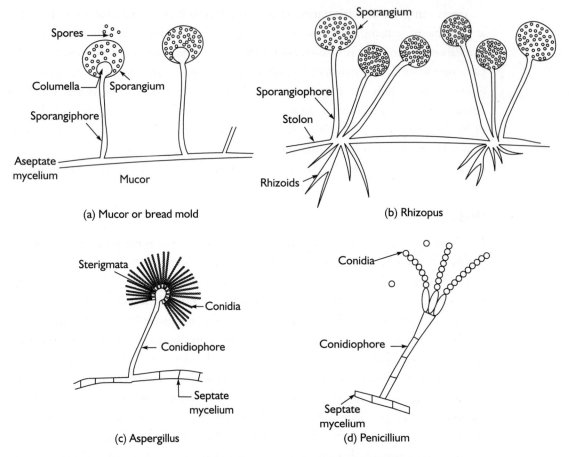

Fig. 10.5   Molds of economic importance

Parasites

Parasites are microorganisms which are dependent on a living host for growth and reproduction. Parasites can be in the form of single-celled animals in the case of protozoa, *Entamoeba histolytica* which causes amoebic dysentery in humans, or multi-celled animals such as intestinal worms, e.g., *Taenia solium* or pork tapeworm. They vary in shape and size from two micrometres to many feet. Intestinal worms are included as microorganism because their cysts or eggs are of microscopic dimensions and are transmitted through infected food and poor personal hygiene.

Amoebic dysentery or amoebiasis occurs when drinking water is contaminated with sewage or through consumption of salads or root vegetables grown on soil to which un-treated excreta is applied as a fertilizer. Entamoeba forms cysts which require heat treatment for their destruction. Amoebiasis is prevalent in India, while trichinosis is mostly seen in countries where pork is consumed in large quantities. It is caused by the parasitic worm *Trichinella spiralis.* Parasitic larvae occur in the muscles of infected pigs. If undercooked pork is consumed, these larvae develop into small round worms in the individual's intestines causing a gastrointestinal illness resulting in fever, muscular pain, and general weakness. After sometime, the worms migrate to the muscles of the patient to form cysts and cause muscle spasms.

FACTORS AFFECTING THE GROWTH OF MICROBES

Microorganisms need certain conditions for growth and reproduction. They are as follows:

1. Food
2. Warmth
3. Moisture
4. Time
5. pH
6. Osmotic pressure
7. Oxygen

Food

Microorganisms use our food supply as a source of nutrients for growth. Since bacteria, yeasts and molds are saprophytic, they need a source of carbon and nitrogen as well as growth factors and trace elements to grow and multiply. Some can synthesize the growth factors or vitamins essential for growth. Green algae can manufacture their own food like plants, while viruses, some bacteria, and protozoans are parasitic and feed on living host cells. In the laboratory, they are cultivated on culture media which is specially prepared to meet their growth requirements. When bacteria are inoculated on culture media or on potentially hazardous foods, they multiply rapidly by binary fission. In 24 hours, visible colonies appear on the media. When the food supply gets exhausted or conditions get unfavourable, the bacteria form spores or die.

Warmth

Microorganisms thrive in warm temperatures. They grow and multiply best in the temperature range between 5°C to 63°C (41°F to 145°F). This temperature range is called the danger zone. High and low temperatures have a marked influence on microbial growth. Microorganisms are destroyed if exposed to temperatures above 63°C for several minutes. Their growth is retarded at temperatures below 5°C. They are not killed when they are refrigerated or frozen but merely become dormant. Different microorganisms have minimum, maximum, and optimum temperatures for growth. They cannot grow below their minimum temperature or above their maximum temperature. They grow best at their optimum temperatures for growth. On the basis of temperature required for growth, they are classified as follows:

1. Psychrophiles: Microorganisms having an optimum temperature below 20°C, e.g., *Pseudomonas* which grows at refrigeration temperature and spoils frozen food.
2. Mesophiles: Microorganisms having an optimum temperature between 20°C to 45°C, e.g., human pathogens which grow best at human body temperature and cause diseases such as typhoid, bacillary dysentery, and most lactic acid fermenting bacteria like Lactobacilli are mesophiles.
3. Thermopliles: Microorganisms having an optimum temperature above 45°C, e.g., spore forming microorganisms, such as *Bacillus* and *Clostridium*, which grow best in improperly heat-treated canned and bottled food and cause food poisoning and food spoilage.

Moisture

All microbes need water in the air and in the substrate to grow. Water accounts for a large percentage of the weight of the microbial cell. Water and moist conditions encourage the growth of all microbes. In general, bacteria need more moisture than fungi, and growth of microbes does not depend on total moisture but it depends on available moisture in food. Water activity is the amount of water that is available to microbes. Salt and sugar when present in food, bind the water making it unavailable for microbes to grow. Surface spoilage is seen in foods when relative humidity is high during the monsoons or in coastal areas, as the surface gets hydrated permitting the growth of microbes even if the food has a low water activity.

Time

Microorganisms need time to grow to numbers, large enough to harm us. When the environment is favourable in terms of temperature, moisture, and food, they multiply rapidly and in a short span of time they are in numbers large enough to cause spoilage or illness. Bacteria multiply by a process called binary fission by dividing into two every 20 minutes. Foods often contain small number of pathogenic microorganisms which multiply rapidly and cause foodborne illnesses after such food is consumed. Food which is consumed as soon as it is cooked has lesser chances of causing foodborne illnesses. No potentially hazardous food should be allowed to remain within the danger zone for more than 4 hours total.

pH level

The pH value tells us the acidity or alkalinity of the medium and pH of a medium ranges from 0 to 14. A pH value of 7 is neutral, pH values below 7 are acidic, and values above 7 are alkaline. Most microorganisms prefer a neutral pH to grow and multiply. Molds and yeasts grow better in an acidic medium of pH 4 to 4.5, as compared to bacteria. In general, foods with an acidic pH have a better shelf life as compared to foods with a near neutral pH. Acids, such as acetic and citric, are added to preserve foods. Foods containing buffers, i.e., substances which resist a change in pH, e.g., milk, will permit microbial activity and will spoil faster. Molds can tolerate a wider difference in pH as compared to yeast and bacteria.

Osmotic pressure

The osmotic pressure of food depends on the kind and amount of solute, e.g., sugar and salt, dissolved in it. The bacterial cell wall is semi-permeable and if it is kept in a hypotonic solution (solution having an osmotic pressure lower than that of the bacterial cell) water from the surrounding media will enter the cell resulting in bursting of the cell. If it is kept in a hypertonic solution (solution having an osmotic pressure higher than that of the bacterial cell), water from the cell will enter the surrounding media resulting in shrinking of the cell. Bacteria cannot grow in high concentrations of sugar or salt, whereas yeasts and molds grow at high osmotic pressures. This is the reason for yeast and mold spoilage seen in preserves such as jams and pickles.

Oxygen

On the basis of oxygen requirements, microorganisms are classified into aerobic, anaerobic, and facultative organisms. Oxygen is necessary for all aerobic microorganisms. Anaerobic microorganisms do not need it and it may be toxic to some anaerobes. Facultative microorganisms can respire either aerobically or anaerobically. Molds and most yeasts need oxygen while bacteria may be aerobic, anaerobic, or facultative. All microbes grow well in inadequately ventilated areas and dark humid places where ultraviolet (UV) rays do not reach.

Danger Zone

Temperatures between 5°C to 63°C (41°F to 145.4°F) are the range in which microorganisms grow and multiply best. This temperature range is known as the danger zone. Multiplication is maximum between 15°C to 49°C and slows down towards both ends of the danger zone. Figure 10.6 shows the effect of temperature on bacterial growth. Pathogenic microorganisms grow and multiply best at normal body temperature of 37°C, which is within the danger zone. Potentially hazardous foods should not be kept in the danger zone for more than 4 hours. As foods move in and out of the danger zone during cooking, cooling, storage, and reheating, they should be monitored carefully. While holding food, hot food should be kept at temperatures above 63°C and cold food should be kept at temperatures below 5°C.

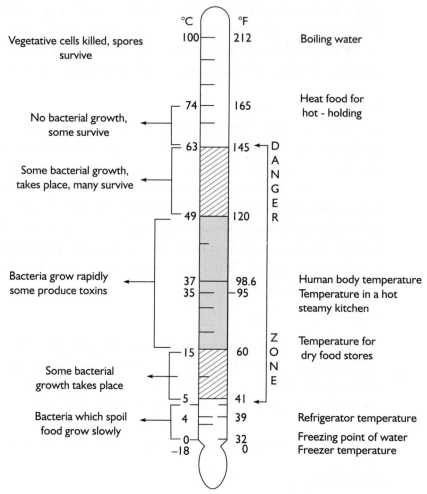

Vegetative cells killed, spores survive

No bacterial growth, some survive

Some bacterial growth, takes place, many survive

Bacteria grow rapidly some produce toxins

Some bacterial growth takes place

Bacteria which spoil food grow slowly

°C   °F
100 — 212   Boiling water

74 — 165   Heat food for hot - holding

63 — 145 D
          A
          N
          G
49 — 120 E
          R

37 — 98.6   Human body temperature
35 — 95   Temperature in a hot
             steamy kitchen

             Z   Temperature for
             O   dry food stores
15 — 60   N
             E
5 — 41

4 — 39   Refrigerator temperature
0 — 32   Freezing point of water
−18 — 0   Freezer temperature

Fig. 10.6 Effect of temperature on bacterial growth and survival

Useful and Harmful Microbes

Some microorganisms are beneficial to human beings. Most, in fact are useful to humankind and to our environment in general. Microorganisms bring about the decay of living organisms which have perished. They are an important part of the life cycle, returning the nutrients of dead matter back to the soil, and conserving the fertility of the soil. Algae and mold, including mushrooms, are used as food. Yeast is cultivated on a large scale referred to as microbial farming. Food yeast is rich in B-complex vitamins and is also used for enzyme production. Vitamins and antibiotics are produced by different bacteria and species of the mold *Penicillium*. They play an important role in the food industry and form part of our daily diet, e.g., curds, bread, cheese, idli, and alcoholic beverages all require some type of microorganisms for their preparation.

FOOD FERMENTATIONS

Alcoholic fermentations

$$\text{Sugar from grape juice} \xrightarrow[\textit{Saccharomyces cerevisiae var. ellipsoideus}]{\text{YEAST}} \text{Wine} + CO_2$$

$$\text{Sugar from malted grains of barley} \xrightarrow[\textit{Saccharomyces carlsbergensis}]{\text{YEAST}} \text{Beer} + CO_2$$

Fermentation of milk

$$\underset{\text{Lactose (milk sugar)}}{C_{12}H_{22}O_{11} + H_2O} \xrightarrow{\textit{Lactase enzyme}} \underset{\text{Glucose + Galactose}}{2C_6H_{12}O_6} \xrightarrow{\textit{System of enzymes}} \underset{\text{Lactic acid}}{2CH_3CHOHCOOH}$$

Manufacture of vinegar

Step 1

$$\underset{\text{Sugar}}{C_6H_{12}O_6} \xrightarrow[\text{fermentation}]{\text{YEAST}} \underset{\text{Ethyl alcohol}}{2C_2H_5OH} + \underset{\text{Carbon dioxide}}{2CO_2}$$

Step 2

$$\underset{\text{Ethyl alcohol}}{2CH_3CH_2OH} + 2O \xrightarrow[\text{action}]{\text{Bacterial}} \underset{\text{Acetic acid}}{2CH_3COOH} + 2H_2O$$

Fermentation is a chemical process that breaks down organic materials. This process is carried out by microorganisms such as bacteria, yeasts, and molds. The microorganisms that bring about food fermentations may be added as a culture, e.g., cheese manufacture, or they may be naturally present in adequate numbers in the food, e.g., no culture needs to be added to idli batter for fermentation to take place. In bread dough, sugars are fermented by the yeast *Saccharomyces cerevisiae* to ethanol and carbon dioxide which give flavour and a light spongy texture to bread. Table 10.1 describes the beneficial role of microorganisms in some food products.

TABLE 10.1   Beneficial role of microorganisms in some food products

S. no.	Food product	Raw material	Microorganisms involved
1	Idli	Rice + black gram	*Leuconostoc mesenteroides, Streptococcus faecalis, Pediococcus cerevisiae*
2	Soya sauce	Soya beans and wheat bran	*Aspergillus oryzae, Streptococci, Lactobacilli*
3	*Tamari* sauce	Soya beans + rice	*Aspergillus tamari*
4	*Tempeh*	Soya beans	*Rhizopus stolonifer*
5	*Poi*	Corms of taro plant	Lactic acid bacteria, yeasts, molds

Contd

Table 10.1 Contd

S. no.	Food product	Raw material	Microorganisms involved
6	Coffee	Coffee berries	*Pectinolytic* bacteria, *Leuconostoc mesenteroides*, *Lactobacillus brevis*, *Lactobacillus plantarum*, *Streptococcus faecalis*
7	Cocoa	Cocoa beans	*Candida yeast enzymes*
8	Vinegar	Starchy vegetables, malted grains, sugars, and fruit juice	*Saccharomyces cererisiae var ellipsoideus* (alcoholic fermentation), *Acetobacter aceti and Gluconobacter* (acidic fermentation)
9	*Sauerkraut*	Cabbage	*Enterobacter, Leuconostoc mesenteroides Lactobacillus plantarum*
10	Pickles	Cucumber, dill, olives	*Pediococcus cerevisiae*
11	Curds	Milk	*Streptococcus lactis, Streptococcus cremoris, Leuconostoc cremoris*
12	Cheese: Hard	Milk	*Streptococcus lactis, Lactobacillus casei*
	Swiss		*Propionibacterium freudenreichii*
	Roquefort		*Penicillium roqueforti*
	Camembert		*Penicillium camemberti*
	Cheddar		*Streptococcus thermophilus, Streptococcus faecalis*
	Yoghurt		*Streptococcus thermophilus, Lactobacillus bulgaricus*

Some microorganisms on the other hand are not beneficial and cause disease and wastage of our food supplies and water bodies. The disease-causing microorganisms are known as pathogens, and they cause diseases in humans and plants. Certain microorganisms cause food spoilage resulting in off-odours, off-flavours, or changes in the colour and texture of food. Others do not alter the appearance, colour, odour, or taste, but are capable of causing foodborne illnesses. Table 10.2 shows the harmful effects of microorganisms with special reference to foodborne illnesses.

TABLE 10.2 Harmful effects of microorganisms with special reference to foodborne illnesses

S. no.	Illness	Causative agent	Foods commonly involved
1	Staph food poisoning (food poisoning)	*Staphylococcus aureus*	Protein-rich foods that have been handled by bare hands and cooked food that cannot be reheated
2	Botulism (food poisoning)	*Clostridium botulinum*	Inadequately processed canned foods
3	Salmonellosis (food infection)	*Salmonella enteritidis*	Contaminated animal products such as meat, poultry, and eggs

Contd

Table 10.2 Contd

S. no.	Illness	Causative agent	Foods commonly involved
4	Shigellosis (food infection)	*Shigella sonnei*	Sewage-contaminated food and water
5	Listeriosis (food infection)	*Listeria monocytogenes*	Milk and meat of infected animals and contaminated cold foods which cannot be reheated
6	Trichinosis (food infestation)	*Trichinella spiralis*	Insufficiently cooked pork and pork products
7	Giardiasis (food infestation)	*Giardia lamblia*	Cysts in contaminated food and water
8	Amoebiasis (food infestation)	*Entamoeba histolytica*	Cysts in contaminated food and water
9	Gastroenteritis (food infection)	*Enteropathogenic Escherichia coli*	Sewage-contaminated food and water
10	Cholera (food infection)	*Vibrio cholerae*	Fish and shellfish from polluted water, contaminated food and water
11	Hepatitis (food infection)	*Hepatitis A virus*	Contaminated food and water
12	Brucellosis (food infection)	*Brucella abortus*	Contaminated milk
13	Flat sour spoilage (food spoilage)	*Bacillus coagulans*	Inadequately processed canned food
14	Sulphide stinker (food spoilage)	*Desulfotomaculum nigrificans*	Inadequately processed canned corn and peas in brine
15	Bloated leaky cans (food spoilage)	*Clostridium thermosaccharolyticum*	Inadequately processed canned food
16	Blue rot (food spoilage)	*Penicillium*	Citrus fruits
17	Ropy milk (food spoilage)	*Alcaligenes viscolactis*	Milk contaminated with non-potable water
18	Yellow to greenish discolouration in fish (food spoilage)	*Pseudomonas fluorescence*	Spoilt fish, improper storage
19	Aflatoxin moldy grains (food spoilage)	*Aspergillus flavus*	Improperly dried peanuts and cereal grains

CONTAMINATION OF FOOD

Foods can get contaminated by microorganisms at any stage in processing right from the farm to the table. Food handlers can carry microorganism that can cause illness in people who eat the food prepared by them. People are the most common source of food contamination.

Hands, hair, breath, sweat, coughs, and sneezes transmit harmful microorganism. Even if a food handler does not show any signs or symptoms of illness, he or she could still be carrying microorganisms that can cause illness if they get into prepared food. The disease-causing microorganisms are transmitted to food either directly by the food handler or indirectly by a contaminated vehicle, resulting in contaminated food. Figure 10.7 shows how food is contaminated directly by a food handler who may be suffering from symptoms of the disease or does not show any signs or symptoms of the disease but excretes live pathogens and is a carrier of the disease. Figure 10.8 shows the various routes by which food can be contaminated indirectly.

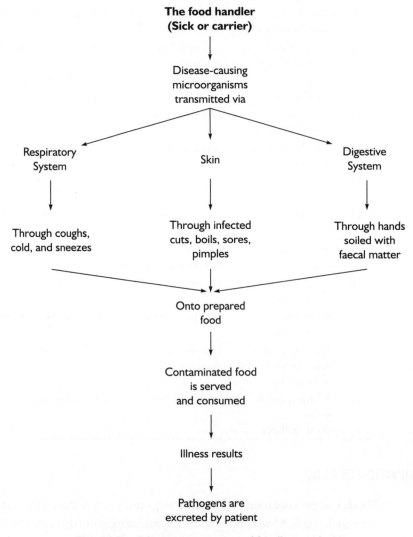

Fig. 10.7   Direct transmission of foodborne disease

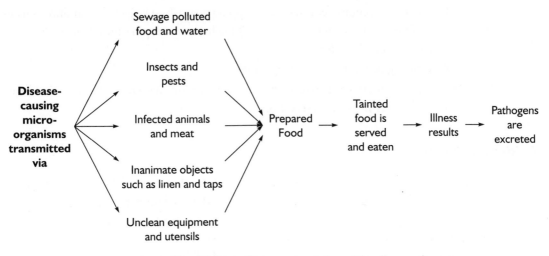

Fig. 10.8 Indirect transmission of foodborne disease

Cross-contamination

Harmful microorganisms present in one food can contaminate other foods if hygienic practices are not observed in the food-preparation area. This process is known as cross-contamination and is defined as the transfer of microbes from raw food products to finished food products through non-food vehicles, such as chopping boards, equipment, clothing, and hands of the food handler, and occurs when clean and dirty operations are mixed.

Cross-contamination occurs when the same equipment is used for raw and cooked foods without cleaning and sanitizing it between operations. Raw food items, such as meat, fish, and root vegetables, contain millions of microorganisms and the same are likely to be transferred onto cooked foods if the same chopping board is used.

Cross-contamination takes place when clean and dirty operations are mixed. For example, when

1. A dishwasher places soiled plates on a table reserved for clean and sanitized plates
2. A busboy brings used plates to the dishwashing machine and picks up clean plates without washing his hands
3. The chef places a dirty cardboard carton on the food preparation table, the table gets contaminated and subsequently any food placed on the table will get contaminated

Other examples of cross-contamination are through the same work surfaces, dish cloth, knives, chopping boards, equipment, utensils, and storage space used for raw and finished food items.

Cross-contamination can be prevented by

1. Segregating raw and finished foods and preparing as well as storing them separately.

2. Colour coding equipment, such as chopping boards and knives, for handling only one type of food, e.g., green for vegetables, blue for seafood, pink for raw meat, brown for cooked meat and poultry

3. Not mixing up clean and dirty operations

Scientific principles to control growth of microorganisms have been discussed in Chapter 11 on Food Processing and Preservation.

FOODBORNE ILLNESSES

A foodborne illness is a general term applied to all types of illness caused through consumption of contaminated food or water. The contaminant may be a pathogenic organism, a toxin (or poison or harmful chemical), or an allergen which is present in food and gains entrance into the body when such food is consumed.

Food may transmit disease in one or more of the following ways:

1. By acting as a vehicle of disease transmission if handled carelessly by unhygienic or ill handlers, e.g., diseases such as tuberculosis, typhoid, or tonsillitis can be transmitted in this way

2. By serving as an ideal medium for growth and permitting microorganisms to grow and multiply in food resulting in food poisoning or in food infection, e.g., Staph food poisoning and Salmonella food infection

3. Food poisoning may be caused by agents other than microorganisms. These include toxic chemicals, poisonous plants such as poisonous mushrooms, insecticides, and pesticides. Toxic metals, such as lead, arsenic, and zinc, or excessive use of *aji-no-moto* in food may lead to severe reactions. Some individuals show abnormal sensitivity to certain foods and develop allergic reactions, e.g., egg white, gluten, and shellfish.

Microbial foodborne illnesses occur due to unhygienic handling of food, poor personal hygiene on part of the food handler, and sewage contamination of water. Microorganisms which cause foodborne illnesses are bacteria, viruses, protozoans, and nematodes. Bacterial contamination is the most common cause of foodborne illnesses in the food industry and results in either food poisoning or food infection. These illnesses are characterized by a severe disturbance of the stomach or intestines which occurs after consuming food in which the offending bacteria were given a chance to multiply.

Food Poisoning

Food poisoning or food intoxication is an illness caused by toxins present in contaminated food. The toxin may be a poisonous chemical which is accidently or intentionally added to food, a naturally occurring toxin in food such as solanine in green potatoes or a toxic metabolite excreted by bacteria. In this section, we will discuss illnesses resulting from microbial action only.

In bacterial food poisoning or intoxication, the toxin is produced when the cells multiply in the contaminated food. When such food is consumed, the toxin already present in the food irritates the lining of the stomach and causes vomiting. If the toxin reaches the intestine, it may cause abdominal pain and diarrhoea. The incubation period is quite short since the toxin is already formed and ranges from 1 to 6 hours. Living bacteria need not be present. Toxins need much higher temperatures to be destroyed than the bacteria which produce them and are often present in foods that are inadequately reheated, although living bacteria may be killed.

Food Infection

Food infection is an illness caused by microorganisms. It results from the consumption of food that contains living bacteria which are multiplying and capable of producing disease. The illness which results is the reaction of the body to the presence of the living microorganisms or their products of metabolism. When food is consumed, the acid in the gastric juices destroys some bacteria. If the number of living bacteria is high, when food reaches the intestine where the pH is neutral, bacteria multiply rapidly. The metabolites irritate the lining of the intestines resulting in nausea, diarrhoea, and abdominal pain. The incubation period for an infection to occur is at least 12 hours. Living bacteria need to be present in sufficient numbers for an infection to develop. Approximately one million or more bacteria need to be in food for an infection or intoxication to develop. Some of the microorganisms causing food poisoning and food infections and an example of foods likely to cause illness, have been listed in Table 10.3.

TABLE 10.3 Difference between bacterial food poisoning and food infection

Food poisoning	Food infection
Caused by toxin produced by bacteria	Caused by living organisms
Incubation time: 1 to 6 hours	Incubation time: 12 to 36 hours
Symptoms: nausea and vomiting, diarrhoea, usually no fever	Symptoms: diarrhoea, abdominal pain, vomiting, fever
Duration: 1 day; sometimes longer	Duration: 1 to 7 days; sometimes longer

Control of Foodborne Illnesses

Foodborne diseases are generally transmitted through careless food handlers, who are either suffering from the disease or are the carriers of microorganisms. A healthy food handler may transmit microorganisms indirectly through cross-contamination. These diseases are a constant threat to the food industry. They can be prevented by practicing the basic principles of hygiene listed here.

1. High-risk foods such as meat, poultry, eggs, and milk should be purchased from certified dealers only.

2. Food should be handled in a hygienic manner by all food handlers and infected handlers should be kept away.

3. Frozen foods should be thawed carefully at temperatures between 10 and 15°C and frozen food should not be cooked till it has thawed. Foods once thawed should not be refrozen unless it has been cooked well after thawing.

4. Food should be prepared in quantities required and quantities for which adequate refrigerated storage space is available. This will prevent perishable or high-risk items from spoiling.

5. Cross-contamination from raw to cooked foods can be prevented by washing hands and all equipment or surfaces in contact with raw food.

6. The time gap between preparation and service of food should be reduced to avoid long storage in a warm environment.

7. Large masses of food, which have to be reheated later, should be cooled quickly to 15°C and refrigerated immediately.

8. Food should be reheated thoroughly so that the centre of the food gets heated to temperatures high enough to destroy bacteria.

9. Cooked foods which are to be served hot should be stored above 63°C. Avoid cooling and heating food repeatedly.

10. Leftover food should be refrigerated immediately to keep it out of the danger zone.

11. Suspect food should be discarded immediately without tasting it.

12. The kitchen and cooking equipment should be cleaned daily and regular pest control measures should be taken.

13. Adequate toilet and wash basin facilities with a continuous supply of water should be provided.

Table 10.4 presents the common temperature-related problems contributing to foodborne illnesses.

TABLE 10.4   Common temperature-related problems contributing to foodborne Illnesses

Problem	Precaution
Frozen foods not solidly frozen	Packets should be intact and food should be solidly frozen when purchased with no ice crystals inside the packet and temperature not higher than (−15°C) when delivered.
Thawing frozen food at room temperatures	Thaw or defrost frozen foods under refrigeration at temperatures below 4°C (40°F), under potable running water, in a thawing cabinet or in the microwave oven if it is going to be cooked immediately.
Internal temperatures not high enough	Metal stemmed thermometers must be used to check temperatures of the food product. Internal temperatures of solid food should be checked using a probe thermometer and the probe should be sanitized between uses.
Inadequate hot-holding	Keep the temperature of food to be served hot, above 63°C (145.4° F), until it is served and ensure that all parts of the food, specially the surface, is exposed to a safe holding temperature.

Contd

Table 10.4 Contd

Problem	Precaution
Inadequate chilled display	Potentially hazardous foods that are to be served cold over an extended meal timing should be held at temperatures below 5°C and should not be held in the 15°C to 49°C range for more than 2 hours.
Delayed cooling time	All cooked perishable foods which are not going to be consumed immediately, should be chilled to an internal temperature of 4°C (39.2° F) within 4 hours.
Frequent and uneven re-heating	Food to be reheated must be brought rapidly to an internal temperature of at least 74°C (165.2°F) or greater. Microwave ovens do not heat food evenly. Solid food heated in microwave ovens are subject to cold spots which may not receive proper heat treatment. Liquids must be stirred periodically.

SUMMARY

Many different types of microorganism, such as viruses, bacteria, fungi, algae, and parasites, are present in food which may be useful or harmful to humans. Various factors, such as food, warmth, moisture, time, pH, osmotic pressure, and oxygen, affect their growth. The food handler needs to understand how the growth of microorganisms can be controlled to prevent the spread of foodborne illnesses. Foods can get contaminated by microorganisms at any stage in processing right from the farm to the table. Food handlers can carry microorganisms that can cause illness in people who eat the food prepared by them. People are the most common source of food contamination. Microorganisms are transmitted to humans directly by the unhygienic food handler or indirectly through various routes of contamination. Some microorganisms cause food spoilage and foodborne illness, but others are beneficial in food processing and preparation. Harmful microorganisms present in one food can contaminate other foods if hygienic practices are not observed in the food preparation area. This process is known as cross-contamination and is defined as the transfer of microbes from raw food products to finished food products through non-food vehicles such as chopping boards, equipment, clothing, and hands of the food handler, and occurs when clean and dirty operations are mixed. Microorganisms which cause foodborne illnesses are bacteria, viruses, protozoans, and nematodes. Bacterial contamination is the most common cause of foodborne illnesses in the food industry and results in either food poisoning or food infection. These illnesses are characterized by a severe disturbance of the stomach or intestines, which occurs after consuming food in which the offending bacteria were given a chance to multiply. These diseases are a constant threat to the food industry. They can be prevented by practising the basic principles of hygiene.

KEY TERMS

Aerobes   These are microorganisms that need oxygen for growth.

Anaerobes   These are microorganisms that do not need oxygen for growth; and sometimes oxygen may be harmful to them.

Antibiotics   They are substances produced by microorganisms that are capable of either inhibiting the growth or killing other organisms. For example, the molds *Penicillium notatum* and

Streptomyces gricens produce antibiotics that destroy certain bacteria.

Autotrophs They can synthesize their own food by converting simple inorganic substances into complex protoplasm.

Bound water It is the water that is not available to microorganisms for their growth as it is bound to solutes, such as sugars and salts, dissolved in water.

Carrier A carrier is a person who harbours a specific infectious agent in the absence of specific signs and symptoms of the disease and serves as a potential reservoir of infection for others. Carriers may be temporary during incubation period, or convalescence or healthy carriers who do not exhibit any symptoms but excrete the disease-causing agent for variable periods. Chronic carriers may harbour and excrete the disease-causing agent for years, e.g., typhoid and dysentery.

Cleaning It is the removal of matter from a surface on which it is not acceptable

Contaminated food The term contaminated is used for those foods that are not fit to be eaten for sanitary reasons. Although food may look, smell and taste good, it may contain harmful chemicals, non-food matter, and bacteria.

Contamination The term contamination means the entry and multiplication of an infectious agent into or onto inanimate objects such as food and equipment.

Cross-contamination It is defined as the transfer of microbes from raw food products to finished food products through non-food vehicles, such as chopping boards, equipment, clothing, and hands of the food handler and occurs when clean and dirty operations are mixed.

Encapsulation It is a process in which some rod-shaped bacteria form a dense, slime-like protective case over its cell wall that makes it more resistant to destruction by heat, chemicals, etc.

Facultative These microorganisms can grow either in the presence or in the absence of oxygen. For example, the microbes present in the human intestinal tract such as *Escherichia coli*.

High-risk food These are ready-to-eat foods that can easily support the growth of food-poisoning bacteria if not handled carefully and will not be cooked any further before being served but may be reheated, such as meat pâté, cooked egg dishes, and cooked fish.

High temperature short time (HTST) pasteurization It is a process in which a food product is heated to 72°C (161.6°F) for 15 seconds, then immediately cooled to 10°C (50°F) or less.

Hygiene The term hygiene derived from the Greek word *Hygieia* (the goddess of health) means using sanitary principles to maintain health.

Infection Infection is the entry and multiplication of an infectious agent in the body resulting in a response in the form of symptoms such as fever, vomiting, and stomach cramps.

Infestation An infestation denotes the presence of parasites in or on the body such as head lice and intestinal worms.

Microaerophilic These bacteria are basically aerobic but oxygen requirement is less, e.g., *Lactobacilli* species.

Micrometre or micron (μm) A micrometre or a micron is a unit of length equal to one thousandth of a millimetre or 10^{-3} mm. A millimetre (mm) is the smallest marking on a foot ruler.

Microorganisms Any microscopic or ultramicroscopic animal or plant organisms that are too small to be seen with the unaided eye are called microorganisms. They include viruses, bacteria, fungi, algae, and protozoas.

Osmophilic These are organisms, specially yeasts, that can grow at high osmotic pressure. For example, *Zygosaccharomyces* species grow in high concentrations of sugar, while *Saccharomyces rouxii* can grow in high concentrations of salt causing spoilage of pickles.

Parasite It is a plant or animal that lives on or in another living organism, at the cost of the organism without any benefit to the host, usually causing disease or harm.

Pasteurization It is a method of high temperature food preservation in which food is heated to 63°C (145.4°F) for 30 minutes or 72°C (161.6°F) for 15 seconds and immediately cooled to 10°C (50°F) or less.

pH level It is the degree of acidity or alkalinity of a food measured by the hydrogen ion concentration. The higher the hydrogen ion concentration lower will be the pH and vice versa. It is measured on a pH scale of pH 1 to pH 14 by a pH metre or by pH papers.

Psychrophiles These are cold-loving microorganisms that can survive at temperatures as low as -28°C (−18.4°F) and can multiply at temperatures as high as 20°C (68°F).

Putrefaction It is the anaerobic decomposition of proteins by bacteria with the development of foul-smelling compounds.

Sanitation The word sanitation comes from the Latin word *sanus* which means 'sound and healthy' or 'clean and whole'. In the food industry, sanitation means creating and maintaining hygienic and healthful conditions.

Sanitize It means to reduce the number of disease-causing bacteria to safe levels

Saprophyte Any organism that lives on dead or decaying organic matter for its survival is called saprophyte.

Sewage It is the waste matter from the toilets, bathrooms, kitchen, and other drains carried off by sewers. Liquid waste from above sources is also called grey water.

Spore A bacterial spore is a resistant structure formed in some rod-shaped bacterial cells that can withstand unfavourable conditions. It remains dormant till conditions become favourable and germinate into a vegetative cell that can multiply and grow.

Thawing It is the stage when a frozen food reaches an unfrozen state, i.e., when the ice crystals that were formed during the freezing process, melt.

Thermophiles Microbes that grow better at temperatures from 45°C to 60°C and sometimes higher.

Ubiquitous Present everywhere in our environment, in and on humans, plants, animals, water, air, soil, and inanimate objects.

Vaccination It is the introduction of any kind of dead or weakened microbes into the body of a living being to develop resistance or immunity against that specific disease.

Water activity (a$_w$) It is the amount of water in food that is available to microorganisms for their growth. Some water is bound to other substances and hence does not support microbial growth.

Wholesome food It is food that is healthful, at the right stage of maturity, free from pollutants, and contaminants and is fit for consumption.

REVIEW EXERCISES

1. Why does a food handler need to have knowledge about food microbiology?
2. Classify the different microorganisms which are present in our food.
3. Discuss the beneficial effects of microorganisms.
4. Explain the terms cross-contamination, sanitation, foodborne illnesses, and danger zone.
5. Differentiate between food poisoning and food infection.
6. List the various factors which affect microbial growth and explain any two factors.
7. Define the following terms:
   (a) Anaerobes
   (b) Infestation
   (c) Thermophiles
   (d) Saprophytes
   (e) Contamination
   (f) Endospores
   (g) Thawing
   (h) High-risk foods
8. With the help of a line diagram, explain how diseases are transmitted directly and indirectly.
9. Discuss the harmful effects of microorganisms with respect to food spoilage and foodborne illnesses.

ASSIGNMENT

Visit the kitchen of your college canteen and list measures you would suggest to the caterer to ensure service of safe and wholesome food.

CHAPTER 11

Food Processing and Preservation

LEARNING OBJECTIVES

After reading this chapter, you should be able to
- understand the need for processing food
- know the different methods by which food is preserved
- describe the advantages and disadvantages of the different methods
- select the appropriate method for preserving a foodstuff
- understand the limitations of irradiation of food
- appreciate the benefits of using a combination of methods instead of a single method
- understand the effect of processing on food constituents

INTRODUCTION

In Chapter 1 on Introduction to Food Science, we have read about the intimate relationship of food chemistry and food microbiology with food processing. The chemical composition of food and its microbial load will dictate the processes food needs to be subjected to if its shelf life has to be extended. Without adequate processing, food cannot be stored indefinitely. Unless natural foods are processed or preserved, they will deteriorate. Most foods are easily decomposed by microorganisms and every food handler should be familiar with the principles underlying food spoilage. This knowledge would enable one to handle food correctly and extend its keeping quality.

Food can spoil at any stage in its preparation or storage. In fact, spoilage in food begins as soon as

1. Vegetables and fruits are harvested
2. Eggs are laid
3. Fish is caught
4. Animals are slaughtered for meat
5. Milk is drawn from milch animals

This spoilage continues till food is consumed.

Spoilage Spoilage can be defined as decomposition or damage causing undesirable changes in food. It is caused due to various agents making food unsuitable for consumption. A spoiled food looks, smells, and tastes bad.

Contamination The term contaminated is used for those foods which are not fit to be eaten for sanitary reasons. Although contaminated food may look, smell, and taste good, it may contain harmful chemicals, non-food matter, and bacteria. Contamination of food results in its spoilage.

CAUSES OF FOOD SPOILAGE

Foods spoil because of any one or more of the following reasons:

Growth and activity of bacteria, yeast, and mould Microorganisms can cause visible changes in the food. Milk turning sour, mould growth on bread, and fruit juices fermented by yeast are some examples of visible signs of spoilage. The kind of microorganisms which spoil the food will depend on the composition of food, i.e., its pH, moisture content, nutrients, temperature, etc.

Insect infestation Insects such as worms, weevils, and moths infest cereal grains and make grains unfit for consumption. Weevils bore holes into grains and multiply, destroying the flavour and the grain.

Enzymatic changes Natural enzymatic changes by autolysis, such as overmaturing, softening, browning, and sprouting, damage the food. Sprouting of potatoes, browning/darkening of bananas, and softening of fruits and vegetables are seen after harvesting if cool temperatures are not maintained.

Chemical action Chemical reactions which are not catalysed by enzymes or microorganisms can also result in chemical spoilage of food. Oxidative rancidity in fats and hydrogen swell in canned foods are examples of this type of spoilage.

Physical changes Physical changes in food caused by freezing, dessication, absorption of moisture, etc. can spoil food. Mechanical damage such as bruising or cracked egg shells can accelerate spoilage by microorganisms or by enzymes. Bruised apples which are brown when cut, freezer burn in deep frozen foods, or cracked eggs are signs of spoilage in foods.

Spoiled food cannot be rectified by any processing method. It results in wastage and should be discarded immediately. To prevent spoilage and ultimately wastage of food, any surplus food should be processed and preserved immediately. Only food which is wholesome, i.e., at the desired stage of maturity, free from pollution, and any objectionable changes resulting from microbial or enzyme action should be preserved.

Markets are flooded with a vast array of processed foods, which are processed using latest technology, to meet the ever-changing demands of the customer. The glut or surplus produced is preserved to meet the year round demand during the lean period.

OBJECTIVES OF FOOD PROCESSING

The main objectives of food processing on a home scale, institutional scale, or in the food industry are similar. They include the following:

Removal of unwanted matter from the food   Unwanted matter may be inedible, indigestible, or harmful to health, such as husk from grains, rind from oranges, cherry stones, and coconut shells. Unwanted matter is removed by appropriately designed gadgets. The processes include shelling, destoning, milling, peeling, etc.

Making food safe for consumption   Some foods contain natural toxins which need to be inactivated, e.g., trypsin inhibitors in soya beans and goitrogens in the red skin of groundnuts. Fungal toxins such as aflatoxin in moldy groundnut and grains, infected portions of food material, and green portion in potatoes are removed by visual examination, and chemical toxins and poisons are discarded. Ensure safety of food by using processes to remove toxins, and heat to destroy microorganisms and their toxins. Develop safe processes to prevent contamination at any stage.

Increasing digestibility   Most foods are difficult to digest unless they are cooked. Cooking softens fibre, gelatinizes starch, denatures protein, and makes food easier to digest. With the exception of fruit, all other foods need some kind of processing to make them more digestible.

Enhance flavour, colour, and taste   The acceptability of food depends to a large extent on its organoleptic or sensory qualities. Processing techniques enhance the appearance of food and many techniques make food more appetizing and tasteful such as baking of cakes and bread. The brown crust is formed due to Maillard reaction which gives bakery items its characteristic baked flavour, aroma, and taste. Processes such as caramelization of sugar, fermentation of idli batter, and alcoholic fermentations produce a superior taste as compared to unprocessed foods.

Improving texture and consistency   Processes such as emulsification, aeration, gel formation, and increase in viscosity are aimed at improving the texture and consistency of ready-to-eat, cook-chill, and cook-freeze operations. Processing prevents changes in consistency of such operations during the freeze-thaw process. Special starches which do not retrograde or show syneresis are used for setting gels. Crystal formation in fondants, jams, and ice cream can be retarded in processed foods and desirable texture can be obtained.

Minimizing nutrient loss Nutrients are better retained by controlled processing conditions such as autoclaving, freeze drying, and controlled heat. Nutrients lost during processing are generally compensated by adding synthetic vitamins. Processed margarine, a substitute for butter, is fortified with 30 IU vitamin A and 2 IU vitamin D per gram of fat. Processed foods are often enriched with vitamins, minerals, and lysine.

Extending the shelf life Processing extends the shelf life because apart from removing unwanted, spoilt, and harmful matter and subjecting the food to temperatures outside the danger zone, all processes such as dehydration, cold storage, canning, and pasteurization are aimed at preservation of food.

Increasing acceptability through fabricated foods New products of uniform size and shape are being introduced in the market. They are made from low-grade commodities which are plentiful or good for health.

Extruded ready-to-eat snacks, soya meat substitutes, non-dairy whiteners, and creamers have flooded the market. Tapioca, maize, dried fish, etc. are blended into tasty snacks. A health drink such as aloe vera juice is blended with its tastier counterparts, such as blackcurrant and blueberry, to which aloe vera pieces are added.

METHODS OF FOOD PRESERVATION

Use of Low Temperatures

Low temperatures preserve food by retarding chemical reactions, enzymatic action, and growth and activity of microorganisms. The lower the temperature, the better the food will be preserved. At low temperatures, microorganisms are not killed and since foods already have a microbial load, microorganisms will multiply once the temperatures become favourable.

Refrigeration/chilling

Temperatures of 1 to 4°C prevent food from spoiling for short periods. It merely retards the decay but frozen foods kept at −18°C preserve food for a year and at −28°C food can be preserved for upto two years.

Chilling temperatures retard microbial growth and biochemical changes which affect colour, texture, flavour, and nutritive value. Most perishable foods such as eggs, dairy products, chicken, meat, and seafood are held at chilling temperatures for a limited time without affecting their condition. They need to be consumed by the 'best before date'. The relative humidity (RH) in refrigerator storage is another important factor which needs to be controlled. A low RH results in loss of moisture and wilting and shrinkage in fruits and vegetables. A high RH favours surface spoilage by microorganisms.

Cook–chill

In this system, food is cooked in the kitchen in advance and rapidly chilled and stored at 0–3°C. It is reheated just before it is served. The cook–chill system is used for almost all kinds of foods and is popular in airlines and institutional catering. Proper cooking procedures and hygienic standards need to be followed to ensure safety and quality. The steps in cook–chill process are presented in Fig. 11.1.

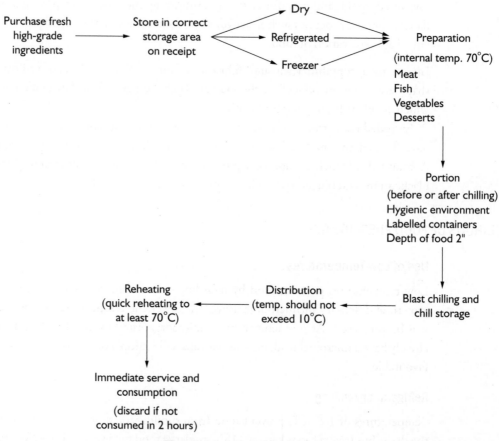

Fig. 11.1 Steps in cook–chill process

Precautions for cook–chill foods

1. Food should be properly cooked to destroy microorganisms and complete the cooking process.
2. Cooked food should be portioned and chilled in a blast chiller unit within 30 minutes of cooking.
3. Chilling temperature of 3°C must be reached within 1½ hours after cooking.
4. Chilled storage temperature should be between 0–3°C.

5. While distributing cook–chill foods, temperature should be as low as possible.
6. During reheating, the temperature must reach 70°C (internal temperature) and it should be held at that temperature for at least 2 minutes.
7. Food should be reheated just before it is consumed and it should not be consumed after 2 hours of reheating.
8. The critical safety limit for chilled food is 10°C and if the temperature during storage or distribution exceeds this limit the food should be discarded.
9. Recipes should be suitably modified for cook-chill foods to prevent curdling or changes in consistency of soups, sauces, and crispness of batter-fried products.
10. The storage life of cook–chill meals should not exceed 5 days.

The caterer should know that even at chilling temperatures, bacterial, chemical, and enzymatic reactions are taking place but at a more slower rate than room temperature. Chilling temperatures only help to prolong shelf life.

Freezing

Food is preserved for long periods by reducing its temperature to −18°C or lower. At this temperature, water present in food is converted to ice and microbial growth stops. Freezing retains colour, flavour, and nutritive value. However, the texture of some foods is adversely affected. If properly stored, frozen food has a shelf life of 3–12 months. Fruits, vegetables, meat, fish, and poultry can be preserved in this way.

Food to be frozen should be frozen quickly so that small ice crystals form in the cells of the food which is desirable. Slow freezing causes large irregular shaped ice crystals to form in the cells. These contain the flavour and nutrients. When food is thawed, flavour and some nutrients are lost as large ice crystals pierce the cells. Food is quickly frozen by using any one of the following equipment.

Blast freezers   In this cold-air at −18°C to −34°C is vigorously circulated over food while it passes through an insulated tunnel.

Plate freezers   Food to be frozen is placed in contact with a metal surface which is cooled by a refrigerant. It is used for ice creams, juices, etc., both packaged and unpackaged foods.

Immersion freezers   Packaged or unpackaged food is frozen by immersing it or spraying it with a freezing agent. It is used for freezing poultry.

Spray freezers   This is the quickest freezing method in which liquid nitrogen or carbon dioxide is used. It is called cryogenic freezing. The food to be frozen is placed on a conveyor belt which passes through an insulated freezing tunnel. Liquid nitrogen or carbon dioxide is injected into the tunnel through a spray which changes its state and vaporizes, resulting in instant freezing.

Freeze flow

In this system, food freezes but does not harden.

A wide variety of frozen foods, both cooked and uncooked, are available in the market. They should be thawed/cooked as per manufacturer's instructions. Some are to be cooked in the frozen state. Frozen foods once thawed should never be refrozen. This is because when food is thawed its temperature is within the 'danger zone' in which bacteria present in food multiply rapidly.

Cook-freeze

It is a specialized method of a food processing system in which food is cooked and immediately blast frozen at −18°C or below, and stored at that temperature till it has to be served. Such food has a shelf life of 3 to 6 months. The food should be frozen immediately so that large ice crystals do not form and freshness is retained and should be accomplished within one to one and a half hours. Table 11.1 presents the steps in cook–freeze system.

TABLE 11.1   Steps in cook–freeze system

Steps	Precautions
1. Purchasing and storing	Licensed suppliers; temperature control
2. Pre-preparation	Clean kitchen and equipment; wholesome ingredients
3. Cooking	Use proper method of cooking; use a probe thermometer; check internal temperature
4. Portioning and packaging	Use clean sanitized containers of correct size; accurate portion size filled to 5 cm depth; cover/seal container
5. Labelling	Label should state production date, best by date, name of preparation, number of portions, and shelf life
6. Freezing	Freeze immediately below −5°C within 1½ hours. Once frozen, shift food to deep freeze storage.
7. Storing	Record temperature of freezer regularly (at least −18°C. Destroy outdated packages. Follow first in, first out (FIFO) and keep door well shut.
8. Transporting	Distribute in refrigerator vans in insulated containers. If temperature increases, use up the food and do not refreeze
9. Thawing and reheating	Thaw in thawing cabinet. Reheat to at least 70°C for 2 minutes. Serve immediately and discard food unconsumed for 2 hours.

Once the foods are frozen they should be stored at −18 °C, and transported as and when required in insulated containers and refrigerated transport. Before service, foods should be thawed in a thawing cabinet at 10°C and reheated in a combination oven or in a microwave oven if quantity is less.

Advantages of cook–freeze

1. Complete utilization of staff time
2. Complete utilization of equipment
3. Portion control and minimal wastage
4. Less frequent deliveries from commissary
5. Food can be prepared, when in season and prices are low, days or weeks in advance during lean periods
6. Menus can be planned and prepared in advance
7. Lesser staff required with more variety in menu
8. Overall savings in staff, equipment, space, fuel, and food costs.

Follow proper instructions while preparing and storing food to prevent loss of flavour and texture. Avoid slow freezing and freezer burns due to prolonged storage and badly packaged food.

Use modified starches such as waxy maize starch along with regular starches to prevent syneresis and retrogradation of starch-based dishes.

Vacuum cooking   Also known as *sous-vide,* it is a form of cook–chill using a combination of processes. The food is first sealed in a plastic pouch. It is then cooked by steam and quickly chilled in ice-water. It can be used by many catering establishments. The steps in vacuum cooking are given in Fig. 11.2.

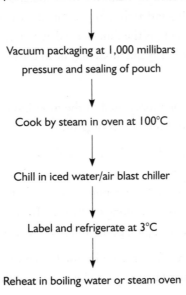

Fig. 11.2   Steps in vacuum cooking

Although this system has many advantages, its main disadvantages are uneven cooking if size of cut food varies, longer cooking time, and extra cost of vacuum pouches and packing equipment.

Creating a Vacuum

Removal of oxygen can stop aerobic microorganisms from growing. This can be done by packing foods in airtight containers or vacuum packing of foods as in canned foods. However, anaerobic microorganisms can still grow in such foods if these have been inadequately processed.

Vacuum Packing

Vacuum packing of prepared food in vacuum packs of special plastic pouches is an excellent means of preserving food. Vacuum-packed food does not get oxidized, there is minimal weight loss or drip, and once packed chances of cross contamination is reduced. Packs should be stored at appropriate storage temperature, well labelled, and FIFO must be followed strictly. If the contents of the pack are discoloured or if pack is bloated or leaking, it should be discarded immediately. Strict hygiene needs to be followed for such processed food.

Use of High Temperatures

High temperatures destroy microorganisms by denaturation of cell proteins and inactivation of enzymes needed by them for their metabolism. At temperatures above 63°C, bacteria stop multiplying and as the temperature increases, they are gradually destroyed. The thermal death time (TDT) is the time needed at a given temperature to kill a number of microbes. Heat used to destroy microbes may be in the form of wet heat or dry heat.

Wet heat

This is more commonly used in the food industry. If carefully administered, it is a useful method of controlling microorganisms.

Blanching   Foods which are to be frozen, dried, or canned are immersed in hot boiling water for a few minutes prior to processing. Blanching helps in removal of peel, inactivation of enzymes that oxidize vitamin C, removal of gas in tissue spaces, and wilting of the tissue which helps in proper filling of the can. The enzymes which bring about discolouration or browning seen in apples, pears, and potatoes are also inactivated.

Pasteurization   This method is used to control microorganisms in milk, fruit juices, and wines. Food may be pasteurized by any one of the three methods:

1. Low temperature holding (LTH) method at 62°C for 30 minutes.
2. High temperature short time (HTST) or flash method at 72°C for 15 seconds.

3. Ultra high temperature sterilization (UHTS) at temperatures above 135°C for 2 seconds. This method makes foods commercially sterile. Such foods are packed under aseptic conditions and can be stored at room temperature for three to six months.

Canning   In this process, temperatures used are above 100°C. All microorganisms that could spoil food under normal conditions of storage are destroyed by heating the food in an autoclave at temperatures between 115°C and 125°C. The exact temperature and time required for canning depends on the type of food to be canned. Acidic foods such as fruit are heated to 100°C only because acid also helps in preventing microbial growth. A vacuum is created inside the can or the air in the headspace may be replaced by nitrogen gas to prevent growth of aerobic bacteria.

This is the most common method of food processing in developed countries. It is used to preserve fruits, vegetables, fish, meat, poultry, etc. In this process, no preservative is added to the food which is sealed in airtight containers. These are then heated to sterilize the food.

The following basic steps need to be followed while canning or bottling food:

Cleaning and preparing   The food to be canned is cleaned thoroughly and prepared for canning. For example, fruits and vegetables may be cut, peeled, sliced, or stoned. Some foods may be blanched.

Filling   Raw prepared food is filled into cans or bottles either mechanically at the rate of 1,200 containers a minute or by hand. Filling should be carefully controlled to ensure that the headspace, i.e., the amount of empty space in the can is neither too little nor too large.

Exhausting   A partial vacuum is created in the can by removing part of the air. As oxygen is reduced, bacterial spoilage is retarded. Exhausting prevents the ends of the can from bulging during heating.

Sealing   Cans and bottles are sealed with airtight lids by sealing machines.

Processing   The sealed containers are heated at a controlled temperature for a specified length of time. The time and temperature depend on the food being processed and the size of the container. Cans are processed in containers called retorts. They are commercially sterilized using steam under pressure.

Cooling   As soon as processing is over, cans are cooled immediately to stop further cooking. Cans are cooled by dipping them in cold water, spraying them with cold water, or partially cooling them by water as well as air-cooling.

The cans are then labelled and packed in cartons to be marketed.

Disadvantages of wet heating:

1. Heat labile nutrients are lost
2. Heat required for processing affects the texture, colour, and flavour of the product
3. Cost of canned food is high in India

4. Once opened, canned food should be treated like fresh food and consumed within stipulated period.

Advantages of wet heating:

1. Convenience
2. Long shelf life
3. Needs little preparation
4. No chemical preservatives
5. Variety of food is available

Cooking (boiling, steaming, stewing, and poaching)   In these methods of cooking, wet or moist heat is used. The temperature attained is 100°C. At this temperature, most microorganisms are destroyed but spores survive. Foods cooked by these methods cannot be stored for long periods.

Dry heat

It is used in the following methods.

Sun drying, smoking, and freeze drying   One should also make use of heat to preserve food. In these methods, dry heat is used to control microorganisms. Dry heat brings about dehydration of the foods or of the surface of food. It destroys molds, yeast, and most bacteria and spores.

Cooking (baking, roasting, grilling)   In these methods of cooking, food is cooked by dry heat. The temperature reached on the surface is approximately 115°C. Most bacteria are destroyed. Internal temperature of food is generally lower.

If food has to be kept for sometime, it should be cooked thoroughly. Foods cooked by dry heat methods do not spoil as fast as moist heat methods as they have a lower moisture content.

Figure 11.3 shows the temperatures used in the food industry and their effect of microorganisms and Fig. 11.4 presents the classification of methods of food preservation.

Removal of Moisture from Food

Microorganisms need moisture for their growth. If foods are dried or dehydrated, i.e., if the moisture is extracted from food, they will not be spoilt by bacteria, yeasts, or molds.

Moisture can be removed by sun drying, mechanical dryers (spray or roller driers), and freeze drying.

Sun drying   It is used for certain fruit, such as grapes, figs, and apricots, which are placed on trays. The fruit may be turned during drying. Light coloured fruit is sulphured to prevent enzymatic browning.

Disadvantage: It can be used in hot dry climates only.

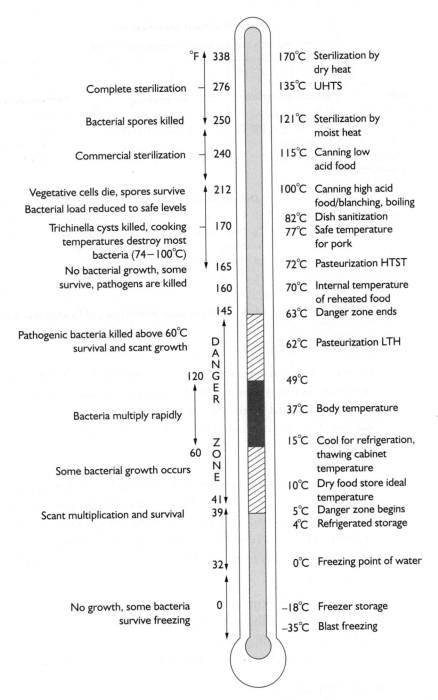

Fig. 11.3   Temperatures used in the food industry and their effect on microorganisms

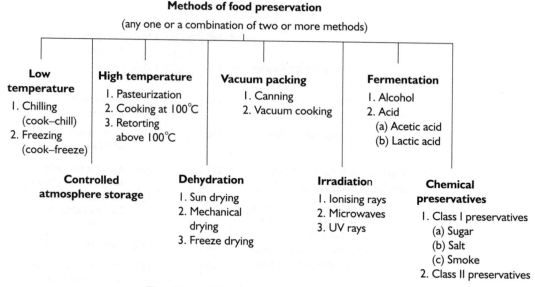

Methods of food preservation

(any one or a combination of two or more methods)

Low temperature	High temperature	Vacuum packing	Fermentation
1. Chilling (cook–chill) 2. Freezing (cook–freeze)	1. Pasteurization 2. Cooking at 100°C 3. Retorting above 100°C	1. Canning 2. Vacuum cooking	1. Alcohol 2. Acid (a) Acetic acid (b) Lactic acid

Controlled atmosphere storage	Dehydration	Irradiation	Chemical preservatives
	1. Sun drying 2. Mechanical drying 3. Freeze drying	1. Ionising rays 2. Microwaves 3. UV rays	1. Class I preservatives (a) Sugar (b) Salt (c) Smoke 2. Class II preservatives

Fig. 11.4   Classification of methods of food preservation

Use of mechanical dryers

The food to be dried is passed on conveyor belts through hot air with controlled relative humidity, or hot air is passed through the food. Liquid food such as milk is dried either by passing it over heated rollers or by spraying the liquid into a current of dry heated air. Dried food should be packed in airtight containers immediately.

Freeze drying

In this process of dehydration, the food to be dried is first frozen in a cabinet. A vacuum is created by pumping out the air in the cabinet and by the process of sublimation, ice turns into vapour. Freeze-dried food needs no further refrigeration or preservation. It is light in weight and retains its size and shape, and when soaked in water, regains its original size and flavour. It is used to dry fruits, vegetables, meat, poultry, and seafood.

Advantages of drying:

1. Dried food is easy to transport and store.
2. It has a long shelf life provided it remains dry.
3. It occupies less storage space.
4. It is a cheap method of preservation and is convenient to use.

Use of Preservatives

A preservative is any substance which retards deterioration of food. There are two groups of preservatives used in food.

Class I preservatives

This class includes sugar, common salt, glucose, fructose, alcohol, spices, vinegar or acetic acid, honey, and wood smoke. There is no restriction by law on the addition of these substances in food.

Class II preservatives

This class includes chemicals which inhibit microbial growth and can be added to certain foods only in definite permitted limits. They are usually added at the end of the processing operation and their presence has to be mentioned on the label, i.e., there is a restriction on the use of these preservatives in food by law. They include salts of benzoic acid, fumaric acid, sulphurous acid, nitrates and nitrites of sodium and potassium, sorbic, propionic, and acetic acid. Nisin, an antibiotic, is used in the preservation of cheese.

They are used to preserve food in the following ways.

1. They may be added to food, e.g., sodium benzoate in tomato sauce and potassium metabisulphte in lemon squash.
2. They may be applied on the surface of foods. Sulphur dioxide is used on dry fruits and borax is used to wash vegetables and whole fruit.
3. Wrappers may be impregnated with sorbic acid to prevent surface spoilage of cheese.
4. The ice used to chill foods like fish may contain tetracycline, an antibiotic which is a permitted preservative.
5. They may be used as gases around food. Fruits and vegetables are stored in an atmosphere containing two to three percent carbon dioxide to retard the ripening process.

Table 11.2 shows the uses of various chemical preservatives.

TABLE 11.2 Uses of chemical preservatives

Class I	Class II
They include sugar, salt, vinegar, spices, smoke, and oil.	*They include salts of various acids.*
(a) Sugar: A high concentration of sugar prevents molds, yeast, and bacteria and is used to preserve jams, jellies, marmalades, fruit preserves, candied fruit, glaced fruit crystallized fruit, and chutneys.	(a) Benzoic acid and its salts, e.g., sodium benzoate in tomato sauce, squashes, and syrups.
(b) Salt: Microorganisms cannot grow in high concentrations of salt. Meat is pickled in salt solution, e.g., ham and ox tongue. Salt is used for pickling and curing. Mango, lime, and vegetable pickles are preserved by salt. Salt and sugar preserve food by binding water and making it unavailable for microbial activity.	(b) Sulphurous acid and its salts, e.g., potassium metabisulphte in fruit beverages such as lime cordial, before dehydration of fruits and vegetable, and in bulk storage of fruit pulp.

Contd

Table 11.2 Contd

Class I	Class II
(c) Smoke: It is a complex mixture of alcohols, acids, phenols, and toxic substances which inhibit microbial growth. Meat to be smoked is first salted and then smoked. Temperature control during smoking is essential to maintain the texture.	(c) Nitrates and nitrites of potassium and sodium are used in the preservation of meat and for colour retention in pork.
(d) Vinegar: 4 per cent acetic acid in water is used for pickling vegetables such as onions, gherkins, red cabbage, shallots, and to preserve chutneys.	(d) Propionic acid and its salts such as sodium and calcium propionate are used as mold inhibitors on cheese surface and to prevent rope in bread.
	(e) Sorbic acid and its salts such as potassium sorbate is used in fruit juice, sauces, jam, flour confectionery, and in magarine to prevent yeast and mold growth.

Controlled Atmosphere Storage

When fruits and vegetables are harvested, they are still alive and respire using up oxygen and giving out carbon dioxide, water vapour, and heat. The faster the rate of respiration, the quicker the ripening process. The ripening rate can be reduced by

1. Lowering the temperature
2. Reducing available oxygen
3. Increasing the carbon dioxide concentration.

All three methods are used in controlled atmosphere storage.

Fruits can be stored for varying lengths of time under controlled conditions, thus extending their shelf life.

Modified atmosphere storage is also used for food storage. It differs from controlled atmosphere storage because in controlled atmosphere storage the percentage of gas is monitored, while in modified atmosphere the air is initially replaced with gas, but no further measures are taken to check the percentage of gas in the atmosphere. The concentration and proportion of gases used varies with the kind and variety of fruit. The carbon dioxide concentration is usually increased and oxygen concentration is decreased for fresh fruits and vegetables stored in cold rooms. Modified atmosphere packaging is another technique of enhanced preservation based on gas storage (refer Chapter 13 on New Trends in Food).

Table 11.3 shows the composition of the atmosphere.

TABLE 11.3 Composition of the atmosphere

Gas	Normal atmosphere	Controlled atmosphere
Oxygen	20.95%	2.5–5%
Carbon dioxide	0.3–0.4%	2–5%
Nitrogen	79%	90–95%

Preservation by Fermentation

Select microorganisms act on certain foods such as milk, soya beans, cereals, pulses, and cabbage, and give it a distinctive taste, better acceptance, higher nutritive value, and a longer shelf life. Examples of food fermentations are:

1. Alcoholic beverages such as beer and wine

$$C_6H_{12}O_6 \xrightarrow[\text{anaerobic conditions}]{\text{yeast}} 2C_2H_5OH + 2CO_2\uparrow$$

Simple sugar   Ethyl alcohol

2. Acetic acid fermentation in vinegar manufacture

$$C_2H_5OH + O_2 \xrightarrow[\text{Acetobacter}]{\text{aerobic}} CH_3COOH + H_2O$$

Ethyl alcohol   Acetic acid

3. Lactic acid fermentation in curds and yoghurt

$$C_6H_{12}O_6 \xrightarrow[\text{Lactobacilli}]{} 2C_3H_6O_3$$

Lactose   Lactic acid

It is also seen in sauerkraut and dill pickles.

Preservation by Radiation

Radiation of various frequencies ranging from low-frequency microwaves to high-frequency gamma rays are being used to preserve various foods. Radiations can be classified into two categories on either side of the light spectrum.

1. Low-frequency, long wavelength, and low-energy rays—from radio waves to infrared rays.
2. Higher frequency, shorter wavelength, and higher energy rays on the other side of the light spectrum are of two types:
   (a) Shorter wavelength, lower frequency, and lower energy rays, e.g., ultraviolet (UV) rays
   (b) Higher frequency, short wavelength, and high-energy rays, e.g., ionizing rays that are capable of breaking molecules into ions.

Ultraviolet irradiation

This type of radiation is most widely used in the food industry. Ultraviolet rays are an invisible form of light. They lie just beyond the violet end of the visible spectrum. They are present in sunlight. They can be produced artificially by low pressure mercury vapour lamps.

Ultraviolet rays are effective in killing bacteria and viruses. They have poor penetrating power and can be used for surface sterilization of food, or for sterilizing the air in storage and processing rooms. They are used to control mold growth on the surface of bakery products and to prevent spoilage of meat while tenderizing and aging. Treating knives for slicing bread, treating water for beverages, and sanitizing of food service utensils are some of other successful uses of UV rays.

Microwave oven   Microwaves are short radio waves which heat food by penetrating it. These waves cause molecules in food to vibrate rapidly. The friction caused by the rapidly moving molecules creates heat which cooks the food (Fig. 11.5).

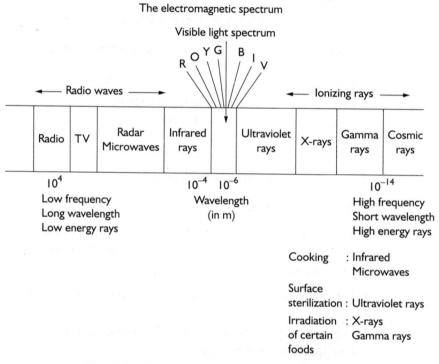

Fig. 11.5   Types of radiation used for cooking food

Microwaves are produced by an electronic vacuum tube called a magnetron. They penetrate food to a depth of $1\frac{1}{2}$ inches. Cooking is faster in a microwave oven because heat is produced inside the food and no heat is lost. Natural flavour is better retained if correct cooking procedures are followed.

Ionizing rays or cold sterilization   Foods are exposed to ionizing radiation to extend its shelf life. These rays transfer some of their energy as they pass through food killing pathogenic and spoilage causing microorganisms.

Food irradiation in low doses of 0.05–70 kilo grays is used for the following purposes.

1. To inhibit sprouting, e.g., potatoes, onions, garlic, ginger, and shallots

2. To control insect infestation, e.g., rice, wheat, and dry fruits
3. To reduce microbial load, e.g., spices, meat, chicken, and frozen fish
4. To extend shelf life and delay ripening, e.g., mango, papaya, and banana
5. To sterilize food, e.g., packaged food and food in hermetically sealed containers
6. For treatment of water

Ionizing radiation is electromagnetic like radiowaves, infrared light, or ultraviolet light. Its controlled use can protect food without making it radioactive. It is more powerful than UV rays. The advantages of irradiation are follows:

1. It can be used for heat sensitive food and frozen food as it does not increase the temperature.
2. Nutritive value and chemical changes in foods are minimal as compared to any other method of preservation.
3. Food can be sterilized after it is packed.

Milling

Whole grains of cereals, pulses, and nuts are often crushed or ground into flours of various particle size. For example, wheat is ground into whole wheat flour, refined flour, semolina, and dalia.

Whole grains are made up of an outer most covering of bran which encloses the endosperm and the germ. Bran is rich in cellulose and resists the action of water and heat. Crushing helps in absorption of water and heat and in cooking the grain. A number of flours are available in the market. The processing quality and the nutritive value depend on the quality of grain used and the rate of extraction. Since wheat is the most popular cereal in the world, milling will be explained with reference to wheat grain. Figure 11.6 gives the structure of a wheat grain.

The extraction is the percentage of whole wheat grain present in the flour. Whole meal flour is 100 per cent extraction and it retains all the grain components. Lower extraction rates mean most of the bran and the germ have been removed. Refined flour or maida has an extraction rate of 70 per cent and is almost pure endosperm. Removal of the bran and the germ can improve the processing quality and the shelf life of the cereal. The lower the extraction rate, the lighter is the colour of flour.

But the nutritive value of the cereal depends on the amount of bran and germ retained when the cereal is milled. Bread made from whole wheat flour is dark in colour and coarse in texture as compared to white bread, but more nutritious.

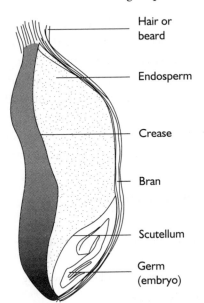

Hair or beard

Endosperm

Crease

Bran

Scutellum

Germ (embryo)

Fig. 11.6 Structure of a wheat grain

Modern milling processes are carried out using steel rollers, and the bran and germ can be removed producing a flour which is purely endosperm. The complex process involves many steps. The grains are cleaned to remove extraneous matter and conditioned or brought to the optimum moisture content before it is milled. The grain is passed through a series of rollers which break the grains which is then sifted to obtain flour of different extraction rates.

Effect of milling on nutrient content　Bran is made up of cellulose, B-complex vitamins and contains 50 per cent of the minerals present in the grain. It constitutes 15 per cent of the grain.

The germ is rich in vitamin E, B-complex vitamins, proteins, iron, and oil, and is approximately 20 per cent of the grain.

Starch is the major constituent of the endosperm along with protein.

The scutellum or membrane which separates the germ from the endosperm is very rich in vitamin B_1 or thiamine.

When refined flour is extracted, practically all the bran, germ, and scutellum are removed during milling. Since wheat germ is rich in oil, which can turn rancid, removal of the germ increases the shelf life of flour.

EFFECT OF PROCESSING (HEAT, ACID, AND ALKALI) ON FOOD CONSTITUENTS

The term processing is very vast and includes a number of treatment food is subjected to while making it ready for consumption.

Processing helps preserve surplus food so that it can be made available at a later date. While food is being processed, some loss of nutrients does occur, but if we see the overall benefits of processing, this loss is minimal and can be replaced by restoring, enriching, or fortifying food. Colour pigments present in fruits and vegetables are affected by heat, acid, alkali, and metals, and these need to be controlled (refer Chapter 6 on Fruits and Vegetables).

Effect of processing (see Table 11.4) has been dealt with under the different nutrients as effect of heat, acid, and alkali on nutrients, specially the water soluble, heat labile vitamin B-complex and ascorbic acid.

TABLE 11.4　Effect of some processes on food constituents

Process	Food	Effect
Heat	Soya bean	Trypsin inhibitor destroyed; digestibility increases
	Egg white	Avidin is destroyed, hence biotin is available
	Egg yolk	Iron availability increases

Contd

Table 11.4 Contd

Process	Food	Effect
	Starch and protein	Digestibility increases; bioavailability of niacin increases
	Fruits and vegetables	Loss of B1, B2, and C vitamins
		Leaching loss of minerals and water-soluble vitamins while washing and cooking in water.
	Sugar	Caramelization
	Bakery products	Maillard browning with aroma
Freezing	Vegetables and fruits	Loss of vitamin C minimal
		Loss of B1, B2, and C vitamins during blanching prior to freezing and while thawing.
Freeze drying	Meat, vegetables, and fruit	Loss of pyridoxine
		Loss of vitamin C in unblanched foods.
Sun drying, dehydration	Carrots	Loss of carotene due to oxidation. Loss of vitamin C.
Fermentation	Milk and cereals	Digestibility increases. B-complex increases. Bioavailability of minerals increases
Smoked foods	Meat and fish	Fat oxidation is retarded. Carcinogens may be present.
Milling	Cereal, pulses, and nuts	Varies with rate of extraction of flour

FOOD ADDITIVES

A variety of chemicals may be found in our food which have gained entry either intentionally or unintentionally. Intentional additives are those chemical substances which have been purposefully added to food to perform a specific function such as increasing its shelf life, modifying its texture, improving its flavour, etc. They are generally added in small specified quantities. This chapter deals with intentional food additives.

Unintentional additives are those chemical substances which find their way into food through a certain stage in manufacture or handling of food. Examples of unintentional additives are fertilizer and pesticide residue from the farm, lubricants from food processing equipment and chemicals from packaging materials. They are also called accidental additives. They have no specific function in food and their presence is undesirable.

Definition Food additives are chemical substances which are not food items by themselves but are intentionally added to food to improve the overall quality.

Food additives are not new to the food industry. Some additives have been used by our ancestors; e.g., salting bacon, preparing pickles with vinegar/acetic acid, and using sulphur dioxide for wine making. With the booming food processing industry, many new additives have been added to the list of permitted additives.

Food additives are grouped into different categories on the basis of the functions they perform. The different categories are as follows:

1. Preservatives	10. Non-nutritive sweeteners
2. Antioxidants	11. Humectants
3. Emulsifying agents	12. Firming agents
4. Stabilizers	13. Clarifying agents
5. Thickening agents	14. Gases and propellants
6. Food colours	15. Leavening agents
7. Flavouring agents	16. Sequestrants
8. Nutrient supplements	17. Bleaching agents
9. Anti-caking agents	

Food additives should be used only if they perform at least one of the following functions.

1. Preserve flavour	4. Maintain nutritional quality
2. Enhance taste	5. Enhance keeping quality
3. Improve acceptability and appearance	6. Aid in food processing

All additives should be added with caution and mentioned on the label. They should be used only when the desired effect cannot be achieved through good manufacturing practices (GMP). It should not be used to cover up faulty processing practices.

Numbering of Additives

Each additive is assigned a unique number called 'E number'. This has been introduced to regulate the use of food additives and keep the consumer informed about the same. All approved additives in Europe have an E number. Countries outside Europe use only the number. For examples, sulphur dioxide is written as E 220 on products sold in Europe, but is known as additive 220 in some countries.

The numbering scheme has been adopted by the Codex Alimentarius Commission to internationally identify all additives, both approved and non-approved. Each additive has to be named and numbered, the numbers being the same worldwide. The additive must be mentioned on the label as a number. For example, a popular brand of instant soup in India mentions the following additives

- Flavour enhancers 627 and 631
- Acidity regulator 330

While a seafood starter mentions both the name and number of the additives.

- Baking soda   –   E500

- Sorbitol   –   E420
- Paprika   –   E160c
- Glycine   –   E640
- MSG   –   E621
- Polyphosphate   –   E451
- Thickener and binder   –   E415, E410, E412, E417

Laws relating to mention of name or number of additive on the label may vary from one country to another, but the universally accepted number remains the same.

Food additives can be divided into several groups as shown in Table 11.4.

Some additives perform more than one function, e.g., acids which may be categorized as preservatives and antioxidants as well.

Types of Additives

The different types of additives are listed in Table 11.5.

Preservatives

Foods deteriorate because of microbial action, enzyme action or chemical reactions. The main function of preservatives is to inhibit the growth and activity of microorganism. Preservatives have been discussed earlier in this chapter under the section on the use of preservatives.

TABLE 11.5 Some examples of food additives and their description

S. no.	Additive	Description	Examples
1	Acids	Food acids are added to give sour or tart flavours to food. They also act as preservatives and antioxidants.	Vinegar, citric acid, tartaric acid, malic acid, fumaric acid, and lactic acid.
2	Anti-caking agents	Anti-caking agents keep dry food powders such as instant idli mix from forming lumps or caking.	Calcium phosphate, magnesium carbonate
3	Antioxidants	Antioxidants inhibit the effects of oxygen on food. Some prevent the fatty phases of food from turning rancid due to oxidative rancidity.	BHA(Butylated hydroxy anisole), EDTA(Ethylene diamine tetraacetic acid)
4	Anti-foaming agents	Anti-foaming agents reduce or prevent foaming in foods.	Mineral oil
5	Food colours	Artificial colours are added to food to replace the colour lost during preparation, or to make food look more attractive.	Ponceau 4 R, curcumin
6	Emulsifiers	Emulsifiers stabilize emulsions and ensure that water and oils remain mixed together in an emulsion, as in mayonnaise, ice cream, and homogenized milk.	Stearyl tartarate, polyoxyethylene monostearate

Contd

Table 11.5 Contd

S. no.	Additive	Description	Examples
7	Flavouring agents	Flavouring agents are additives that give food a particular taste or smell, and may be derived from natural ingredients or created artificially.	Synthetic fruit flavours, essential oils
8	Bleaching agents	Bleaching agents are added to flour to improve its colour.	Hydrogen peroxide, potassium bromide
9	Humectants	Humectants help in binding and retaining water and prevent foods from drying out.	Propylene glycol, glycerol, sorbitol
10	Gases and propellants	Both reactive gases and inert gases are used in food processing and for packaging and to prevent foods from being exposed to atmosphere, thus guaranteeing shelf life.	Carbon dioxide, Nitrous oxide, Argon, Helium
11	Preservatives	Preservatives increase shelf life by preventing or inhibiting microbial spoilage of food.	Sodium benzoate, potassium metabisulphite
12	Stabilizers and thickeners	Stabilizers, thickeners, and gelling agents increase its viscosity without substantially modifying its other properties. The change in consistency gives foods a firmer texture. While they are not true emulsifiers, they help to stabilize emulsions.	Dextrin, modified starch
13	Non-nutritive Sweeteners	Non-nutritive sweeteners are added to foods for flavouring, to keep the calorie content low, or because they have beneficial effects for diabetics and help reduce incidence of tooth decay.	Acesulfame K
14	Nutrient supplements	Foods are fortified or enriched with vitamins, minerals and aminoacids in which they are deficient.	Iodine, ascorbic acid, lysine
15	Glazing agents	Glazing agents provide a shiny appearance or protective coating to foods.	Bees wax, rice bran wax, paraffin wax
16	Flavour enhancers	Flavour enhancers enhance a food's existing flavours. They may be extracted from natural sources or created artificially.	MSG, Disodium inosinate, maltol
17	Acidity regulators	Acidity regulators are pH control agents used to change or otherwise control the acidity and alkalinity of foods.	Sodium potassium tartarate, Sodium fumarate
18	Sequestrants	Sequestrants or chelating agents immobilize metal contaminants and prevent clouding in beverages.	Disodium EDTA, sodium gluconate

Antioxidants

These compounds are used to prevent oxidative rancidity of fats in food. They preserve organoleptic qualities and nutritive value. For example, butylated hydroxyanisole (BHA), Butylated hydroxy toluene (BHT) or tertiary butyl hydroquinone (TBHQ) are added to the oil in which snacks are fried to prevent the unsaturated fatty acids from turning rancid.

While selecting an antioxidant, care should be taken to ensure that it is heat stable and fat soluble. Fumaric acid is used to prevent rancidity in butter, cheese, and wafers. Other antioxidants used are EDTA (Ethylene diamine tetra acetic acid), tocopherol (vitamin E), and ascorbic acid (vitamin C)

Emulsifying agents

Emulsifying agents (EA) or emulsifiers are added to stabilize emulsions by enhancing the formation of small droplets and reducing the rate at which the droplets coalesce or come together. Emulsifying agents have both hydrophilic (H_2O loving) and hydrophobic (H_2O repelling) groups and get attracted to water and oils at the interphase of the two liquids, thereby preventing the emulsion from breaking or water and oil from separating out . EA may be natural or synthetic. Commercially used EA are glyceryl mono stearate (GMS), stearyl tartarate and polyoxyethylene mono-stearate.

Examples of natural emulsifying agents present in food are lecithin in egg yolk and caseinogens in milk.

Stabilizers and thickening agents

These additives are used to increase the viscosity of food and to stabilize the texture of food systems like foams, emulsions, and suspensions. A number of hydrocolloids are used in the food industry to maintain the texture and consistency of foods.

CMC, gums, starch, dextrins, agar, gelatin and pectin are used in ice creams, jellies, puddings, salad dressings, and chocolate beverages. They stabilize the food system by increasing the viscosity of the system.

Humectants

1. Humectants are also known as water binding and retaining agents. They prevent food from drying out.
2. They are used in food to control crystallisation, water retention, and improve softness and rehydration of dehydrated foods.
3. Glycerol, sorbitol, propylene glycol, mannitol, and polyethylene glycol have water-binding properties.
4. In intermediate moisture foods (IM foods) such as fruitcakes, jams, and jellies, glycerol is used to retain moisture, IM foods are foods which contain 15 to 30 per cent moisture.

Gases and propellants

Reactive gases such as sulphur dioxide, ethylene, hydrogen, and chlorine are used for specific functions during food processing. For example, SO_2 is used on green grapes to prevent enzymatic browning, ethylene gas is used under MAP for ripening fruit such as bananas and mangoes, hydrogen is used for converting oil into fat and chlorine is used as a bleaching agent for flour.

Inert gases, such as CO_2, are used in aerated soft drinks, beer, champagne, and fruit juice for the fizz and tang. Other gases such as nitrous oxide and CO_2 are used as propellants to dispense liquid, foam, or spray products Freon C 318 and Freon 115 are liquidfied propellants used to dispense whipped creams and foam toppings.

Food colours

Colouring agents used in the food processing industry include natural colouring matter, certified food dyes, and derived colours. Natural colour pigments such as anthocyanin, carotenoid, betalins, curcumin, chlorophyll, and caramel are safe to use in any amounts. Disadvantages of natural colours are poor stability, high cost, and limited range of shades. These colours are extracted from fruits and vegetables but have very low pigment content.

Certified food dyes are synthetic colours which are non-toxic and have been approved by the Food and Drug Administration (FDA). They are stable, easy to blend, and economical. However, they cannot be used in large amounts as their safety is doubtful.

Permitted synthetic colours

1. Red   –   Ponceau 4, carmoisine, erythrosine
2. Yellow –   Tartrazine, sunset yellow FCF
3. Blue   –   Indigo carmine, brilliant blue FCF
4. Green   –   Fast green FCF

Non-nutritive sweeteners

They are used in foods for diabetics, or for obese individuals requiring weight loss as they do not contain any sugar or calories. They are required in very small quantities to sweeten food. Refer the section on artificial sweeteners in Chapter 4. They may be beneficial to prevent tooth decay and during diarrhea.

Anti-caking agents   They are added to keep products dry, prevent caking, and maintain the free flowing nature of granular and powdered food materials which are normally hygroscopic such as table salt. For example, calcium silicate is used in table salt and baking powder and calcium stearate is used in dehydrated vegetable products.

Flavouring agents These include natural and synthetic flavours as well as flavour enhancers. Fruit essences like orange, lemon, etc, are volatile oils in an alcohol base. In citrus drinks, fumaric acid is used as a flavouring agent and for cloud retention. Synthetic flavours are used to overcome the loss of flavour in processing or to add a new flavour. Refer to Chapter 7 on flavour for flavour enhancers.

Nutrient supplements Vitamins, minerals, protein isolates, amino acids, etc. are sometimes added to fortify convenience foods or add value to commonly consumed food items like salt and bread. They are used extensively in infant foods and in foods during convalescence. Iodised salt, lysine enriched bread, ascorbic acid in fruit juices are some examples of nutrient supplements.

Bleaching agents These chemicals are used to lighten or whiten the colour of food. Nitrous oxide is used for bleaching refined flour and hydrogen peroxide and potassium bromide is used to impart a white colour to cheese.

Sequestrants or chelating agents

Metals, such as iron and copper are, present in traces in foods and bring about discolouration of processed beverages. Sequestrants or chelating agents are metal scavengers.

These chemicals combine with metal contaminants and set it aside so that it can be removed from solution.

Examples of sequestrants are Ethylene diamine tetra acetic (EDTA) acid, polyphosphates, citric acid and phosphoric acid.

Clarifying agents These are added to prevent haze formation, sedimentation, and deterioration of beverages such as, wines, beer, and fruit juices. Haze is formed because of phenolic substances, proteins, and pectin present naturally in the beverage. the phenolic substance tannin in apple juice is precipitated out by adding gelatin. Other clarifying agents include bentonite, polyvinyl pyrrolidone (PVP), and physical filtration.

Acids and acidity regulators

Food acids, both organic and inorganic, may occur naturally in some foods or may be added to give a sharp or tart flavour to food. Apart from flavour, acids perform many functions such as preservation, preventing discolouration or browning, as an antioxidant, etc. Benzoic acid and sorbic acid are antimicrobial agents, adipic acid is used to improve gel formation in marmalades and jellies and lactic, butyric, and acetic acid are used as flavouring agents and to modify and intensify the taste perception of flavouring agents.

Acidity regulators change or control the acidity or alkalinity of foods. They include organic acids, bases, buffers, and neutralizing agents.

SUMMARY

Food, unless processed or preserved, is bound to spoil. The spoilage rate depends on the composition of food, the temperature at which it is stored, and the time for which it is held at a specific temperature. Food needs to be protected from spoilage and contamination at all stages till it is consumed. Food spoils for various reasons and a wise food handler should be able to protect food from spoilage by subjecting it to various processes.

The objective of food processing is to remove unwanted matter from food, make it safe for consumption, increase its digestibility, enhance its flavour, colour, and taste, minimize nutrient loss, extend the shelf life, and increase the overall acceptability of the food.

Food is preserved by use of low temperature, high temperature, adding chemical preservatives, vacuum packing, modified atmosphere packaging, aseptic packaging, irradiation, fermentation, etc. A single method or a combination of methods may be used. All these processes have some effect on the constituents of food which must be borne in mind. If the losses of nutrients are significant, these could be replaced by restoring, fortifying, or enriching the food.

Food additives may enter our food intentionally or accidentally. They are added to perform a specific function to improve the overall quality of the processed food product. All additives have a number which is universally accepted. It is mandatory to mention the additive used on the label.

KEY TERMS

Blast chillers   Use of rapidly moving cold air to chill food evenly and rapidly. This may be fitted with temperature probes.

Commercially sterile   Packaged food which has been subjected to sufficient heat to prevent any growth of microorganisms that may cause spoilage under normal storage conditions.

Commissary   A central food production kitchen from which food is distributed to other food-service outlets.

Controlled atmosphere storage   Storage of fruits and vegetables in a cold modified atmosphere in which percentage of CO_2 and O_2 are controlled to preserve the food.

Danger zone   The temperature range of 5–63°C in which microorganisms multiply rapidly in food. At temperatures below 5°C they become dormant, and at temperatures above 63°C they start getting killed.

Enrichment   Addition of nutrients which are present in limited quantities in a food to enrich it.

Fortification   Addition of nutrients to a food which were not originally present, e.g., iodized salt.

Freezer burn   Dehydration and discolouration of foods which are frozen for long periods without being packaged.

Gray (Gy)   A gray is equal to 100 rad. A kilogray is equal to 1,000 gray.

Kilogray (kGy)   A unit for measuring radiation. A kilogray (kGy) is equal to 100 kilorads (krad).

Microwaves   Short radio waves which can be used to cook food. Its wavelength ranges from 1 mm to 30 cm.

Millibar   A unit for measuring atmospheric pressure equal to $1/_{1,000}$ bar or 1,000 dynes/sq.cm.

Pasteurization   A process to destroy the pathogens in milk and extend its shelf life. Two methods: low temperature holding (LTH) method at 62°C for 30 minutes, and high temperature short time (HTST) method at 72°C for 15 seconds.

ppm   Parts per million, a measure for concentration. 200 ppm means 200 mg of a substance in 1 kg or a million parts of water (1 kg = 1,000,000 mg).

Rad (rad)   A rad is that quantity of radiation which results in absorption of 100 erg/g at the point of application.

It is the unit of radiation dosage. A kilorad is 1,000 rad and a megarad is equal to 1 million rads (1,000,000 rad).

Restoration   Addition of nutrients to a food which were originally present but were lost in processing, e.g., addition of vitamin C to canned orange juice.

Retorting   An autoclave used for processing cans and bottles by using steam under pressure. The time and temperature for processing will depend on the microbial load, the pH, the size of the can, the type of food, etc.

UHTS   Ultra high temperature sterilization of food stored in tetrapacks packed under aseptic conditions and heated to 135°C for 2 seconds.

IM foods   Foods which contain 15 to 30 per cent moisture and have a water activity of 0.7 to 0.85 and can be stored without refrigeration without being spoiled by microbes, for e.g., dried fruits, jams, jellies, and fruitcakes, due to sucrose, glucose, salt, and polyhydric alcohols present in them.

REVIEW EXERCISES

1. Why is food processing necessary? Explain with suitable examples.
2. What type of undesirable changes in food can be controlled by food processing?
3. Describe the steps in the cook–chill process.
4. How can irradiation be used to preserve food?
5. Discuss the effect of heat processing on the nutritive value of food.
6. How do sugar and salt help in preserving food?
7. List five Class II preservatives which are permitted in food and name the food in which they are used.

8. Write notes on
   (a) Types of freezers
   (b) Types of radiation in food
   (c) Advantages of cook-freeze system
   (d) Steps in canning food
9. Discuss the role of food additives in the food processing industry.
10. What is E numbering and why is it necessary?
11. Classify the different additives used in the food industry with one example for each of category.

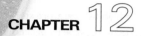
Evaluation of Food

LEARNING OBJECTIVES

After reading this chapter, you should be able to
- understand the importance of evaluating food before it is formally launched in the market
- know the different types of evaluation and the various tests conducted
- define and differentiate between different tests
- select the proper test or technique for evaluating specific characteristics
- appreciate the special environmental conditions and precautions to be followed for accuracy in test results
- understand the limitations of both subjective and objective tests

INTRODUCTION

Food is constantly being rated for its quality either consciously or sub-consciously by all people. Consumers choose food on the basis of its quality and their individual likes and dislikes. The attractiveness of food is clearly a quality which is important both to the manufacturer and to the consumer. When consumers make a selection, they basically look for food that is attractive in terms of colour, flavour, and texture, apart from other psychological and social factors which they may associate with food. The nutritional quality and shelf life or keeping quality and cost factor are other criteria which may affect their selection.

The distinctive and attractive colours of food are not only pleasing but an indicator of good quality and freshness. The senses of taste and odour help us in detecting and appreciating different flavours and deciding on whether we like the food. The feel and texture of food entering the mouth be it firm, juicy, crisp, or bland are extremely important characteristics that dictate the acceptance of a food. Today's consumers are discerning, demanding, and more knowledgeable about food. They expect products that are safe, of good value, and of high sensory quality. Therefore, knowing consumer's preferences and perceptions of the sensory characteristics of food and beverage products is vital to food manufacturers as well as caterers.

Without appropriate evaluation, there is a high risk of market failure.

Importance of evaluation to the food industry

1. The food industry depends on evaluation in developing new products and maintaining quality in existing products.
2. How the consumer reacts to a particular food dictates the quality to be produced.
3. Catering supervisors in institutional food service depend on evaluation to identify changes in menus to make food acceptable.
4. Studies of plate waste provide valuable information regarding food acceptability.
5. To assist in determining the shelf life of a product.
6. To understand how their product performs against competitors products.
7. To determine whether or not consumers can detect differences between products due to recipe modification.

METHODS OF EVALUATION

Scientific methods of evaluation of food are gaining importance in assessing the acceptability of food products. Methods of evaluation can be broadly categorized into two categories: subjective evaluation and objective evaluation. These categories are further classied in Fig. 12.1.

Subjective Evaluation

This is carried out by a panel of individuals who are given a scoring system based on various characteristics that can be judged by using the senses. This evaluation is also called sensory, organoleptic, or psychometric evaluation. In subjective evaluation, distinctions among foods, i.e., either differences or preferences are obtained by our senses. Preference testing is valuable in developing new foods and in evaluating quality. Difference testing can be used to test the sensitivity of judges and to determine whether an inexpensive ingredient could replace an expensive ingredient in a recipe, e.g., if saffron essence could replace pure saffron strands in the sweet *shrikhand*. The type of information which is required should be clear as this will determine the type of test which needs to be conducted.

Preference tests

These tests are designed to provide information on selected characteristics and to indicate preference or acceptability of products.

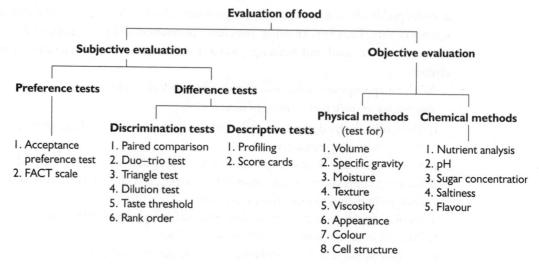

Fig. 12.1   Classification of methods of evaluation

Acceptance preference test

In this method, a single sample or two samples may be tested. It is used to find out whether a product will be used by consumers and this also shows their preference for the sample being tested. If a new food is introduced, only one sample is offered to the consumer panel, but if a food is modified then two samples are offered and their preference is requested.

The consumer panel is made up of untrained, inexperienced judges who represent a segment of the population for whom the product is being introduced, e.g., if the product is ready-to-eat chicken biryani, the panel would consist of housewives and young working professionals. The size of the panel should be about 50 to 100 people to avoid any experimental error.

The hedonic scale is most commonly used for evaluation. Hedonic relates to pleasant and unpleasant states of an organism. In this scale, ratings of preference or liking and disliking are measured. This scale is generally used with untrained assessors. The verbal hedonic scale consists of a nine point scale with phrases such as like extremely to dislike extremely (Fig. 12.2).

1	2	3	4	5	6	7	8	9
Dislike extremely	Dislike very much	Dislike moderately	Dislike slightly	Neither like nor dislike	Like slightly	Like moderately	Like very much	Like extremely

Fig. 12.2   Verbal hedonic scale

The facial hedonic scale consists of 5, 7, or 9 faces depicting varying degrees of pleasure and displeasure. It may be used when young children with limited reading ability form the panelist (Fig. 12.3).

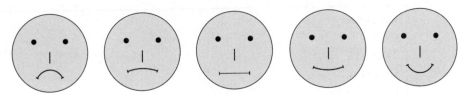

Fig. 12.3 Facial hedonic scale

Disadvantages The hedonic scale indicates likes or dislikes for a specific characteristic of food such as colour, flavour, or texture. It does not indicate change in intensity of that characteristic.

Food action rating scale (FACT scale)

The fact test is a more sensitive method made up of a nine point food action rating scale. The codes used clearly indicate the action the panelist would take regarding the food being tested, i.e., how often the subject would like to eat the food.

In addition, the respondent may indicate that a food was never tried.

Preference frequency scales are of two types. One scale uses verbal categories of frequencies, as shown in Fig. 12.4, and the other uses quantitative categories, as shown in Fig. 12.5.

These tests should supplement the hedonic scale.

Difference testing

These tests are designed to determine whether the difference in two or more food products can be detected. The results of these tests are more precise and reproducible.

Name _____   Department _____
Date _____   Booth _____
Code
I would eat this at every opportunity
I would eat this very often
I would frequently eat this
I like this and would eat it now and then
I would eat this if available but would not go out of my way
I do not like it, but would eat it on occasion
I would hardly ever eat this
I would eat this only if there were no other food choices
I would not eat this even if I were forced to
Never tried
Comments _____
Code _____

Fig. 12.4 Food attitude rating form for FACT method

Categories
Often
Twice a day
Once a day
Every other day
Twice a week
Once a week
Every other week
Once a month
Every 3 months
Once a year
Never

Fig. 12.5 Quantitative categories

Difference tests are basically of two types: discrimination tests and descriptive tests.

Discrimination tests The discrimination tests are explained below.

Paired comparison In this test, two samples are presented together and one has to judge the difference in the samples regarding a specific characteristic and identify the sample with the greater level of characteristic being measured. For example, a sweeter piece of cake in comparison with a standard cake. The judge has a 50 per cent chance of being right.

Duo–trio test In this test, three samples are to be tested of which two are control samples and one is the variable sample (Fig. 12.6). One of the control samples is presented first, followed by two other samples, and the judge is requested to identify which of the two samples is different from the control. The chances of guessing correctly is 50 per cent.

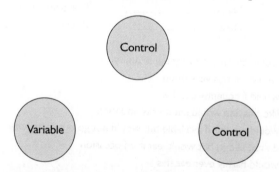

Fig. 12.6 Presentation of samples in a duo–tri test

Triangle test Three samples are given, and all the three are presented together (see Fig. 12.7). The judge is asked to identify the odd sample. Chances of guessing correctly is 33 per cent. The judge may be asked to indicate any distinguishing feature in the odd sample. Of the three samples, two are similar and one is different.

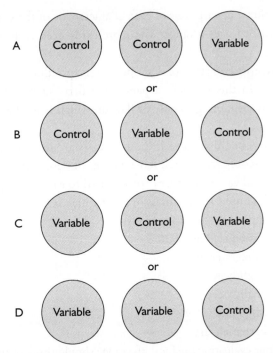

Fig. 12.7 Presentation of samples in a triangle test

Dilution test This test is used to measure the quality of an ingredient which has been substituted. A standard sample is presented to the judges followed by other samples which may or may not contain the unknown at a definite level of dilution, e.g., use of dried egg powder with fresh eggs. Higher the quality of the dried egg powder, greater will be the difficulty in detecting it. A poor-quality product would be detected at low concentration or high dilution.

Taste threshold test This test determines the lowest concentration of a substance that can be detected. It also indicates the lowest concentration of a substance required to be able to identify it. The taste threshold of sweet, salty, sour, and bitter tastes can be detected.

Rank order In this test, a series of samples are ranked in increasing or decreasing order of intensity for a specific characteristic. This test is done when several samples need to be evaluated for a single characteristic, e.g., pineapple flavour in pineapple souffle. Ranking gives the direction for the difference, but does not measure the degree of difference. Numerical values may be given to ranks and the highest value indicates the best product.

Descriptive tests These tests describe the sensory attributes of food in exact words and the judge/evaluator is asked to select the exact word description from the score card which matches with the sample. These tests are superior to preference tests which provide information about acceptability of a food sample and discrimination tests which detect deviations between samples.

Accurate descriptions of each characteristic of the sample to be evaluated by the judges is described over a range. The score cards need to be carefully designed for descriptive testing.

There are two types of descriptive tests: profiling and score cards.

Profiling In this method, a panel of experts sit together and formulate a very detailed word description, generally of flavour, which is used as a standard for evaluating further products.

Score cards In this method, food samples are individually evaluated by judges with the help of score cards which have a series of descriptive terms or levels of a characteristic. Numerical values or scores are assigned to each descriptive term.

For example, the juiciness of meat which is a textural characteristic is evaluated on the basis of one of the following terms:

- Extremely juicy   –   6
- Moderately juicy   –   5
- Slightly juicy   –   4
- Slightly dry   –   3
- Moderately dry   –   2
- Extremely dry   –   1

While evaluating the food, the judge should think of the appropriate descriptive adjective and take a decision and not decide on the basis of the score. It is preferable not to mention the numerical score on the score card which is given to the evaluator. All score cards should have columns to fill the name of the judge and date of evaluation, and this should be filled in advance.

Score cards need to be designed for all recipes which use descriptive terms.

The following are the points to be kept in mind while preparing score cards.

(i) Select the different characteristics of a food product which need to be evaluated, e.g., appearance, colour, flavour, and texture.

(ii) Select appropriate descriptive terms pertaining to the characteristics chosen, and arrange in sequence.

(iii) Give numerical values to the descriptive terms.

(iv) All products which are to be evaluated should be given a code. Codes should be in the form of geometric shapes, such as △, ○, and □, colours, or randomly selected three digit numbers such as 519, 267, or 483. Avoid codes such as 123 or ABC as they suggest first choice.

(v) Standard specifications for a standard high-quality product should be described. The standard specifications for a soup, cream of tomato, are listed in Fig. 12.8.

(vi) Score cards could be descriptive (Fig. 12.9) or they could utilize hedonic ratings (Fig.12.10) as depicted in sample score cards.

Appearance	Steaming hot garnished with a swirl of cream/croutons/parsley
Colour	Light orange red
Texture	Croutons crisp and bite size
Consistency	Smooth thin cream consistency should lightly coat the back of the spoon
Flavour/taste	Distinct tomato flavour, well seasoned

Format for tabulation of scores

Characteristic	Max score	Evaluated score	Comments
Appearance			
Colour			
Texture/consistency			
Flavour/taste			

Fig. 12.8 Specifications for a standard product—cream of tomato

Product: Cream of tomato

Name: ....
Date: ....

Characteristic	Descriptive rating			
	(encircle the term that best describes each characteristic)			
Presentation/ appearance	No garnish	Fat floating on surface	Well garnished/ bite-sized croutons/swirl of cream/parsley	Heavy garnish large croutons
Colour	Pale	Orange	Light orange red	Bright red
Texture	Croutons light in colour	Croutons soggy	Croutons golden brown crisp	Croutons dark brown burnt
Consistency	Thin and watery	Curdled	Smooth thin cream	Thick and lumpy
Flavour	Raw flour taste	Mild tomato flavour	Distinct tomato flavour	Strong flavour
Taste	Less seasoning	Excess pepper	Well seasoned	Excess salt

Note: The numerical scores are not mentioned on the score card but have been assigned and are tabulated after evaluation is over.

Fig. 12.9 Score card using descriptive ratings

Product: Cream of tomato

Name: ....
Date: ....

Characteristic	Sample		
	□	△	○
Presentation/ appearance			
Colour			
Texture/consistency			
Flavour/taste			

Scale   5 – Very good
         4 – Good
         3 – Fair
         2 – Poor
         1 – Very poor

Fig. 12.10 Score card using hedonic ratings

The environment for conducting sensory tests is detailed here.

1. Separate sensory booths should be provided so that judges do not interact with each other except when preparing profiles because judges work together to develop vocabulary needed to describe food samples.
2. Controlled air and lighting so that food is correctly visible and booth is free from odours other than those from the sample. Temperature should be comfortable and non-smoking zone observed.
3. Small sinks should be provided for spitting out samples or rinsing ones mouth when meat is to be evaluated for tenderness.

The sample preparation and presentation process is described below.

1. Samples should be of identical size.
2. They should be identical in shape or from identical portions, e.g., edge of cake from one sample and centre slice from another sample should not be taken.
3. It should be served at the customary serving temperature, e.g., a soup should be served hot.
4. Sample plates should be marked with a wax pencil.
5. Plates or containers used should be of identical size, and colour.
6. Necessary cutlery, glass of water at room temperature should be provided.
7. Only a limited number of samples should be evaluated at a time to avoid fatigue and for efficient judging. If possible a control sample should be evaluated.

The requirements of the members of the panel are described below:

1. The judge should neither be too hungry or too well fed.
2. Smoking, chewing gum, or nibbling snacks 20 minutes prior to the test should not be permitted.
3. The judges should be healthy and not suffering from a cold as this will affect their senses of taste and smell.

Objective Evaluation

Objective methods of evaluation of food consist of various physical and chemical tests to measure physical features, such as volume, viscosity, and specific gravity, and chemical composition such as nutrients present and pH of food. These tests supplement the data obtained through sensory evaluation. These tests are necessary because sensory tests rely on panelists who may sometimes present highly variable results. Personal problems related to health or emotional upsets may have a major influence on the individuals ability to evaluate food. To overcome the human error in evaluation, additional data in the form of objective tests is necessary.

Plate 1

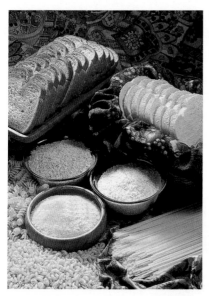

Cereals and cereal products include a variety of bread, wheat, rice, and pastas (Chapter 4, page 53).

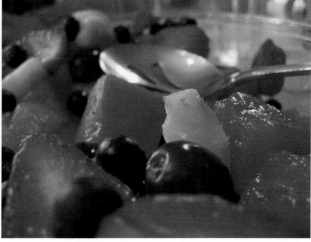

Natural colouring pigments flavonoids and carotenoids present in strawberries, black grapes, melons, and pineapples add colour to our meals (Chapter 6, page 97).

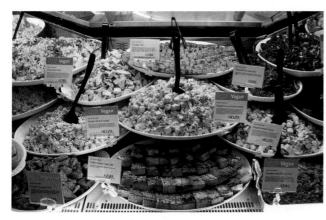

Tofu prepared from soya bean is a good alternative to *paneer* and chicken in a vegan diet (Chapter 13, page 211).

Plate 2

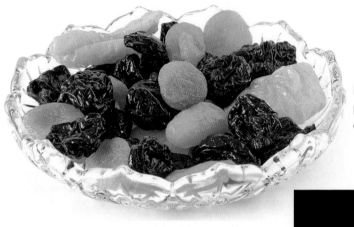

Dry fruits such as apricots and prunes are rich in fibre and prevent constipation (Chapter 15, page 243).

Luncheon meat, cheese, cakes, biscuits, doughnuts, wafers, and crispy snacks are all high-fat foods (Chapter 17, page 273).

All fresh citrus fruits are excellent sources of vitamin C (Chapter 19, page 295).

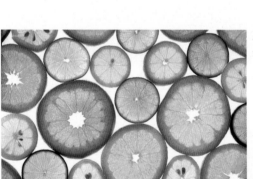

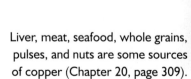

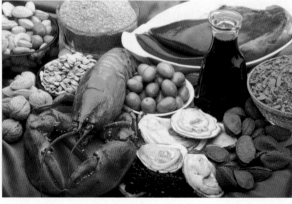

Liver, meat, seafood, whole grains, pulses, and nuts are some sources of copper (Chapter 20, page 309).

Plate 3

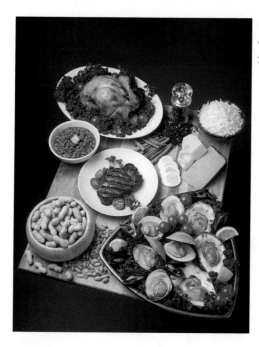

Liver, peanuts, cheese, oysters, seafood, eggs, and wholegrains are sources of zinc (Chapter 20, page 309).

Fats, butter, and oil should be used sparingly by an obese individual (Chapter 21, page 326).

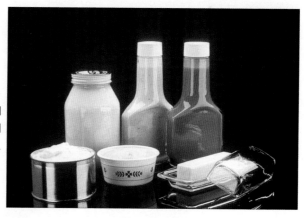

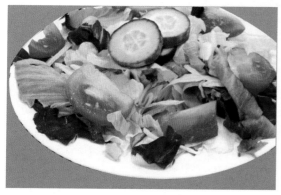

A salad platter is part of a low-energy-density meal recommended for all individuals. It is specially included in a weight-reduction diet (Chapter 21, page 326).

Plate 4

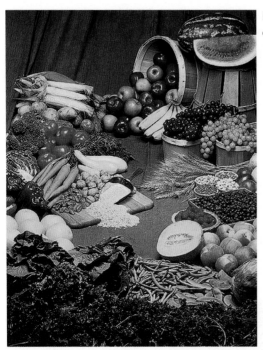

Include a variety of fresh foods in your daily diet (Chapter 22, page 330).

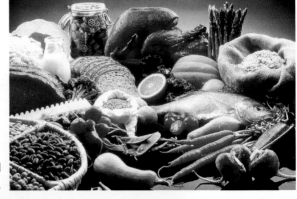

A balanced diet includes foodstuff from all food groups (Chapter 23, page 345).

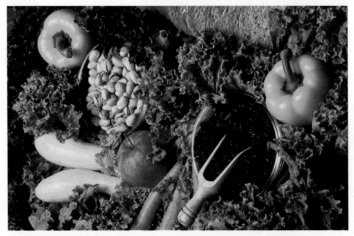

Carotene-rich fruits and vegetables are important sources of vitamins, fibre, and nutraceuticals in a vegetarian diet (Chapter 25, page 394).

Objective tests are important because of the following:

1. They do not depend on human senses.
2. They are more reliable as they are less subject to error.
3. If the test chosen is appropriate, then the results will agree with those of sensory evaluation.
4. Well-maintained, accurate testing devices are necessary.

Physical methods

These methods include the following tests.

Test for volume

Seed displacement Volume of firm food products can be determined by displacement. The volumeter is used for measuring volume by seed displacement (see Fig. 12.11). In the volumeter, the volume of seeds in a closed system is determined with and without the sample. The actual volume of the sample is the difference between the two measurements. This method is used mainly for baked products such as cakes and bread.

Volumeter

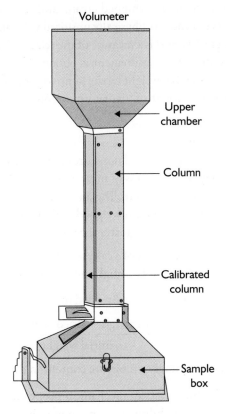

Upper chamber

Column

Calibrated column

Sample box

Fig. 12.11   Volumeter

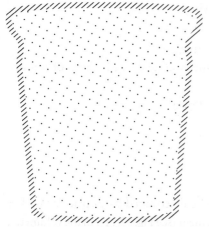

Fig. 12.12   Imprint of the inked sample of bread on paper

Disadvantage: The test can be conducted only after the product is 24-hours old.

Index to volume   This is an indirect means of comparing volume by measuring the circumference of a cross-section of the product. It is essential that the slice be taken from exactly the same portion on each sample. A detailed outline is traced by a pointed pencil or by making an inkblot or a photocopy of the slice. A planimeter is then used to trace the entire outline of the sample making sure that all indentations and protrusions are recorded, and the final measurement on the planimeter represents the exact circumference of the slice.

The inkblot is made by pressing the food sample onto an inkpad and making the imprint of the inked sample on paper (see Fig. 12.12).

Specific gravity test   This test indicates the amount of air incorporated into products such as egg white foam, whipped cream, and cake batters. This test is used for comparing the lightness of products physically unsuited to volume measurements.

Specific gravity (SG) is a measure of the relative density (RD) of a food sample in relation to that of water. The measurement is obtained by weighing a given volume of the sample and then dividing that weight by the same volume of water. Low specific gravity and density indicates larger amount of air incorporation and is associated with good volume of the product.

Test for Moisture

Press fluids   The juiciness and moisture content of a food sample can be judged subjectively and objectively. The juiciness of meat, poultry, and fish is measured by the succulometer, a machine that applies pressure. The amount of pressure applied and length of time applied for is measured. The sample is weighed both before and after pressure has been applied. The greater the weight loss, the greater the juiciness of the sample.

Wettability   It is the ability of a cake or other food to absorb moisture during a controlled period of time (5 seconds). High moisture retention means good wettability.

Drying oven   Food is gradually dried in an oven till its weight is constant.

$$\text{Moisture content} = \frac{\text{initial weight} - \text{dried weight} \times 100}{\text{initial weight}} = \text{moisture \%}$$

This gives percentage of moisture content in the sample.

Texture   Texture refers to mechanical properties of tenderness, hardness, cohesiveness, adhesiveness, fracturability, viscosity, gumminess, springiness, and chewiness. Objective methods for determining texture should reflect the action of the mouth in ingesting the food, action of tongue and jaw in moving food, action of teeth in cutting, tearing, shearing, grinding, and squeezing food.

Penetrometer   It is used to measure tenderness of some foods, e.g., meat. The instrument is provided with a heavy cone, the action of which stimulates the biting action of the teeth. The force required to shear the meat sample which is cylindrical in shape is recorded on a scale and this determines the texture. The tenderness of gels and baked products may also be measured this way (see Fig. 12.13).

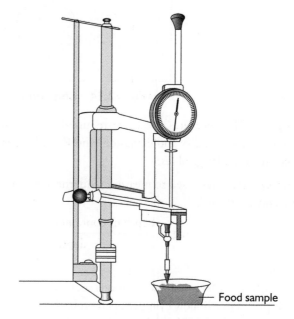

Food sample

Fig. 12.13   Penetrometer

Tensile strength   This is the amount of force required to pull apart a small sample of meat.

The force required to pull apart the meat sample when the fibres are parallel to the force gives the strength of the muscle fibre.

Puncture testing   This determines the texture of fruits and vegetables, i.e., the firmness of the tissue. It measures the amount of force required to penetrate a sample to a specific depth.

Shortometer   This determines the texture of a baked product, e.g., cookies, crackers, and pastries. The pastry or wafer is placed across two horizontal bars. A single horizontal bar is brought down by means of a motor until it breaks the wafer and the force is recorded. Shortometer values are highly correlated with sensory values for tenderness (see Fig. 12.14).

Compressimeter   The firmness or softness of a cooked product can be measured by this instrument. The force required to compress a food sample to a predetermined amount is measured. The greater the force, the firmer is the product.

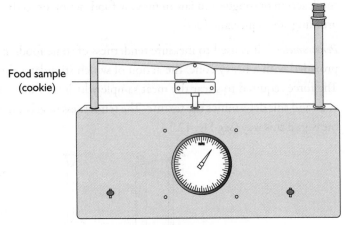

Food sample
(cookie)

Fig. 12.14   Shortometer

Shear press   This measures the force required to cut through a baked product. It also measures compressibility and extrusion, and is used for measuring textural characteristics of some fruits and vegetables.

Percent sag   It is a test used to measure tenderness of a gel. The greater the percent sag, the more tender is the gel.

$$\text{Percent sag} = \frac{\text{depth in container} - \text{depth on plate} \times 100}{\text{depth in container}}$$

Viscosity

Line spread test   This is suitable for foods such as white sauce, starch puddings, and batters. Food is placed in a hollow cylinder open on both ends in the centre of the template. When the food has reached the desired temperature, the cylinder is lifted and the product is allowed to spread for a specific period of time (30 seconds to 2 minutes). Consistency is measured in distance (centimetre) spread in a fixed period of time on all four lines, i.e., at 90° intervals, and the mean of all four values is the line spread (see Fig. 12.15).

Amylograph   This is used for determining the viscosity of starch pastes at controlled, selective temperatures.

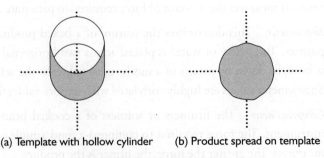

(a) Template with hollow cylinder   (b) Product spread on template

Fig. 12.15   Line spread test

Farinograph It determines the consistency of a dough, thereby predicting the quality of the final product.

Viscometer This is a device for measuring viscosity of liquids that flow.

Jelmeter It measures the adequacy of the pectin content of fruit juices used to make jams and jellies.

Test for appearance   This includes photograph, photocopy, and ink print method.

Photograph This furnishes a record of size if scales are included in the picture (Fig. 12.16). The grain of the baked product is visible if lighting has been carefully controlled.

Photocopy This furnishes actual size and shape of a sliced or halved baked product. It also indicates grain. The sliced samples are arranged on a clear plastic film placed on the glass plate of the photocopying machine.

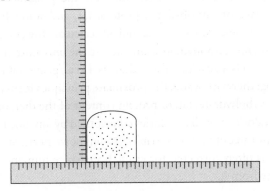

Fig. 12.16   Test for appearance (photograph)

Ink print method Refer the index to volume method.

Test for colour   The colour of the food sample is tested against a colour sample to match the colour of the food being identified.

A spectrophotometer and the Hunter colour difference metre is commonly used to identify food colours.

Test for cell structure   The cell structure of baked products is an important characteristic which can be measured by making photocopies of cross-sectional slices. The uniformity, size, and thickness of cell walls are revealed three dimensionally.

Chemical methods

Nutrient analysis   This is an important measurement of the nutrient content of food in terms of kilocalories, proteins, fat—saturated, trans fats, cholesterol; kilocalories from fat; carbohydrates, sugar, fibre, all vitamins, and minerals. The nutrients in the pack are chemically analysed using specific tests for each nutrient. The values are mentioned on the label as nutritive value per serving.

pH   pH paper or pH meter shows degree of acidity or alkalinity of the food.

Sugar concentration   Light is refracted as it passes through sugar solutions and is measured in degrees Brix. Refractometers can be used to determine the concentration of a sugar solution, which is a useful index while preparing preserves.

Saltiness   This can be analysed by flame photometry to measure sodium content.

Flavour   This is identified by measuring numerous volatile and non-volatile substances by chromatography, i.e., separation of discreet chemical compounds, although sensory tests are more suitable for flavour evaluation.

Proximate Composition of Food Constituents

Protein, carbohydrate, and fat are sometimes referred to as proximate principles. They are oxidized in the body to yield energy to meet the body's need.

For most foods, analytical data for the proximate composition is available, i.e., the percentage of carbohydrate, protein, fat, and water found in a typical food sample. By knowing these values, one can quickly calculate the energy value of a food.

Proteins, carbohydrates, and fats are the only nutrients which yield energy. Energy value of protein is 4 kcal/g, carbohydrate is 4 kcal/g, and fat is 9 kcal/g.

Together with water, the proximate principles form the bulk of the diet. By knowing the total carbohydrate, fat, or protein content of the diet, one can determine the percentage of total calories as well as calories contributed by any one nutrient. By knowing the sample size and any three of the four variables, the unknown nutrient can be calculated. The carbohydrate value is often corrected for crude fibre, since humans cannot digest fibre and do not get energy from it.

Proximate Analysis of Food Constituents

The proximate principles, namely, proteins, fats, and carbohydrates are chemically analysed. The value for fat in a food can be assessed directly by extracting the lipid chemically in ether, which is a fat solvent. Protein value is estimated by measuring the nitrogen content and the factor used is 6.25 for all foods as proteins contain 16 per cent nitrogen. The carbohydrate content given is the difference between 100 and the sum of moisture, protein, fat, crude fibre, and ash content.

SUMMARY

The consumer today is more well read and demanding about high-quality food and looks for products which are not only safe and wholesome but appealing and attractive. Evaluating foods for its sensory characteristics is of importance to both food manufacturers and caterers, and food likes and dislikes or preferences of consumers have to be considered to eliminate the risk of market failure.

Food is evaluated both subjectively as well as objectively. Subjective evaluation is done by a panel of individuals who are given a scoring system based on various characteristics such as appearance, texture, and flavour which can be judged by using the senses. Subjective tests include preference and difference testing methods. In difference testing methods, the judges are asked to discriminate between the samples offered or they may be based on a detailed description of the food being evaluated, and numerical values or scores are awarded to the descriptions. The environment for conducting these tests as well as selection of the judges and presentation of the samples should be as per set norms.

Objective tests are often conducted to supplement subjective analysis as they help in eliminating the human error which may arise in subjective tests. Objective tests require specialized techniques and equipment for each test. These tests are of two types, namely physical tests that test the volume, texture, viscosity, etc. and chemical tests that measure nutrient content, sugar concentration, etc. This information is necessary for nutrition labelling. Both subjective and objective tests have their own advantages as far as measuring food quality is concerned. The proximate principles namely proteins, carbohydrates, and fats along with water form the bulk of our food. By knowing these values, one can quickly and conveniently calculate the energy value of any food.

KEY TERMS

Farinograph   An instrument used for measuring the physical properties of a dough, i.e., time taken to make standard dough, time it can maintain consistency, and extent to which it falls on further mixing.

Hedonic   Pertaining to pleasure. Hedonic rating measures the degree of pleasure provided by the characteristic of food being evaluated.

Objective evaluation   Evaluation of various characteristics of food such as texture, viscosity, and colour by accurate testing devices, often used to supplement sensory evaluation.

Organoleptic   Affecting an organ or the senses; used to evaluate the taste and aroma of a food.

Used interchangeably with the term sensory or subjective evaluation.

Profiling   Detailed description of characteristics of food developed by trained panel experts, which is used as a standard for quality product evaluation.

Proximate analysis   Analysis of protein, fat, and ash content of food, and calculating carbohydrate content by subtracting the value obtained from the total. Carbohydrate value may be corrected for crude fibre.

Score card   Numerical evaluation of various characteristics of food on cards which are specific for each recipe with appropriate descriptive terms for which numerical scores are assigned.

REVIEW EXERCISES

1. Why is sensory evaluation of importance to the food industry?
2. Describe the environment necessary for conducting sensory tests.
3. What precautions should you take while
   (a) Selecting the panel
   (b) Preparing and presenting the sample
4. Differentiate between
   (a) Subjective evaluation and objective evaluation
   (b) Preference testing and difference testing
   (c) Profiling and scoring
   (d) Duo–trio test and triangle test

5. Design a score card for any recipe you have prepared in the food production practical class.
6. Which technique would you select for measuring the following?
   (a) Volume of cake
   (b) Tenderness of meat
   (c) Crispness of biscuits
   (d) Tenderness of lemon souffle
   (e) Sugar concentration in jam
7. Why should objective evaluation of food supplement subjective or sensory evaluation?

CHAPTER 13

New Trends in Foods

LEARNING OBJECTIVES

After reading this chapter, you should be able to
- understand the importance of evaluating food before it is formally launched in the market
- identify trends in food selection
- understand the benefits of the present-day techniques of food processing
- list various products made from soya beans and their benefits
- understand the exaggerated claims made with respect to certain foods
- describe the latest packaging techniques available in the food industry

INTRODUCTION

Our eating habits have changed dramatically in the last decade. Food is no longer just a source of energy but a sensory, cultural, and social phenomenon. With the number of working couples on the rise, the trend to prepare elaborate menus at home is fast fading away. We look for food which is enjoyable, healthy, tasty, convenient to purchase, and quick to prepare. It should be available all year round in the nearest supermarket and reasonably priced.

Technological developments in the food processing industry and recent research has made it possible to choose from an enormous variety of high-quality food products to suit every budget and group or community.

Our lifestyle and eating habits have undergone a radical change, creating an imbalance between calorie intake and physical activity. Medical science is emphasizing the increased risk for chronic illnesses and debilitating diseases particularly cardiovascular diseases, obesity, osteoporosis, diabetes, and cancer striking at an earlier age. In this backdrop, the common man has realized the importance of certain food ingredients in influencing our body functions, and we hear people discussing things such as cholesterol, whey proteins, omega-3 fatty acids, and fibre. These discoveries are having an impact on our eating habits, and the trend is towards health foods and natural foods. Market analysis of consumer forecasts that in the next few years special health-enhancing foods will form a part of every product group. For example, cooking oil with natural antioxidants such as vitamin A, carotene, and vitamin E, which imparts a natural golden yellow colour to fried foods and is devoid of trans fats, being 100 per cent natural and 100 per cent vegan. Priced at a much higher rate than cooking oil, it will be used by affluent societies because it is natural, healthy, environment friendly, and packaged in an attractive bottle.

Plants with a fat composition beneficial for health are being bred, e.g, rapeseed oil with a low erucic acid content. The fatty acid composition of oils can be selectively modified with health enhancing effects. The health conscious consumer today demands lighter dishes, less fat, sugar, and salt. Food additives, especially added colours and flavours, are viewed suspiciously and natural foods are chosen. There is also an increasing trend towards vegetarianism.

Vegan diet is 100 per cent plant-based vegetarian diet, which if well planned may offer protection against many degenerative disenerative diseases. It excludes all dairy products as they are derived from animal soures.

SOYA FOODS

Soya bean, the golden bean, is used to prepare soya milk, soya *paneer* or tofu, herbal tofu, *shrikhand*, *amrakhand*, patties, kebabs, cheese spread, and textured vegetable protein (refer Chapter 5 on Proteins). With extrusion techniques, good-quality meat analogues can be produced from textured vegetable protein. Tofu is a good alternative to *paneer* and chicken in a vegan diet (see Plate 1). Soya milk is the basis for manufacturing the wide range of dairy products mentioned previously. Soya milk is extracted from soya beans by processing in an equipment called soya cow.

Benefits of consuming soya products

1. Soya milk is lactose free and can be digested by people who are lactose intolerant.
2. Soya milk has twice the protein of cow's milk and half the fat content.
3. Soya milk is cholesterol free.
4. It contains isoflavones which provide the following benefits.

   (a) Facilitate absorption of calcium and prevent osteoporosis
   (b) Retard the aging process
   (c) Raise HDL cholesterol and reduce LDL cholesterol levels
   (d) Protect the heart
   (e) Provide protection against growth of cancer cells

Soya milk can replace whole milk in preparations such as curds, *raita*, *lassi*, or *kadhi*. The meal left after extraction of soya milk can be used in cutlets, *koftas*, etc. Soya beans should always be processed prior to use to destroy the trypsin inhibitor present in the raw bean. The beans may be boiled whole in their green pod, or sprouted and used in dishes. Soya beans are classified as oilseeds as they contain approximately 20 per cent oil.

Lecithin, a phospholipid and an emulsifying agent, is extracted from soya bean and used as a thickening agent in yoghurt and as an emulsifier in mayonnaise. It has many applications in the food industry.

FOOD FADS

The consumer today is more health conscious and aware of the consequences of eating junk food, and does not mind spending more for foods available in special stores in posh shopping malls which make tall claims in curing diseases and maintaining vigour and vitality.

Millions of people around the globe fall prey to food faddists and quacks who ascribe special curative properties to foods. Foods such as raw milk, yoghurt, stone-ground wheat flour, wheat germ, sea salt, and vegetable juices are said to have miraculous properties for promoting good health. The food faddist criticizes the food available in the market as being inferior in nutritive value because of being subjected to chemical fertilizers, pesticides, different processing methods, and added chemicals in the form of additives. The use of health foods, live foods, natural foods, and organic foods available at an added premium is being widely promoted. If we compare the nutritive value and shelf life of pasteurized milk vis-à-vis unpasteurized raw milk, the former will be superior. Similarly, stone-ground wheat flour and whole meal flour milled with 100 per cent extraction would be comparable; the latter being readily available to the consumer.

The foods with exaggerated claims which are available in the market today are organic foods, health foods, natural foods, and live foods.

ORGANIC FOODS

Organic foods in Europe are those foods which are produced in accordance with legally regulated standards. For plant foods, it means crops grown on soils that have been treated only with organic matter, i.e., manures and plant compost. It also means that no conventional pesticides, artificial fertilizers, or sewage sludge has been used, and that they have been processed without ionizing radiations or food additives.

For animal food, it means milk or meat obtained from animals that have been fed no antibiotics or hormones.

Organic food initially was the produce obtained from small family run farms and was available only in farmers' markets. Now special stores in supermarkets and malls sell organic foods to the health-conscious affluent consumers at higher prices as compared to the conventional fare. The sales at organic food stores are growing rapidly every year.

Consumers are gradually turning towards organic foods because they are environment friendly. Apart form health concerns, it is also a social priority. The organic foods market lacks a good distribution network, the quality of organic produce is variable, and the cost of organic food is high, which make it difficult for the caterer to incorporate these products in their day-to-day menus.

The consumer selects organic produce because it contains fewer contaminants and not for its nutritional value. A better approach for the future would be towards environment friendly food products and processes, rather than emphasizing on organic foods, live foods, or health foods. Environment friendly practices would include

1. Converting biodegradable waste into vermicompost by vermiculture
2. Limiting the use of fertilizers and pesticide sprays
3. Using environment friendly packaging material
4. Using processes which save electricity and water.

HEALTH FOODS

Health foods are defined as foods which are believed to be highly beneficial to health, especially foods grown organically and free from chemical additives.

NATURAL FOODS

Natural foods are those foods which have come straight from the farm. They have not been processed or refined in any way and contain no additives. They may or may not have been organically grown. They are similar to live foods.

LIVE FOODS

Live foods are raw foods which have not been heated above a certain temperature and include raw fruits, vegetables, seeds, unpasteurized dairy products, eggs, meat, and honey. These foods contain enzymes which are released in the mouth when vegetables are chewed. These enzymes along with the enzymes from our digestive system enhance the process of digestion.

Fruits and vegetables are physiologically active even after they are harvested. Enzymatic and respiratory processes continue to take place. This can be seen by the ripening of green fruits and the moisture which collects if vegetables are stored in unperforated plastic bags. This loss of moisture from fruits and vegetables is called transpiration. Whole grains and seeds are also live foods. When they are soaked in water and sprouted, we see signs of life in them.

The caterer should understand that the additional virtues ascribed to these foods does not justify the additional price which one has to pay to obtain these foods. Modern techniques of food processing retain most of the nutritive value of food and restore the losses of vitamins due to processing. Food substitutes like margarine instead of butter is fortified with vitamins A and D. Modern processing techniques increase the safety of food, e.g., pasteurization of milk and other dairy products destroys pathogenic bacteria and increases the shelf life of milk. Processing prevents wastage of food by preserving excess for later use.

Good nutrition and balanced meals which include a variety of foodstuff is a better and economical option for all caterers.

NEW TRENDS IN PACKAGING

Safe and attractive packaging today is as important as the contents of the pack. Along with advances in the field of food processing, new convenient methods of packaging are available which meet all the criteria of a package, namely, to contain, preserve, protect, present, and dispense the product while maintaining quality, and being easy to transport and store. The consumer today is looking for an elegant pack which is light in weight, unbreakable, easy to store or transfer contents from, maintains freshness, and has a good shelf life. The desirable attributes of a package are:

1. It should be attractive.
2. It should be easy to open and close without requiring an additional opener.
3. It should have a tamper-proof seal.
4. It should be easy to dispense.
5. Instructions for use should be clearly spelt out.
6. Warnings, ingredients, and preservatives, if any, should be clearly mentioned.
7. Nutritive value of the contents should be listed with number of servings and serving size.
8. Percentage of recommended dietary allowances (RDAs) provided by a serving is a desirable feature.
9. The package should be recyclable.
10. The package should be convenient to carry.

Aseptic Packaging

This is the most popular form of packaging used today. In this process, the food to be packed is sterilized and then packed in a sterile container. Such packages can be stored without refrigeration for one to three months. This method is superior to canning because of the following reasons

1. Natural flavour and nutrients are better retained as heat treatment time is much lesser.
2. Cost of the container, i.e., foil lined cartons, plastic cups, and plastic bags is less.
3. Weight of the pack is also less.
4. It is cheaper than canning.
5. Convenience in storage and opening the pack.

The food to be packaged is subjected to rapid heating in a heat exchanger. Fluid products are pumped continuously through heat exchangers so that the desired temperature is reached very quickly. The liquid food is held at the temperature recommended for commercial sterilization for a prescribed time and cooled rapidly. It is immediately filled into sterile containers in an aseptic filling zone.

Some foods are sold in modern flexible and semi-rigid packaging made of plastic paper board and aluminium foil. Milk and fruit juices packaged by this technology are available in tetrapack containers which have an ambient shelf life of three to six months. Once opened, the pack must be refrigerated and used within five days. The most recent additions are homogenous and particle containing desserts, several brands of soups, sauces, and ready meals containing meat and vegetables.

If aseptic conditions are not maintained, the major potential hazard for acidic food is spoilage by yeast and mould, and for low-acid foods. The microorganism *Clostridium botulinum* could grow causing botulism food poisoning.

Modified Atmosphere Packaging (MAP)

Modified atmosphere packaging is defined as 'the replacement of air in a pack by a mixture of different gases' such as oxygen, nitrogen, and carbon dioxide, whose proportion is fixed when introduced but no further measures are taken to control the percentage during storage.

Originally known as controlled atmosphere packaging, it is used to extend the shelf life of fresh food by two to three times. In this method, the atmosphere within food packages is replaced by a gas or a specific mixture of gases to inhibit the growth of harmful micro-organisms. Mixtures of purified carbon dioxide, nitrogen, and oxygen are used to extend the length of refrigerated storage time. The percentage of various gases depends on the food being preserved.

Carbon dioxide inhibits the growth of pathogenic bacteria if stored at a temperature below 8°C. It is used for bakery products as it prevents the product from drying up and spoilage by mould.

Nitrogen gas is used in 100 per cent strength in packages containing dairy products.

Oxygen is used to prevent growth of anaerobic bacteria.

Because of increased consumer demand for fresh and chilled convenience foods with fewer preservatives, there has been a significant increase in the range of products packaged in modified atmospheres. These include raw and cooked foods such as red meat, fish, poultry, bacon, cheese, bakery products, fresh pasta, potato crisps, tea, and coffee.

The advantages of MAP are

1. Enhanced shelf life
2. Economic losses are minimized

3. Chemical preservatives need not be added or are used in small amounts
4. Improved presentation—customer has a clear view of product
5. High-quality product is available.

The further developments in MAP are

1. Development of smart films which have the ability to absorb or emit gases and vapour
2. Combination of other preservation methods along with MAP
3. Designing retail packs which are resealable and microwave proof
4. Use of indicators which change colour to indicate if package has been opened or damaged.

EDIBLE FILMS

Food materials need to be protected from loss of volatile flavour and reaction with other food ingredients, moisture, and oxygen when they are stored in intimate mixtures. Edible film forms a protective package or coating around the food particle or piece. It forms a primary package or part of the food itself.

The film could be in the form of a thin layer of maize protein zein, starch, gelatin, or gum arabic which is flavoured, or in the form of confectionery glaze used on desserts or coating nuts with monoglyceride derivatives to prevent oxidative rancidity.

Edible films have a wide variety of applications. The films may be cast into small packets which can hold ingredients and which dissolve on addition of water to release the ingredients. Edible films require an outer wrapper to protect it from contamination.

 ## SUMMARY

The food processing industry is growing at a rapid pace to provide meals to the millions in a variety of packages available off the shelf. With food products being available all year round because of innovative processing and packaging techniques, the health conscious consumer is offered an array of health foods, organic foods, natural foods, or live foods. These foods are claimed to have curative properties and special health benefits. Most of these are natural, with minimum processing and use of pesticides or chemical additives. The consumer does not mind paying an additional price for the benefits it claims to offer. However, the educated consumer should be able to select cost-effective foods as these special foods do not have added nutritive value but reduced contaminants. By selecting a meal wisely and ensuring variety in selection, a balanced wholesome meal can be planned without spending extra on organic or natural foods purchased from select stores.

In the packaging industry, there has been a revolution as it is now possible to store perishables such as whole milk at room temperature safely for a couple of months. By modifying the atmosphere inside the food package, it is possible to extend the shelf life further. Edible films are extensively being used to retain flavour, moisture, and crispness in ready-to-eat foods.

KEY TERMS

Aseptic packaging   Filling aseptic packages with commercially sterilized food under aseptic conditions which can be stored at ambient temperature.

Edible film   A thin protective coating around food particles or small pieces which keep the packed contents intact when food is stored in intimate mixtures.

Food fad   A style of eating which remains in vogue for a short time.

MAP   Modified atmosphere packaging in which air in the package is replaced by a mixture of purified gases to prevent microbial spoilage and extend shelf life.

Pathogen   Disease producing microorganism.

Trans fat   A fat having a higher melting point than its cis form because hydrogen is attached to the carbon atoms on either end of the double bond from opposite directions.

Vegans   Strict vegetarian diet which includes only plant foods.

Vermiculture   Conversion of organic waste into a highly enriched biofertilizer by bacteria present in the gut of special species of earthworm.

REVIEW EXERCISES

1. Why are soya-based products recommended in our diet? List the different products available to the consumer.
2. Why do you think food fads occur? What are the present fads among the affluent?
3. Discuss the concept of modified atmosphere packaging.
4. Why does a tetrapack carton of juice not spoil at room temperature?

5. Edible films are used in a vast variety of products. Name any four products you have tasted which use this technology.
6. Define the following terms:
   (a) Live food
   (b) Organic food
   (c) Health food
   (d) Vegan diet

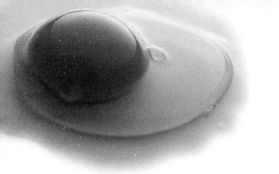

PART TWO

Nutrition

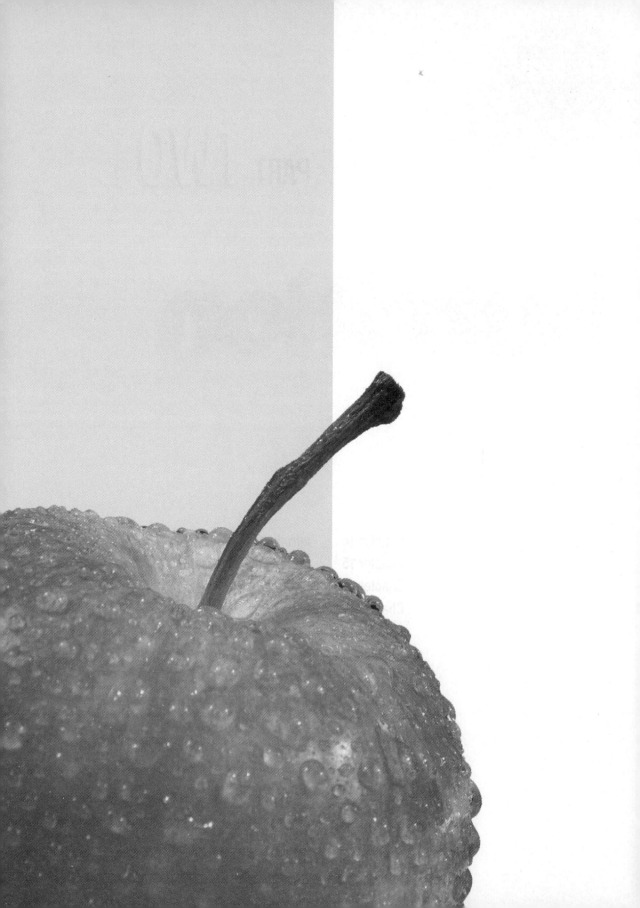

CHAPTER 14

Introduction to Nutrition

Learning Objectives

After reading this chapter, you should be able to
- understand the significance of food in our daily life
- distinguish between the functions of food and various nutrients
- define the terms food, health, nutrition, malnutrition, and nutritional status
- classify the various nutrients into six major categories
- appreciate the need for recommended dietary allowances
- understand the relationship between good nutrition and health

INTRODUCTION

Food is a basic need for all living beings. Just as we cannot live without air and water, we cannot live without food. Food gives us energy to carry out our day-to-day activities and keeps all the systems in our body functioning well. Food supplies the nourishing substances needed by our body to build and repair tissues and to regulate various functions.

Since food has so many functions to perform to keep us in good health, a study of the composition of various foods and the functions performed by these components is essential if one has to enjoy good health.

Food does much more than keeping us alive and healthy. It adds pleasure to life. We enjoy the flavours, aromas, colours, and textures of different cuisines. We use food as a way to celebrate special events and festivals with family and friends. The main functions of food are listed here.

1. Physiological functions
2. Psychological function
3. Social function

Some Important Definitions

Food   Food can be defined as any substance which nourishes the body and is fit to eat. It may be solid or liquid.

Food provides the body with materials for providing energy, growth and maintenance, and regulating various processes in the body. These materials of which food is made up of are termed nutrients.

Six nutrients are of importance in nutrition. They are

1. Proteins
2. Carbohydrates
3. Fats
4. Vitamins
5. Minerals
6. Water

Different foods contain different amounts of nutrients, hence no two foods have identical nutritive value. Some foods contain only one nutrient, e.g., sugar contains the nutrient carbohydrate.

Nutrients   Nutrients are the chemical substances present in food, which the body needs to carry out its functions. Food is the source of all nutrients, except vitamin D. There are six major groups of nutrients, namely proteins, carbohydrates, fats, vitamins, minerals, and water. Each group has several nutrients in it, and each nutrient has specific functions in the body.

Nutrition is the science of nourishing the body. It includes much more than just consuming a balanced diet. Nutrition is a study of various nutrients, their characteristics, functions, requirements, and sources. The effect of deficiency, excessive intake, digestion, absorption, and utilization in the body as well as the interrelationships that occur among some nutrients is an important part of nutrition.

Nutrition   It is a combination of processes by which the human body receives and utilizes nutrients which are necessary for carrying out various functions and for the growth and renewal of its components.

Thus, nutrition refers to the various processes in the body for making use of food. It includes eating the right kind and amount of food, absorption of nutrients into the blood stream, use of individual nutrients by the cells in the body, maintenance and growth of cells, tissues, and organs, and elimination of wastes.

RELATION OF FOOD AND HEALTH

When the diet does not supply all nutrients in required amounts, it results in ill-health or malnutrition.

Malnutrition

Malnutrition (mal means faulty) is an impairment of health resulting from a deficiency, excess, or inbalance of nutrients in the diet. It includes both undernutrition or deficiency and overnutrition or excessive consumption.

Undernutrition

It refers to a deficiency of calories and/or one or more nutrients in the diet. An undernourished person is underweight.

Overnutrition

It refers to an excess of calories and/or one or more nutrients in the diet. An excessive intake of calories results in overweight which can lead to obesity. An excessive intake of fat-soluble vitamins can cause hypervitaminosis or vitamin toxicity.

Diet

A diet means the kinds and amounts of food and beverage consumed every day. A diet may be a normal diet or it may be a modified diet which is used in the treatment of a specific disease or condition.

Kilocalorie (kcal)

It is the unit for measuring the energy value of foods or the energy needs of the body. It is the amount of heat required to raise the temperature of 1,000 g water by 1°C.

$$1 \text{ kcal} = 4.184 \text{ kilojoules (kJ)}$$

Health

The World Health Organization (WHO) defines health as a state of complete physical, mental, and social well-being, and not merely the absence of disease or infirmity.

Health is a positive state of complete well-being and not just the absence of disease. When we are tired or exhausted, we cannot concentrate on our work. To remain healthy a balance between work and rest or recreation is necessary. This improves our work efficiency.

A person must look healthy, feel healthy, and have a balanced mind and be a socially responsible individual.

Nutritional Status

The nutritional status of an individual is defined as the condition of health as influenced by the utilization of nutrients in the body.

The nutritional status of an individual or a community can be assessed by surveying the kind and amount of food being consumed, signs of ill-health or deficiency symptoms if present, height, weight, and other measurements as well as level of nutrients in the blood and excreted in the urine.

Good nutrition and health are closely interlinked. Clean, wholesome, and nutritious food promotes health and keeps away disease.

A balanced diet is one of the essential factors in ensuring good health. The other factors are the wholesomeness of food and a clean environment in which it is prepared and eaten.

The food handler should maintain high standards of personal, food, and environmental hygiene to prevent transmission of foodborne disease.

To ensure that the consumer obtains the maximum health benefits from the food that is served, all food handlers concerned with purchasing, storing, cooking and serving food, and planning meals should have a basic knowledge of nutrition and hygiene.

FOOD AND ITS FUNCTIONS

Food and its various functions (Fig. 14.1) are discussed here.

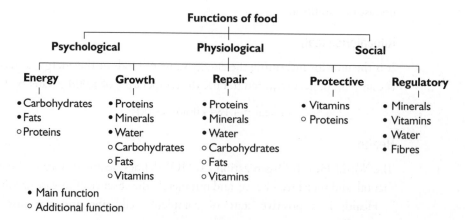

Fig. 14.1   Functions of food

Physiological Functions

Each nutrient in food has specific functions to perform in the body. The physiological functions performed by food are as follows.

Providing energy   The body needs energy to carry out voluntary and involuntary work. Involuntary work includes all processes which are not under the control of our will, such as digestion, respiration, and circulation, and go on continuously irrespective of whether we are asleep or awake. Voluntary activities or activities which we wish to do, such as walking, playing games, and working, require energy, and the amount of energy required will depend on the nature of activity. The energy needed for these activities is supplied by oxidation of the foods we eat, mainly carbohydrates and fats.

Body building or growth   It is one of the most important functions of food. An infant grows into a healthy adult by consuming the right kinds and amounts of food year after year. Our body is made up of millions of cells and when growth takes place, new cells are added to the existing cells and cells increase in size.

Maintenance or repair   In the adult body, worn out cells are continuously being replaced by new ones. The daily wear and tear of cells need to be maintained. Proteins, minerals, and water are the main nutrients required for growth as well as maintenance of all cells and tissues in the body.

Regulation of body processes   Food also regulates numerous activities in the body such as the beating of the heart, maintenance of body temperature, clotting of blood, and excretion of wastes. Each of these processes is controlled and carried out by specific nutrients, e.g., vitamin K and calcium are necessary for clotting of blood.

Protective function   Nutrients keep body cells in a healthy condition to ward off infection. They help in building up the body's resistance to disease and help the body recover rapidly from any infection. These functions are performed by vitamins and proteins.

Psychological Function

We all have emotional needs such as need for love, attention, and security. Food can play an important role in fulfilling these needs. A mother can express her love for her child by preparing the child's favourite meal. Food can be given as a reward for good behaviour or deprived as a punishment for bad behaviour.

People feel comfortable and secure when they are served food they have been used to consuming. Many people eat to relieve anxiety and frustration, while some may eat less or refuse food when they are depressed and lonely.

Certain foods may be associated with sickness, e.g., *sago kheer* and *khichdi* while some others, such as *pedha*, are associated with good tidings. Food is therefore strongly associated with one's emotions and feelings.

Social Function

Food carries a lot of social significance. Warmth and friendship are expressed through sharing one's food or inviting people to dine. Preparing special food or one's favourite food is a way of showing respect or affection.

Food is a significant part of celebrations for occasions such as birthdays, weddings, and other joyous occasions. Festivals such as Diwali, Dussehra, Christmas, and Eid have special menus prescribed for the occassions.

Food also has religious significance. Some foods can be offered to God, while others are avoided on certain days for religious reasons. The type of food prepared and served is a status symbol. Even today, in some communities, adult men are given more and better quality food than women because of their higher social status.

FACTORS AFFECTING FOOD INTAKE AND FOOD HABITS

The kind of food that people eat, varies widely from one country to another and also within the country. This may be because of geographic reasons affecting the availability of certain foods.

This difference in what people consume depends on a number of reasons. These are

1. Geographic reasons
2. Economic reasons
3. Religions reasons
4. Customs
5. Education
6. Social reasons
7. Health
8. Other factors

Geographic Reasons

The location, climate, and physical features of a region will dictate the availability of food in the area. The terrain and soil will determine which staple cereal will grow best, e.g., rice grows best in lowland areas where soil holds water well. People living in coastal areas will depend on seafood and coconuts more than people living away from the sea. However, with the growth of processing industry and improved transportation, all foodstuffs are available globally today, but may not be affordable.

Economic Reasons

Food choices depend to a large extent on what one can afford and on their country's economy. But even in the richest countries, people suffer from malnutrition because of wrong choice of food, while in poorer countries, people may consume a well-balanced diet.

Most developed countries can produce all the food they need and afford to import necessary food items. People can afford to buy a variety of foods both fresh and processed from all food groups. In developing countries, many people suffer from malnutrition and cannot afford three meals a day. Moreover, these meals are mainly cereal based with negligible amounts of protein and protective foods.

Religions Reasons

Foods may be forbidden for religious reasons. Hindus worship cattle, hence eating beef is prohibited. Orthodox Jews and Muslims do not eat pork. Some Hindus do not eat any flesh food or eggs.

Certain days are identified for feasting or fasting, and (food items to be abstained from or) foods served on these days are specified.

Customs influence what people eat and how food should be prepared and served. Each country has its traditional fare and although ingredients may be the same, they taste different because they are prepared differently. Customs also influence the time food is consumed and how it is served.

Anothers factor affecting our eating habits is education. Education plays a vital role in making good food choices, An educated mother will ensure that the family members are served balanced meals, making wise choices within the family budget. Our food preferences begin when we are children and are governed by our early experiences of food served to us by our parents and the overall meal experience.

Social Reasons

The influence of our peers from school to college cannot be denied. Our lifestyle also has a marked effect on our food intake. Travelling long distances for education or work also influences what and where we eat. While school cafeterias, college messes and industrial canteens offer low cost balanced meals, many business travelers need to depend on dining out in restaurants and entertaining clients and guests. The consumption of alcohol and fried snacks during social rituals, often affects consumption of wholesome food.

Health

Our health may pose certain restrictions on what we consume. Diabetics need to avoid sweets, while hypertensive individuals need to control salt and regulate fat intake. Obese individuals look for foods which are low in calories and high in fibre.

Other factors

Several other factors influence what we eat such as our personal choices, advertisements by the media stating health claims, the sensory qualities of a food and the benefits of convenience foods vis-à-vis home-cooked meals. These have a marked influence in today's busy world. Sometimes, instead of knowing the benefits of fresh wholesome food people opt for convenience foods, because of time constraints.

A correct balance in the choice of foods needs to be worked out to combat malnutrition.

CLASSIFICATION OF NUTRIENTS

Nutrients are the essential constituents of food that are required by the body in suitable amounts. There are approximately 50 nutrients which are placed in six categories, namely proteins, carbohydrates, fats, vitamins, minerals, and water.

Classification on the Basis of Amounts Required Everyday

Based on their requirement in the body, nutrients are divided into two major groups: the macronutrients and the micronutrients (Fig. 14.2). Most of the weight of the food we eat is that of proteins, carbohydrates, fats, and water. These are the macronutrients. Vitamins and minerals are required in minute amounts and are also present in food in very small quantities. They are classified as micronutrients. Both macronutrients and micronutrients are equally important for good health, and one cannot enjoy good health without including all nutrients in the diet.

The requirement for macronutrients is in grams, while the requirement for micronutrients is in milligrams and micrograms.

Foods vary widely in their nutrient content. The nutrients are elements that are essential for our body's health. These elements can be classified according to their function, their chemical nature, their essentiality, and the quantity required by the human body.

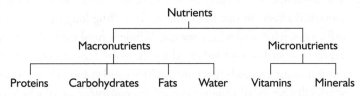

Fig. 14.2   Classification of nutrients

Classification on the Basis of Function

Nutrients can be classified according to their function in the body. Different nutrients have different functions. Foods such as proteins, fats and carbohydrates are called as body-building food. They are the nutrients that form body tissues. Proteins make up 20 per cent or one-fifth of the total body weight. Fat nutrients make up another 20 per cent or one-fifth of the body weight while carbohydrates make up about 1 per cent.

Carbohydrates, fats, and proteins are considered as energy yielding nutrients while the vitamins, minerals and water are called as non-calorie nutrients. The element that is abundant in the body, is water, which makes up about two thirds or about 66 per cent of the entire weight of the body.

Vitamins and minerals are the nutrients that function to regulate body processes. Minerals make up 4 per cent of the body weight and vitamins make up about 28 g of the body weight, considering that they are not really a part of the structural components of the body. Proteins, vitamin A, vitamin C, and iron protect the body against infection and are called protective nutrients.

Classification on the Basis of Chemical Properties

Another way of classifying nutrients is according to their chemical properties. In this classification, the nutrients are further classified as organic and inorganic. Those nutrients that contain carbon such as proteins, carbohydrates, and fats, are called organic nutrients, while those nutrients that do not contain carbon element, such as minerals and water, are called inorganic nutrients.

Classification on the Basis of Essentiality

Nutrients can also be classified according to their essentiality. Some nutrients cannot be synthesized by the body in required amounts and must be included in the diet, e.g., essential amino acids, essential fatty acids, minerals, and most vitamins. While all nutrients are required by the body daily, and all are essential and important, they only differ because the human body is capable of synthesis of some nutrients by interconversion of certain nutrients.

RECOMMENDED DIETARY ALLOWANCES

The amount of food needed to ensure good health will vary from one individual to another. All people do not require the same amounts of nutrients. Requirements vary depending upon age, sex, body size, activity, state of health, etc. For example, a person doing a sedentary job will require lesser energy-giving foods as compared to a farm labourer doing heavy manual work.

The Indian Council for Medical Research (ICMR) has prepared recommended dietary allowances (RDAs) for Indians. These recommendations are revised and updated at regular intervals based on suggestions from experts. This guide tells us the amounts of different nutrients we should consume daily. The allowances are calculated for different age groups for males and females based on activity levels and ensure that good health will be maintained. These tables are based on scientific knowledge and accordingly nutrient intake is recommended for infants, preschool and school children, adolescents, and adults. Additional allowances for some nutrients are included for periods of physiological stress such as pregnancy and lactation.

No two individuals of similar height, weight, and age have the same nutritional requirements, as the actual requirement is influenced by many factors. The RDAs are not actual requirements but allowances that are high enough to take care of almost everyone in that particular group (refer Table 14.1).

DIGESTION, ABSORPTION, AND METABOLISM OF FOOD

The food we eat needs to be broken down into simpler substances which the body can utilize. This is accomplished by the process of digestion. Complex substances, such as carbohydrates, proteins, and fats, are broken down into simpler forms by the mechanical action of the teeth and chemical action of various enzymes in the digestive system. Water, minerals, and vitamins can be absorbed directly without undergoing any

TABLE 14.1   Recommended dietary allowances for Indians

Group	Particulars	Body wt (kg)	Net energy (kcal/d)	Protein (g/d)	Fat (g/d)	Calcium (mg/d)	Iron (mg/d)	Vit. A (μg/d) Retinol	β-Carotene	Thiamin (mg/d)	Riboflavin (mg/d)	Nicotinic-acid (mg/d)	Pyridoxin (mg/d)	Ascorbic acid (mg/d)	Folic acid (μg/d)	Vit. B-12 (μg/d)
Man	• Sedentary work	60	2,425	60	20	400	28	600	2,400	1.2	1.4	16	2.0	40	100	1
	• Moderate work		2,875							1.4	1.6	18				
	• Heavy work		3,800							1.6	1.9	21				
Woman	• Sedentary work	50	1,875	50	20	400	30	600	2,400	0.9	1.1	12	2.0	40	100	1
	• Moderate work		2,225							1.1	1.3	14				
	• Heavy work		2,925							1.2	1.5	16				
	• Pregnant woman	50	+300	+15	30	1,000	38	600	2,400	+0.2	+0.2	+2	2.5	40	400	1
	• Lactation	50			45	1,000	30	950	3,800				2.5	80	150	1.5
	–0–6 months		+500	+25						+0.3	+0.3	+4				
	–6–12 months		+400	+18						+0.2	+0.2	+3				
Infants	• 0–6 months	5.4	108/kg	2.05/kg		500		350	1,200	55 μg/kg	65 μg/kg	710μg/kg	0.1	25	25	0.2
	• 6–12 months	8.6	98/kg	1.65/kg						50 μg/kg	60 μg/kg	650μg/kg	0.4			
Children	• 1–3 years	12.2	1,240	22	25	400	12	400	1,600	0.6	0.7	8	0.9	40	30	
	• 4–6 years	19.0	1,690	30			18	400	1,600	0.9	1.0	11	0.9		40	0.2–1.0
	• 7–9 years	26.9	1,950	41			26	600	2,400	1.0	1.2	13	1.6		60	
Boys	• 10–12 years	35.4	2,190	54	22	600	34	600	2,400	1.1	1.3	15	1.6	40	70	0.2–1.0
Girls	• 10–12 years	31.5	1,970	57			19			1.0	1.2	13				
Boys	• 13–15 years	47.8	2,450	70	22	600	41	600	2,400	1.2	1.5	16	2.0	40	100	0.2–1.0
Girls	• 13–15 years	46.7	2,060	65			28			1.0	1.2	14				
Boys	• 16–18 years	57.1	2,640	78	22	500	50	600	2,400	1.3	1.6	17	2.0	40	100	0.2–1.0
Girls	• 16–18 years	49.9	2,060	63			30			1.0	1.2	14				

change. Glucose needs no further breakdown and is immediately absorbed giving instant energy. Both digestion and absorption take place in the digestive tract in the body.

The digestive tract or alimentary canal in humans comprises the following:

- Mouth
- Oesophagus
- Stomach
- Small intestine (duodenum, jejunum, ileum)
- Large intestine (caecum, colon, rectum, anus)

The liver and pancreas are not a part of the digestive tract, but provide vital secretions, namely, bile, and pancreatic juice, respectively which aid in the digestion of food. Digestive juices are also secreted by all parts of the digestive tract except the oesophagus, rectum, and anus. These juices contain chemical substances called enzymes, which act as catalysts in the breakdown of nutrients.

Digestion of Food

Mouth The process of digestion begins in the mouth. Food is mechanically broken down by the teeth by chewing and is moistened with saliva produced by the salivary glands in the mouth. Saliva contains an enzyme called salivary amylase or ptyalin which acts on cooked carbohydrates and partially digests them into smaller units. If food remains in the mouth for sometime, carbohydrates are further broken down into maltose by the action of salivary amylase, giving food a sweetish taste.

Oesophagus Food passes from the mouth into the stomach through a tube called the oesophagus or food pipe. No digestion takes place in the oesophagus.

Stomach In the stomach the food is mixed with gastric juice. Gastric juice is composed of hydrochloric acid, enzymes, and water. The stomach muscles contract and churn the food to a liquid consistency called chyme. Gastric juice has many important functions. The acidic nature of gastric juice:

1. Destroys harmful bacteria which may be present in food
2. Activates enzyme pepsin
3. Swells proteins so that enzymes can easily act on them
4. Aids in the absorption of calcium and iron

The enzyme pepsin acts on proteins and enzyme lipase has some effect on emulsified fats.

Small intestine Maximum digestion of proteins, carbohydrates, and fats takes place in the small intestine. The small intestine includes the duodenum (which is the first portion), the jejunum, and the ileum. Bile which is produced by the liver and stored in the gall bladder is needed for digestion of fat. Bile is released in the duodenum and it emulsifies fats so that they can be easily attacked by enzymes. Bile is highly alkaline and helps in neutralizing the acidic chyme so that other intestinal enzymes can act. The small intestine secretes intestinal enzymes and the pancreas secretes pancreatic juice and completes the digestion of proteins, carbohydrates, and fats into amino acids, monosaccharides, and glycerol, and fatty acids, respectively. These simple substances are absorbed through the walls of the small intestine into the bloodstream.

Large intestine   The large intestine includes the caecum, colon, rectum, and anus. The food which is not absorbed in the small intestine passes into the large intestine. Water and digestive juices are reabsorbed in the large intestine giving the intestinal contents a solid

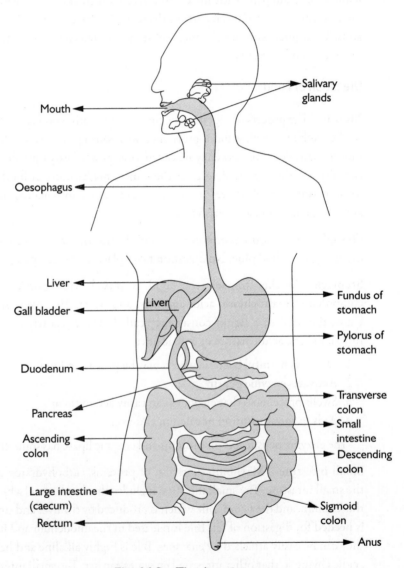

Fig. 14.3   The digestive system

consistency. The unabsorbed material is called faeces, and it contains small amounts of undigested food mainly fibre, bile salts, cholesterol, mucous, bacteria, and broken down cells. It is excreted via the anus.

Figure 14.3 shows the digestive system.

Factors that affect digestion

Consistency, division, and type of food   Foods that are of liquid consistency are more easily digested than food pieces which are solid and big in size. Food which is chewed well is easily acted on by digestive enzymes.

Bacterial action   The normal bacterial flora helps in breaking down food and is desirable.

Chemical factors   Strong acids, spices, caffeine, and meat extracts stimulate the flow of gastric juice. Fats slow down the flow of gastric juice.

Psychological factors   Anger, fright, and worry slow down the secretion of gastric juices. The sight, smell, and aroma of food increases the secretion of saliva and gastric juices. Of all the nutrients, carbohydrates are digested fastest. Glucose needs no further breakdown and is immediately absorbed giving instant energy. A mixture of carbohydrate, protein, and fat gives satiety and remains in the digestive system for a longer time.

Absorption

Absorption is the process in which the end-products of digestion of nutrients are transferred from the intestine into the blood and lymph circulation.

The wall of the small intestine is made up of 4 to 5 million folds or finger-like projections called villi. Each villus has blood vessels and lymph vessels. The presence of villi increases the total area from which absorption can take place. Most nutrients are absorbed in the duodenum and jejunum, and remaining in the ileum.

Nutrients are absorbed across the epithelial cell walls lining each villi by two methods:

1. Passive diffusions, i.e., movement of water and minerals from an area of higher concentration to an area of lower concentration. Sometimes a carrier is required to help ferry water-soluble nutrients across a cell membrane with fat-like material.
2. Most nutrients are absorbed by active transport from an area of lower concentration to an area of higher concentration. Active transport requires energy for transportation. The nutrients absorbed into the lymph are fatty acids, some molecules of fat, and fat-soluble vitamins. Glucose, amino acids, water-soluble vitamins, and minerals are transported by the portal circulation to the liver.

Metabolism

From the blood stream, nutrients are supplied to all the cells in the body where each nutrient performs its specific functions. It is either oxidized to release energy (catabolism), or it is used in the synthesis of complex substances (anabolism).

Anabolism is the term used for all chemical reactions in which simple substances are used to synthesize more complex substances, e.g., amino acids are used for specific protein synthesis.

Catabolism is the term used for all chemical reactions in which complex substances are further broken down to simpler compounds, e.g., glucose is oxidized to produce carbon dioxide, water, and energy.

Glucose and fats are stored as potential energy in the form of adipose tissue. Glucose is also stored as glycogen in the liver. Amino acids are used for synthesis of new cells, enzymes, or hormones. Minerals and vitamins carry out regulatory functions.

The waste products of digestion, absorption, and metabolism are excreted by the bowels, kidneys, skin, and lungs.

SUMMARY

Food is our basic need which we cannot live without. Food gives us energy, builds and maintains our body, and regulates the innumerable functions which take place in our body. Apart from the physiological function, food adds pleasure to our life and helps fulfil our emotional and social needs. There are six groups of nutrients present in food, namely proteins, carbohydrates, fats, vitamins, minerals, and water. Different foods contain different proportions of nutrients and no two foods are alike in their composition.

Nutrition does not only mean consuming a balanced diet, but it is also concerned with the digestion, absorption, and metabolism of various nutrients. The nutrients, we consume, should be utilized by the body and this is reflected in our nutritional status. How much of each nutrient should be consumed everyday varies from person to person. The RDA table gives allowances that are adequate for almost everyone in a particular age group.

The food we consume needs to be broken down into simpler substances which the body can absorb and utilize. The digestive tract is made up of the mouth, oesophagus, stomach, small and large intestines. The digested food is absorbed in the small intestine and sent to the blood circulation via the liver. The cells and tissues in the body are provided nutrients by the blood. Both anabolism and catabolism take place in the body, and waste products of metabolism are excreted via the bowels, kidneys, skin, and lungs.

KEY TERMS

Anabolism   The process in which complex body substances are synthesized from simpler ones in living organisms such as building of body tissues.

Catabolism   The process in which complex substances are progressively broken down into simpler substances generally accompanied by release of energy (opposite of anabolism).

Cell   The smallest unit of life which is capable of functioning independently.

Deficiency   A state or condition caused due to

inadequate dietary intake of one or more nutrients in the diet.

Duodenum   The first portion of the small intestine immediately after the stomach.

Enzyme   Enzymes are made up of proteins and act as catalysts for chemical reactions in the body.

Growth   An increase in the size and number of cells.

Hormone   A secretion of ductless glands into the blood stream which have specific effects on specific organs.

Impairment   Appearance of weakness or damage causing health to deteriorate in quality or lessen in strength.

Infirmity   Physical or mental weakness.

Kilocalorie   The unit of measuring energy in nutrition, i.e., energy value of food or energy needs of the body. It is 1,000 times larger than the physics calorie, and is defined as the amount of heat required to raise the temperature of 1 kg of water by 1°C.

$$1 \text{ kcal} = 4.184 \text{ kJ}$$

Obesity   A condition of overweight in which body weight is 20 per cent or more than desirable weight.

Overweight   A condition in which weight is 10–19 per cent more than desirable weight.

Tissue   A group of similar cells.

Underweight   A condition in which weight is 10–20 per cent less than desirable weight.

 ## REVIEW QUESTIONS

1. What are the functions of food?
2. Classify nutrients into two major categories.
3. Define the following:
   (a) Food
   (b) Nutrient
   (c) Malnutrition
   (d) Kilocalorie
4. What does RDA stand for? Why is it important?
5. List the organs in the digestive tract and state the main function of each.
6. Briefly explain absorption and metabolism of nutrients in the body.

CHAPTER 15

Carbohydrates in Nutrition

LEARNING OBJECTIVES

After reading this chapter, you should be able to
- distinguish between available and unavailable carbohydrates
- identify food sources of sugar, starches, and fibre
- state the functions of different carbohydrates
- understand the importance of selecting the right kinds and amounts of carbohydrate foods for good health
- appreciate the importance of carbohydrates in our daily diet
- describe the process by which carbohydrates are digested, absorbed, and utilized by the body
- know sugar substitutes available and their energy value

INTRODUCTION

Carbohydrates are a major source of energy for humans, providing approximately 45 per cent to 80 per cent of the total caloric intake in different income groups. Since they are a relatively inexpensive source of energy compared to fats and proteins, they form the bulk of the diet of humans throughout the world.

They are mainly present in food in the form of sugars, starches, and fibres. A study of the various types of carbohydrates is necessary because the kind and proportion of different forms of carbohydrate present in food have a direct bearing on our health.

In Chapter 4 on Carbohydrates, we have already studied the definition and general classification of carbohydrates. Three groups of carbohydrates are of importance in our diet from the nutritional point of view, namely sugars, starches, and fibres. The sugar and starch that we consume is ultimately broken down to glucose in the digestive tract and absorbed into the blood circulation. In the human body, glucose is removed from blood by the tissue cells and used as a source of energy. Some glucose is converted to glycogen, also called animal starch, and stored in the muscle and liver as a reserve store of energy.

$$\text{Glucose} \xrightarrow[\text{tissues}]{\text{oxidized in}} \text{Energy} + \underbrace{CO_2 \uparrow + H_2O}_{\substack{\text{Waste products} \\ \text{of metabolism}}}$$

CLASSIFICATION OF CARBOHYDRATES

Carbohydrates, which are of importance in the diet, are classified on the basis of the number of sugar units present in them (see Table 15.1 and Fig. 15.1). They may also be classified as:

Available carbohydrates Carbohydrates which can be digested in the human body and yield energy when they are oxidized in the body.

TABLE 15.1 Classification of carbohydrates

Category	Name of carbohydrate	Sources
Simple carbohydrates or sugars		
1. Monosaccharides (single sugar unit)	Glucose (dextrose) Fructose (levulose)	Fruits, vegetables, honey
	Galactose	On hydrolysis of lactose
2. Disaccharides (two sugar units)	Sucrose (glucose + fructose)	Sugar cane, sugar beet
	Maltose (glucose + glucose)	Sprouted and malted grains, acid hydrolysis of starch
	Lactose (glucose + galactose)	Milk is the only source
Complex carbohydrates or polysaccharides		
1. Available	Starch	Cereals, pulses, roots, tubers, vegetables, and under-ripe fruits
	Glycogen (animal starch)	Liver and muscle of freshly slaughtered animals
	Dextrin	Partial breakdown of starch by dry heat or digestion
2. Unavailable or dietary fibres		
(a) Water insoluble	Cellulose Hemicellulose Lignin*	Structural fibre in whole-grain cereals, nuts, wheat bran, figs, vegetables, etc.
(b) Water soluble	Pectins Gums Mucilages	Non-structural fibres in apples, citrus fruits, guava, oats, barley, pulses, seaweeds, etc.

*Lignin is a fibre but not a carbohydrate.

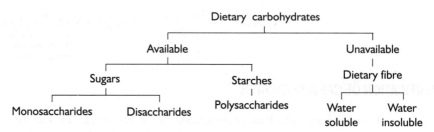

Fig. 15.1 Classification of dietary carbohydrates

Unavailable carbohydrates Carbohydrates which cannot be digested because the human body does not contain the enzymes necessary for their breakdown. Unavailable carbohydrates do not provide any energy to the body but are necessary as they perform some important functions in the body such as regular elimination of faecal waste.

DIGESTION, ABSORPTION, AND METABOLISM

Complex carbohydrates and sugars are too large to be absorbed through the intestinal wall. They need to be broken down into their constituent monosaccharides so that they can be absorbed. Only monosaccharides can be absorbed into the blood stream. The mechanical and chemical digestion of starch begins in the mouth. Ptyalin or salivary amylase in saliva acts on cooked starch and partially breaks it down into dextrin. If ptyalin acts on starch long enough, i.e., if food is chewed well, some maltose may be formed. The stomach does not secrete any starch-splitting enzyme, hence no digestion takes place in the stomach. In the small intestine, pancreatic amylase acts on starch and dextrin, breaking it down into maltose.

The intestinal wall secretes maltase, lactase, and sucrase which acts on maltose, lactose, and sucrose, reducing them to their respective monosaccharides. Some fructose may be converted to glucose. The monosaccharides are absorbed into the blood vessels lining the small intestine and carried to the liver for their further metabolism.

The absorbed monosaccharides, i.e., glucose, fructose, and galactose may be converted into glycogen and stored in the liver, or converted into glucose and released into the blood stream to be oxidized as a source of energy for various tissue cells. In human metabolism, all sugars are converted into glucose. In the muscle cells, some glucose may be stored as glycogen. The fasting level of glucose in blood is maintained at 70–100 mg/100 ml blood. After consuming a meal rich in carbohydrates, it increases to 140–150 mg/100 ml blood. Glucose is taken up from blood by the body cells and oxidized as a source of energy.

In the cells, glucose is first oxidized to form pyruvic acid, and ultimately through the various metabolic cycles, energy is release in the form of adenosine triphosphate (ATP). The waste products of carbohydrate metabolism, i.e., carbon dioxide and water are released from the cell and excreted by the body. The energy released is used by the body for its various voluntary and involuntary processes and to maintain body temperature (Fig. 15.2).

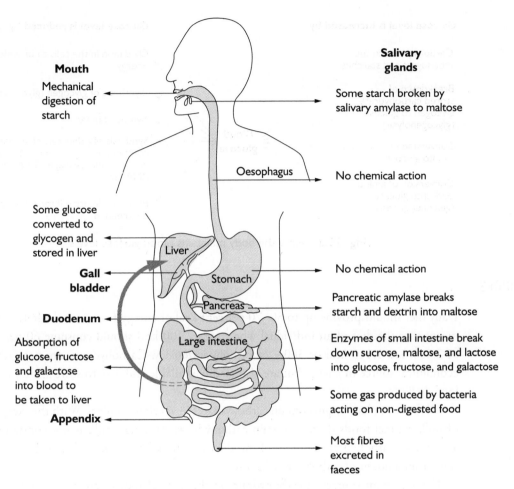

Mouth
Mechanical digestion of starch

Salivary glands
Some starch broken by salivary amylase to maltose

Oesophagus
No chemical action

Some glucose converted to glycogen and stored in liver

Liver

Gall bladder
No chemical action

Stomach

Pancreas
Pancreatic amylase breaks starch and dextrin into maltose

Duodenum

Large intestine
Enzymes of small intestine break down sucrose, maltose, and lactose into glucose, fructose, and galactose

Absorption of glucose, fructose and galactose into blood to be taken to liver

Some gas produced by bacteria acting on non-digested food

Appendix

Most fibres excreted in faeces

Fig. 15.2 Digestion and absorption of carbohydrate

If the level exceeds 170 mg glucose/100 ml blood, it crosses the renal threshold and glucose is excreted in the urine. This condition is observed in diabetic patients. A fasting blood glucose level above 140 mg is called hyperglycaemia and below 70 mg is called hypoglycaemia. The body tries to maintain the normal fasting level by removing glucose from blood when the level is high and adding glucose to blood when the level falls, e.g., when a person is fasting. The hormone insulin, secreted by the cells of the islets of Langerhans in the pancreas, helps in regulating the blood glucose level. Insulin is required for glucose utilization by the cells and synthesis of glycogen from glucose. If insulin is deficient, glucose is not utilized by the cells and blood level of glucose increases. Insulin is the only hormone which lowers blood sugar levels, other hormones, such as the thyroid hormone, increase blood sugar levels (Fig. 15.3).

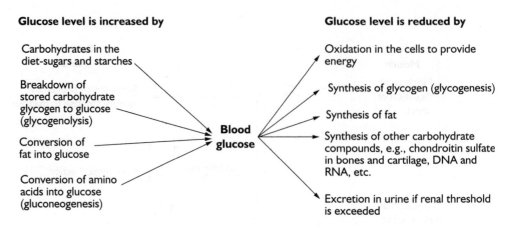

Glucose level is increased by

Carbohydrates in the
diet-sugars and starches

Breakdown of
stored carbohydrate
glycogen to glucose
(glycogenolysis)

Conversion of
fat into glucose

Conversion of amino
acids into glucose
(gluconeogenesis)

**Blood
glucose**

Glucose level is reduced by

Oxidation in the cells to provide
energy

Synthesis of glycogen (glycogenesis)

Synthesis of fat

Synthesis of other carbohydrate
compounds, e.g., chondroitin sulfate
in bones and cartilage, DNA and
RNA, etc.

Excretion in urine if renal threshold
is exceeded

Fig. 15.3   How the body maintains blood glucose levels

SOURCES

Daily diet should provide up to 50–70 per cent kcal of energy from carbohydrate, which means that the diet of an individual who needs 2,400 kcal should consume 60 per cent of 2,400, i.e., 1,440 kcal or 360 g of carbohydrates/day. Carbohydrates are not only an economical source of energy but are also readily available and easy to store as they have a long shelf life.

All foods of plant origin contain carbohydrates in varying amounts. With the exception of milk, animal foods do not contain carbohydrate. Although milk is not consumed as a source of carbohydrate, some milk products, such as khoa and milk powder, contain significant amount of carbohydrate lactose.

The important sources of carbohydrates in the diets of Indians are cereals and millets, roots, tubers, pulses, sugar, and jaggery (Table 15.2).

TABLE 15.2   Some rich sources of carbohydrates

Cereals	Pulses	Fruits and vegetables	Nuts and oilseeds	Miscellaneous
• Wheat	All whole grain and dehusked pulses and their by-products, e.g., *rajma*, bengal gram, whole green gram, lentils, and *besan*	• Mango	• Cashew nuts	• Sugar
• Rice		• *Chikoo*	• Coconut (dry)	• Jaggery
• *Jowar*		• Jackfruit	• Groundnuts	• Honey
• *Bajra*		• Custard apple	• Garden cress	• *Sago*
• *Ragi*		• Banana	seeds	• Tapioca
• Oats		• Green peas	• Niger seeds	• Dates
• Barley		• Beans	• Gingelly	• Raisins
• Corn		• Potato	seeds	• Skimmed milk
		• Yam		powder
		• Colocasia		

All sugars provide 4 kcal/g of energy. The carbohydrate and calorie content of a food can be reduced by using sugars which are sweeter than sucrose so that the quantity of sugar required will be less.

FUNCTIONS

Carbohydrates have many functions in the human body.

1. The chief function of carbohydrate is to provide energy to the body so that it can carry out day-to-day work and maintain body temperature. All carbohydrates except fibre provide 4 kcal/g of energy. It is the cheapest source of energy available.
2. Glucose is the only form of energy used by the central nervous system. When blood glucose levels fall, the brain does not receive energy and convulsions may occur.
3. Carbohydrates spare proteins from being broken down for energy and are used for bodybuilding and repair. In carbohydrate deficient diets, proteins meant for bodybuilding and repair are oxidized to meet the most important and primary need of the body, i.e., energy.
4. They are required for complete oxidation of fat. In a deficiency, fats are broken down rapidly for energy and intermediate products such as ketones are formed in large amounts resulting in a condition called ketosis.
5. Carbohydrates can be converted into non-essential amino acids, provided a source of nitrogen is available.
6. The sugar lactose helps in the absorption of the minerals calcium and phosphorus.
7. Lactose helps certain bacteria to grow in the intestine. This bacterial flora is capable of synthesizing B-complex vitamins in the gut.
8. Dietary fibre plays an important role of increasing faecal mass by absorbing and holding water, stimulating peristalsis, and eliminating faecal waste.
9. Fibre also helps in lowering blood cholesterol levels by binding bile acids and cholesterol.

Deficiency

The daily diet should not contain less than 100 g of carbohydrate. Carbohydrate deficiency is uncommon in our country as diets are cereal based. A deficiency of carbohydrate in the diet results in utilization of fat for energy. In severe deficiency, incomplete oxidation of fats causes ketone bodies to accumulate in the blood.

Excess Carbohydrates

1. Excessive consumption of refined sugars could be one of the causes of dental caries or tooth decay.
2. Excessive sugar depresses the appetite, provides hollow calories, and could result in malnutrition.

3. High intake of sugar and refined carbohydrates increase the blood triglyceride levels leading to heart diseases.

4. When excessive carbohydrates are consumed, they are converted into fat and deposited in the adipose tissue, which could lead to obesity, i.e., body weight of 20 per cent or more than the desirable weight.

5. Excessive fibre could irritate the intestinal lining, causing cramps or bloating due to gas formation.

6. Excessive fibre interferes with the absorption and availability of mineral elements such as iron and calcium.

Role of Dietary Fibre in Prevention and Treatment of Disease

Dietary fibre refers to the total amount of naturally occurring material in plant foods, which is not digested. The terms roughage, bulk, and unavailable polysaccharides are synonymous with fibre. Fibres cannot be digested by human enzymes.

Dietary fibre or roughage does not provide humans with energy but performs many important functions in the body (Table 15.3). Fibre can absorb and hold water thereby increasing faecal bulk. This acts as a laxative and reduces intraluminal pressure in the

TABLE 15.3   Functions and sources of dietary fibre

Type	Functions	Food source
Insoluble fibres		
Cellulose	• Insoluble fibre • Holds water • Increases stool bulk • Reduces intraluminal colonic pressure	Bran, wholegrain cereals, specially wheat, rye, apples, pears, tomatoes, cabbage, beans
Hemicellulose	• Prevents constipation • Binds minerals such as Ca and Fe	Bran, wholegrain cereals, specially millets—jowar, bajra, ragi
Lignin (non-carbo-hydrate source)	• Binds bile acids • Reduces transit time	Wholegrain cereals, pears, peaches, plums, mature vegetables
Soluble fibres		
Pectins	• Soluble fibre • Binds cholesterol and bile acids	Guava, apple, citrus fruits, wood apple, berries, carrots, and green beans
Gums	• Holds water • Fermented in the colon to volatile fatty acids and gas by the normal bacteria flora of the colon	Oatmeal, pulses and beans, *dinkache ladoo,* processed foods
Mucilages, seaweeds, and algae		Thickener in food products, stabilizer, gelling agent in puddings

colon preventing diverticulosis. Insoluble fibre prevents constipation by stimulating peristalsis in the large intestine. The contraction of muscular walls of the digestive tract is stimulated by fibre. Fibre increases water absorption, forming a larger, softer stool that rapidly passes through the colon. Soluble fibre binds bile acids and cholesterol and is beneficial to people suffering from coronary heart disease. Fibre reduces the triglyceride and cholesterol levels in blood. Dry fruits, such as apricots and prunes, are rich sources of fibre and help prevent constipation (see Plate 2).

Fibre is beneficial to people on weight reduction regime. It provides satiety value to the meal because of more chewing required and at the same time does not add to the calorific value of the meal.

It helps in lowering blood sugar levels in diabetic individuals by slowing down carbohydrate absorption and lowers the insulin requirement. Regular intake of fibre may prevent cancers of the colon and rectum.

Although fibre is not a true nutrient, because it cannot be digested by humans, it is nutritionally important. Foods such as wholegrain cereals, fruits, and vegetables, specially when the peel and seeds are edible, are rich sources of fibre.

The fibre content of the daily diet should be approximately 30–40 g/day (Table 15.4).

TABLE 15.4   Fibre and carbohydrate content of food (values in g/100 g)

S. no.	Food	Fibre	Carbohydrate
1	Cereals		
	Bajra	1.2	67.5
	Jowar	1.6	72.6
	Sweet corn	1.9	24.6
	Ragi	3.6	72
	Rice	0.2	78.2
	Wheat	1.9	69
	Bread	0.2	51.9
2	Pulses		
	Bengal gram whole	3.9	60.9
	Moong dal	0.8	59.9
	Lentil	0.7	59
	Green peas	4.0	16
	Rajma	4.8	60.6
	Soya bean	3.7	20.9
3	Roots vegetables		
	Potato	0.4	22.4
	Sweet potato	0.8	28.2
	Tapioca	0.6	38
	Yam	1.0	26
	Colocasia	1.0	21

Cond

Table 15.4 Cond

S. no.	Food	Fibre	Carbohydrate
4	**Other vegetables**		
	Cabbage	1.0	4.6
	Spinach	0.6	2.9
	Fenugreek leaves	1.1	6.0
	Bottle gourd	0.6	2.5
	Cauliflower	1.2	4.0
	Drumstick	4.8	3.7
5	**Fruits**		
	Apple	1.0	13.4
	Banana	0.4	27.2
	Dates (fresh)	3.7	33.8
	Guava	5.2	11.2
	Orange	0.3	10.9
	Papaya	0.8	7.2
	Mango	0.7	16.9
	Sapota	2.6	21.4
6	**Dry fruits and nuts**		
	Almonds	1.7	10.5
	Cashew nuts	1.3	22.3
	Raisins	1.1	74.6
	Apricots	2.1	73.4
	Currants (black)	1.0	75.2
	Dates (dried)	3.9	75.8
7	**Nuts and oilseeds**		
	Gingelly seeds	2.9	25
	Niger seeds	10.9	17.1
	Coconut dry	6.6	18.4
	Groundnut	3	26
8	**Miscellaneous**		
	Sugar	—	99.4
	Honey	—	79.5
	Jaggery	—	95.0
	Sago	—	87
	Sugar cane	—	9.1
	Skimmed milk powder	—	51
	Garden cress seeds	7.6	33

Recommended Dietary Intake for Adults

Fibre

40 g/day is desirable

Available carbohydrates

Minimum: 100 g/day

Maximum: less than 70 per cent of total calories from carbohydrates

ARTIFICIAL SWEETENERS

These are also known as non-nutritive sweeteners. Artificial sweeteners are up to 100–350 times as sweet as sucrose and provide no or very negligible calories. A wide veriety of sweetening agents are available in the market and are used for low-calorie products such as diet coke. These processed products are specially manufactured for obese individuals, weight watchers, and diabetic patients. They are used quite successfully in bakery items such as cakes, biscuits, cookies, Indian sweetmeats, confectionery products, beverages, puddings, and chewing gum. Saccharin, aspartame, sodium cyclamate, and stugar are some of the commonly used substitutes for sugar. Their use is not recommended in soft drinks and other food consumed by children as these foods may be a substitute for essential nutrients.

ALCOHOL

Ethyl alcohol is produced by yeast fermentation of carbohydrates under anaerobic conditions. Different carbohydrates are used to manufacture alcoholic beverages.

Alcoholic beverages do not supply necessary nutrients but contribute significant amount of energy (Table 15.5). Alcohol contributes 7 kcal/g or 5.6 kcal/ml and in people who consume alcoholic beverages, up to 10 per cent of total energy needs may be derived from alcohol. Some chronic alcoholics may consume insufficient food and suffer from malnutrition, while the reverse may be observed in the case of social drinkers who consume large amount of high-calorie foods such as starters, nuts, and wafers along with their drinks. These high-calorie snacks are rich in carbohydrate, fat, and sodium. Alcohol is absorbed rapidly, directly into the blood stream. Drinking on an empty stomach increases the alcohol level in blood twice as fast as on a full stomach. It is a good rule to have some light snacks along with alcoholic beverages.

TABLE 15.5   Calories supplied by alcohol

Beverage	Amount	Calories	Alcohol (%)
Lager beer	240 ml	110	4–15
Ale	240 ml	150	4–12.5
Gin 80 proof	30 ml	65	40
Rum	30 ml	70	42.8
Whiskey 86 proof	30 ml	78	43
Wine red	90 ml	145	12–15
Wine dry	90 ml	90	12–15
Vermouth	30 ml	50	18–22
Martini	90 ml	140	12–13

$$C_6H_{12}O_6 \xrightarrow[\text{anaerobically}]{\text{yeast}} 2C_2H_5OH + 2CO_2 \uparrow$$
$$\text{(sugar)} \qquad\qquad\qquad \text{(ethyl alcohol)}$$

Percentage of alcohol is proof divided by 2

86 proof whiskey = 43% alcohol

Caloric content of one peg or 30 ml of whiskey

$$= \frac{43 \times 30 \times 5.6}{100}$$
$$= 78 \text{ kcal}$$

If alcohol is taken along with antidepressants or tranquilizers, it prolongs the sedative effect of these medicines.

Excessive consumption of alcohol accompanied by decreased intake of other nutrients can lead to malnutrition and serious liver disorders such as cirrhosis of the liver.

SUMMARY

Carbohydrates are nutrients which form the bulk of our diet. They include sugars, starch, and fibre and occur abundantly in the plant kingdom. They are made up of carbon, hydrogen, and oxygen.

Sugars and starches are available carbohydrates and provide 4 kcal/g of energy on oxidation. Sugars are classified as monosaccharides and disaccharides of which glucose is the sugar present in blood, and sucrose or table sugar is consumed in large quantities compared to other sugars. Polysaccharides include starch, the form in which carbohydrate is stored in plants, glycogen, or animal starch stored in the muscles and liver and dextrins, which are formed on partial breakdown of starch. These polysaccharides are made up of glucose units and after digestion and absorption all available polysaccharides are converted to glucose and used as a source of energy by all body cells via the liver and blood. Unavailable polysaccharides play an important role in our diet by regular elimination of faecal matter

and regulating the levels of bile acids and cholesterol.

Carbohydrates are an essential nutrient and a minimum quantity should be consumed daily. They perform many important functions in the body. The diet should not provide more than 70 per cent energy from carbohydrates and at least 25–30 g fibre should be consumed daily. An excessive intake of sugar and starch may lead to obesity and dental caries, while excessive fibre may cause gastric irritability and malabsorption of minerals.

Today, sugar is being replaced by artificial sweeteners, which are many hundred times sweeter than sugar and provide no calories. In people who consume alcoholic beverages, the intake of calories from alcohol needs to be considered because alcohol does not provide any nutrients other than energy. Many beverages and fast foods contain large quantities of refined sugars and starches, which could be detrimental to health if they are not combined with nutrient-dense foods.

KEY TERMS

Agar Unavailable polysaccharide made up of galactose units and obtained from a seaweed (algae).

Bran The outer layers of cereal grain, which are largely removed when the grain is milled.

Dietary fibre   Term used to describe the unavailable polysaccharides, such as cellulose, hemicellulose, pectin, gums, mucilages, seaweeds, and lignin (a non-carbohydrate), which are not digested by humans but are necessary in the diet.

Gluconeogenesis   Formation of glucose and glycogen from non-carbohydrate substances such as glycerol and amino acids.

Glycemic index   The rise in blood glucose produced by the carbohydrate present in a given food as compared with the rise by an equal amount of glucose.

Glycogenesis   Synthesis of glycogen from glucose when excess glucose is present in blood.

Glycogenolysis   Breakdown of glycogen to glucose when energy is required.

Hollow calories or empty calories   Term used to describe foods which only supply energy and have very few or no nutrients.

Insulin   A hormone secreted by the pancreas, which regulates carbohydrate metabolism.

Invert sugar   Mixture of glucose and fructose, sweeter than sucrose, produced by hydrolysis of sucrose, and prevents crystallization in confectionery items.

Lignin   A substance which is not a carbohydrate but present along with carbohydrates in the cell wall of plants and forms part of dietary fibre.

Renal threshold   Blood level of a substance at which it cannot be further reabsorbed by the kidneys and is excreted in the urine, e.g., renal threshold of glucose is 170 mg/100 ml.

REVIEW EXERCISES

1. Describe the important functions performed by carbohydrates.
2. Classify carbohydrates of importance in human nutrition and give one rich food source for each category.
3. List ten rich sources of carbohydrate and fibre in your daily diet.
4. List 10 preparations rich in fibre from the menu card of a typical Indian restaurant.
5. What are hollow-calorie foods? Name any five such foods, which are popular amongst teenagers. Suggest alternate nutrient-dense substitutes for the same.
6. What are the beneficial effects of fibre in the diet of an adult man sedentary worker? How much fibre should be consumed daily?
7. How many calories would the following items provide?
   (a) A peg of whiskey
   (b) A tablespoon of sugar
   (c) A glass of beer
   (d) Artificial sweetener aspartame
8. Briefly describe how the human body utilizes carbohydrates from the diet.
9. How does body regulate the fasting blood glucose level? Explain briefly.
10. What are the negative effects of excessive carbohydrate consumption? How many calories should carbohydrates provide in our diet?

Fill in the blanks

1. Dietary fibre provides _____ kcal/g of energy.
2. The human body stores carbohydrate in the form of _____ in the muscles and liver.
3. The water-soluble fibre _____ is used for setting jams and jellies.
4. The sugar _____ is present in the blood stream.
5. The hormone _____ secreted by the _____ regulates blood sugar levels.

Give one word for the following

1. Disease caused due to insufficient insulin.
2. Elevated blood glucose levels.
3. Disaccharide made up of glucose and galactose.
4. Dietary fibre that is not a carbohydrate.
5. Blood level of a substance at which it cannot be. reabsorbed by the kidneys.

CHAPTER 16

Proteins in Nutrition

LEARNING OBJECTIVES

After reading this chapter, you should be able to
- appreciate the importance of proteins in our daily diet
- describe the chemical nature of proteins
- understand the difference between complete and incomplete proteins
- understand the importance of including proteins of high biological value in our meals
- list rich sources of protein
- improve the protein quality of meals served in catering establishments
- gain knowledge about novel sources of protein available in the market

INTRODUCTION

Protein is the basic material of every living cell and is the most important of all known substances in the organic kingdom. It is the only nutrient that can make new cells and rebuild tissues. Therefore, an adequate amount of protein in the diet is essential for normal growth and development and for the maintenance of health.

Definition   Proteins are large, complex, organic compounds made up of carbon, hydrogen, oxygen, and nitrogen. The presence of nitrogen distinguishes proteins from carbohydrates and fats. Apart from nitrogen, elements such as sulphur, phosphorus, copper, and iron are also found in some proteins.

$$NH_2 \text{ (amino group)}$$
$$R-\underset{\underset{H}{|}}{\overset{|}{C}}-COOH \text{ (carboxyl group)}$$

R – Various groupings because of which amino acids differ from one another

Fig. 16.1   An amino acid

The basic units from which proteins are built are the amino acids. Each amino acid contains a carboxyl group (COOH) or acid group and an amino group (NH_2) or basic group (Fig. 161)

Proteins (Fig. 16.2) consist of chains of amino acids that are linked to each other by a peptide linkage (—CO—NH—).

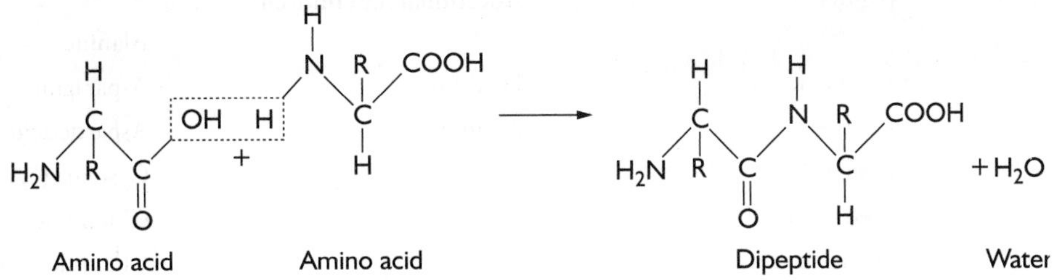

Fig. 16.2   A protein

Twenty-two different amino acids are widely distributed in nature. However, the proteins obtained from plants and animals are quite different both in amounts present and in quality. The proteins that make up the skin, bones, muscles, hair, and nails in the body are obviously very different from each other. Egg, milk, meat, and pulse proteins also differ both in quality and in quantity. This is because the amino acids present in each of these proteins are in different permutations and combinations. Thousands of different proteins exist in nature and vary widely from one another in quality. No two proteins will have an identical amino acid content.

The protein content of any food can be estimated by measuring the nitrogen content of the food. Since proteins contain 16 per cent nitrogen, each gram of nitrogen measured is equal to 6.25 g of protein.

Essential Amino Acids

Those amino acids which cannot be synthesized in sufficient amounts by the body and must be provided by the diet are called essential amino acids. The human adult requires eight essential amino acids, while growing children require ten essential amino acids. Essential amino acids are indispensable to life (Table 16.1).

Non-essential Amino Acids

All amino acids are required by the body for tissue synthesis and repair. Non-essential amino acids (Table 16.1) does not mean that these amino acids are not required by the body. They are termed non-essential because they are not dietary essentials. If they are lacking in the diet, they can be synthesized by the body from other amino acids.

The twenty-two amino acids present in proteins could be compared with the letters of the Roman alphabet and the innumerable words present in our dictionary. Similarly, innumerable proteins can be formed by using the 22 amino acids in varying sequences and quantities.

TABLE 16.1 Classification of amino acids

Essential amino acids		Non-essential amino acids
Adults	Additional for children	
		Alanine
Isoleucine	Histidine*	Asparagine
Leucine	Arginine	Aspartic acid
Lysine		Cysteine (cystine)
Methionine		Glutamine
Phenylalanine		Glutamic acid
Threonine		Glycine
Tryptophan		Hydroxylysine
Valine		Hydroxyproline
		Proline
		Serine
		Tyrosine

Note: Recent studies indicate that histidine may be essential for adults as well.

PROTEIN QUALITY

No two food proteins are identical in their quality, i.e., with the efficiency with which they can be used in the body. The quality of protein depends upon the kind and amount of amino acids present in them in relation to the body needs. Protein quality is an important criterion for tissue synthesis. Each body protein performs a specific function and cannot be replaced by another protein. When a new protein has to be synthesized, all the amino acids, which make up the protein, must be available at the same time and in sufficient quantity. Even if one amino acid is missing or deficient, protein cannot be synthesized just like a word cannot be made if even one of the alphabets of which it is made up of is missing.

Biological Value

It is an index of protein quality. It is defined as the amount of absorbed nitrogen retained in the body. The digestibility factor is not taken into account. Biological value (BV) is a quantitative measure of the nutritive value of a protein food. A protein of high BV will retain more nitrogen than a protein of low BV.

TABLE 16.2 Biological value of some common foods

Food	BV	Food	BV
Egg	100	Rice	73
Milk	85	Wheat	66
Fish	83	Groundnuts	55
Meat	75	Gelatin	00

Cereals and pulses consumed together will have a higher BV than the average value of the individual cereal or pulse. This is because of the complementary nature of proteins. Amino acids deficient in cereals will be compensated by the amino acids present in pulses.

The perfect protein has a BV of 100. The BV of some common food are given in Table 16.2

CLASSIFICATION OF PROTEINS

Proteins may be classified on the basis of their structure or on the basis of their quality, i.e., the amino acids present in them.

Classification by Structure

Simple proteins   These proteins are made up of amino acids only, e.g., zein in corn, albumin in egg white, and gliadin in wheat consist of amino acids only.

Conjugated proteins   These proteins have a non-protein molecule attached to the protein, e.g., blood protein haemoglobin, which contains a haeme (iron) group attached to protein and milk protein casein, which has a phosphate group attached.

Derived proteins   These result from a partial breakdown of a native protein. Proteoses, peptones, and polypeptides are formed when digestive enzymes begin their action on proteins.

From the nutritional point of view, classification of proteins on the basis of their quality is more relevant than classification by structure and is explained in the following section.

Classification by Quality

Proteins are classified into three groups on the basis of their quality.

Complete proteins   These proteins contain all essential amino acids in sufficient proportions and amounts to meet the body's need for growth and repair of tissue cells. A complete protein food has a high BV. Eggs, milk, meat, fish, and poultry are complete protein foods. They are found in animal foods.

Partially complete proteins   These are proteins in which one or more essential amino acids are present in inadequate amounts. They cannot synthesize tissues without the help of other proteins. The value of each is increased when it is consumed in combination with another incomplete protein at the same meal. They can maintain life. They are found in plant foods. Cereals, pulses, nuts, and oilseeds are partially complete protein foods. Cereals contain inadequate amounts of essential amino acid lysine, and pulses are deficient in essential amino acid methionine.

Incomplete proteins   These proteins are incapable of growth and repair of body cells. They cannot maintain life. One or more essential amino acids may be completely lacking in these proteins, e.g., gelatin and zein in corn. Gelatin lacks three essential amino acids and is the only animal protein which is incomplete.

FUNCTIONS IN THE HUMAN BODY

Proteins perform three main functions: structural function, regulatory function, and energy.

Structural Functions

Growth   The primary function of food protein is the synthesis of body cells. All body tissues and fluids, except urine and bile, are made up of protein. Proteins are the major constituent of muscles, organs, endocrine glands, and collagen. Collagen is the main structural protein of bones, tendons, ligaments, skin, blood vessels, and connective tissue. All enzymes and some hormones, e.g., insulin are made up of proteins. Proteins are required for the formation and growth of all these substances. During periods of rapid growth, additional proteins are needed for synthesis of body components.

Maintenance or wear and tear   Protein is required by all age groups for continuous maintenance of all the cells in the body. Cells have a varying lifespan and proteins are needed to replace the old or worn out cells.

Regulatory Functions

All amino acids from food protein are used for growth and maintenance. Certain amino acids and proteins have highly specialized functions in the regulation of body processes and protection against disease. Some of the regulatory functions are as follows:

1. Haemoglobin, an iron containing protein in the red blood cells, performs an important role by transporting oxygen to the tissue cells.
2. Plasma proteins maintain water balance and regulate the osmotic pressure in the body.
3. Antibodies that are protein in nature perform a protective function by increasing the body's resistance to disease.
4. All enzymes and some hormones, e.g., insulin are made up of protein. The hormone insulin regulates blood sugar levels. Enzymes act as specific catalysts to metabolic processes in the body.

5. Some amino acids have specific functions, e.g., tryptophan serves as a precursor for niacin, a B-complex vitamin. The amino acid tyrosine in combination with iodine forms the hormone thyroxine.

Energy

Like carbohydrates, proteins too provide 4 kcal/g when broken down in the body. The basic need of the body is energy and this takes priority over protein synthesis. If the diet does not supply adequate calories from carbohydrates and fats, the proteins from the diet will be oxidized to meet the energy needs of the body.

If the diet is deficient in calories, the body uses up its protein and fat stores. Using protein as a source of energy is not advisable as it puts an extra burden on the body and the pocket. Protein is used by the body as a source of energy only when no other source of energy is available.

DIGESTION, ABSORPTION, AND METABOLISM

To enable proteins to perform their various functions, dietary protein needs to be broken down into its constituent amino acids.

The mechanical digestion of protein begins in the mouth, where the teeth grind the food into small pieces. The mouth does not produce any enzyme to digest proteins. Chemical digestion begins in the stomach. The hydrochloric acid (HCl) in the gastric juice activates the enzyme pepsin, which acts on proteins and reduces them to polypeptides. After the partially digested proteins reach the small intestine, three pancreatic enzymes—trypsin, chymotrypsin, and carboxypeptidase—continue the process of chemical digestion. The peptidases secreted by the intestine finally reduce the smaller peptides and dipeptides into amino acids, which are the end-product of protein digestion.

After digestion, the amino acids in the small intestine are absorbed by the blood and carried to the liver and all body tissues where they are metabolized.

The body needs varying compositions of amino acids to build and repair the different tissues of the body. All essential amino acids must be present if body cells have to be built or repaired. Surplus amino acids are sent back to the liver where they are deaminated by splitting off the amino group. The remaining part of the protein is used for energy or stored as glycogen in the liver and muscles or as fat in the adipose tissue. The end products of the metabolism of amino acids are carbon dioxide, water, and nitrogen. Some of the nitrogen is excreted as urea by the kidneys. Some nitrogen may be retained and used again to synthesize non-essential amino acids as and when required by the body.

TABLE 16.3 Digestion and metabolism of protein

Human body	Fate of protein	Process
Mouth	Food protein	Mechanical digestion
Stomach	Proteoses	Chemical digestion
	Peptones	Enzyme pepsin – gastric
	Polypeptides	juice
Small intestine	Small chain	Pancreatic enzymes
	• Polypeptides	Intestinal juices
	• Dipeptides	
	Amino acids	
Blood	Amino acids	Absorbed into blood circulation
Large intestine	Undigested proteins	Excretion of unabsorbed proteins
Liver	Amino group ⟶ Urea	Deamination

Nitrogen-free residue ↙ Glycogen ↘ Fatty acids — Gluconeogenesis

Body cells	1. Protein — growth, repair → Protein synthesis
	2. Adipose tissue → Storage of fat
	Glycogen (energy) ⟶ Oxidation
Kidneys	Carbon dioxide + Water	Excretion / Urea

METHODS OF IMPROVING PROTEIN QUALITY

Animal proteins contain all essential amino acids in correct proportions and amounts and are good quality proteins. Four essential amino acids are in short supply in plant proteins. They are lysine, methionine, threonine, and tryptophan. Proteins in plant foods are generally deficient in one or two essential amino acids. Cereals are poor in lysine and pulses are poor

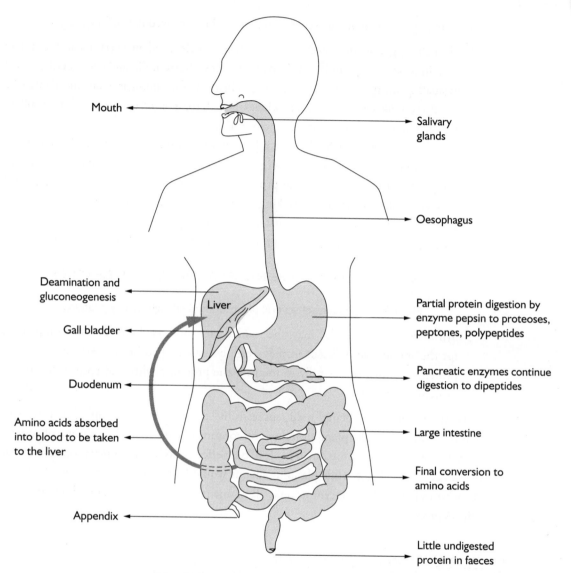

Mouth

Salivary glands

Oesophagus

Deamination and gluconeogenesis

Liver

Partial protein digestion by enzyme pepsin to proteoses, peptones, polypeptides

Gall bladder

Pancreatic enzymes continue digestion to dipeptides

Duodenum

Amino acids absorbed into blood to be taken to the liver

Large intestine

Final conversion to amino acids

Appendix

Little undigested protein in faeces

Fig. 16.3   Digestion and absorption of protein

in methionine. Egg protein has a BV of 100 and is the reference protein as its amino acid composition corresponds most closely to human requirements. Eggs sold in the market are unfertilized and could be included in a vegetarian diet, if acceptable.

We have already read that protein will be synthesized only when all amino acids, which form the protein, are present simultaneously. We have also read that vegetable proteins are partially complete proteins. These two points should be kept in mind while improving the protein quality of a meal.

The protein quality of a mainly vegetarian diet can be improved in the following ways.

1. By including a small quantity of complete protein food in every meal. Complete protein foods such as milk, curds, paneer, cheese, buttermilk, and eggs could be used in small quantities in various preparations instead of including it in one meal only, e.g., cereal and milk, egg or cheese sandwiches, French toast, *raita*, curd rice, or buttermilk at all meals in place of a bowl of curd in one meal.

2. Correct mixtures of plant foods could provide all essential amino acids in suitable proportions and amounts (see Fig. 16.4). Cereal and pulse combinations will complement each other as cereals provide methionine, which is lacking in pulses, and pulses provide lysine, which is lacking in cereals, when cereal and pulses are consumed together in the same meal, e.g., *missi roti, thalipeeth, puran poli*, idli, and *rajma chawal*. This is possible because the same amino acids are not missing from all plant foods.

CEREAL + PULSE + GREEN LEAFY VEGETABLE = FLESH FOODS

Fig. 16.4 Mixtures of several plant foods yield high-quality proteins

3. Synthetic amino acids may be added to processed foods to compensate for the amino acid deficient in them, e.g., lysine-enriched bread. Textured vegetable proteins are used successfully to improve the protein quality and reduce the cost of protein-rich foods.

Plant proteins are being used successfully to stretch the supply of expensive animal proteins. When plant proteins are consumed with a small quantity of animal protein, the quality of the mixture is likely to be as effective as if only animal protein has been consumed. A good rule while planning menus would be to include some animal protein at each meal instead of concentrating it all in one meal. Figure 16.5 shows how the body utilizes protein.

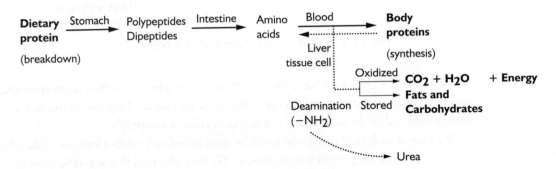

Fig. 16.5 How the body utilizes protein

FACTORS INFLUENCING PROTEIN REQUIREMENTS

Many factors affect the protein requirement of an individual such as

1. Body weight
2. Special physiological needs during
   (a) Growth
   (b) Pregnancy and lactation
   (c) Convalescence
   (d) Infection and fever
   (e) Injury or surgery
3. Adequacy of calorie intake
4. Quality of protein and efficiency of digestion
5. Previous state of nutrition

Body weight   The protein requirement is based on a person's ideal body weight. Adults require 1 g protein/kg body weight from a mixed diet. The Indian reference man weighs 60 kg and requires 60 g protein/day and the reference woman weighs 50 kg and requires 50 g protein/day from a mixed diet.

Special physiological needs   Infants and growing children require additional protein for synthesis of new cells as compared to adults. They need 1.6 to 2 g protein/kg body weight. Whenever new tissue or protein needs to be synthesized, additional protein greater than the amount needed for maintenance should be included in the diet. Protein requirement increases during illness or disease as protein is needed for rebuilding new tissue. In traumatic injury, surgery, burns, and fever, there is breakdown of tissues, which need to be repaired. Extra physical activity does not require any additional intake of protein.

Adequacy of calorie intake   The diet should contain adequate carbohydrates and fats to have a protein sparing effect.

Quality of protein and efficiency of digestion   The quantity of protein required will be more if the protein quality is poor. Plant proteins have a lower digestibility. The method of cooking also affects the availability of protein. Overcooking and toughening of animal proteins affects digestibility.

Previous state of nutrition   Malnourished and underweight individuals require more protein as compared to healthy individuals.

RECOMMENDED DIETARY ALLOWANCES

The amount of protein required depends on the quality of protein consumed, i.e., on the amino acid composition of the protein rather than the quantity of protein present in a

Table 16.4 Recommended protein allowances for Indians

Group	Particulars	Body weight (kg)	Protein (g/day)
Man	Adult	60	60
Women	Adult	50	50
	Pregnancy		+15
	Lactation (0–6 months)		+25
	(6–12 months)		+18
Infants	0–6 months	5.4	2.05 g/kg
	6–12 months	8.6	1.65 g/kg
Children	1–3 years	12.2	22
	4–6 years	19.0	30
	7–9 years	26.9	41
Boys	10–12 years	35.4	54
	13–15 years	47.8	70
	16–18 years	57.1	78
Girls	10–12 years	31.5	57
	13–15 years	46.7	65
	16–18 years	49.9	63

food. On a mixed vegetarian diet, adults require 1g/kg body weight (ideal weight) while infants 0–6 months age need 2g/kg and infants 6–12 months need 1.65g/kg body weight. Requirements are higher in terms of body weight for infants and children because proteins are needed for growth as well as maintenance.

Pregnant women require an additional +15g/day, while lactating mothers need +25g to +18g/day for 0 to 6 months and 6 to 12 months, respectively.

Table 16.4 gives the recommended protein allowances for Indians.

DIETARY SOURCES

Proteins are present in both plant and animal foods.

Animal Food Sources

Animal food sources provide the highest quality or complete proteins such as eggs, milk and milk products (cheese, *paneer, mawa,* milk powder, curds, condensed milk), meat, fish, shellfish, poultry, and organ meat.

Plant Food Sources

Pulses, especially soya bean (43 per cent protein) and its products such as soya milk, tofu, textured vegetable proteins; nuts, and oilseeds—groundnut and gingelly seeds are important sources of protein in the Indian diet. Cereals contain 6–12 per cent partially complete proteins and as they form the bulk of the diet, they contribute significantly to the protein content. Vegetables, with the exception of peas and beans, are poor sources of proteins. Green leafy vegetables contain a small percentage of good quality protein (approximately 1–3 per cent). Fruits do not contribute towards the protein content of the diet. See Fig. 16.6 for protein quality and content of some commonly consumed foodstuff.

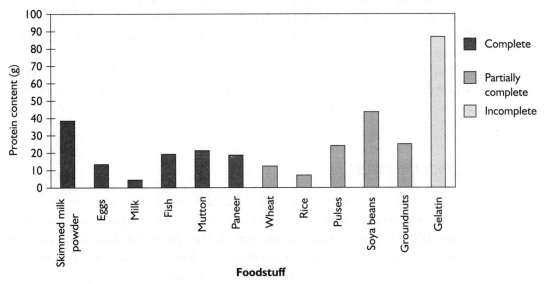

Fig. 16.6 Protein quality and content of some commonly consumed foodstuff in g/100g edible portion

SPECIAL PROTEIN SUPPLEMENTS

Special protein supplements in the form of premix powders or ready-to-consume health drinks are available in a variety of popular flavours and different nutrient compositions. They are used by sportspersons for minimizing muscle catabolism, boosting energy and muscle growth and stimulating greater fat loss. They are recommended by health programmers in gymnasiums to the trainees for maintaining physical fitness and often supplement an exercise regimen on a weight-gain or weight-loss programme.

Protein supplements are available in the form of pure protein isolates, weight gainers or as meal replacements. The protein, carbohydrate, and fat content varies in these supplements depending on what they are being recommended for. The following proteins are used by themselves or as a blend.

1. Whey protein isolate
2. Whey peptides
3. Calcium caseinate
4. Egg albumin
6. Whey protein concentrate
7. Complete milk protein
8. Micellar casein
9. Soya protein isolate

5. Skimmed milk powder

Protein isolates contain 70 to 90 per cent protein of high biological value. They are low in carbohydrates, cholesterol, and fats. Premix powders may be enzymically predigested and one scoop of 33 g can be mixed with a glass of water, milk or juice to provide 24 g of protein. They repair tissues and help in building muscle mass.

Weight gainers are protein supplements which are calorie dense with a ratio of carbohydrates to proteins being at least 2:1. They contain high glycemic index sugars, dietary fibre, omega-3 fatty acids, vitamins, minerals, and may also contain chromium, creatinine and glutamine.

Meal replacements are used instead of a meal and contain high-quality proteins, carbohydrates, fats, vitamins, minerals and fibre in varying proportions. They provide at least half the daily requirement for proteins, vitamins and minerals. They are available as premix powders or as energy bars.

EFFECT OF DEFICIENCY AND EXCESS

A reduced protein intake over a prolonged period of time leads to loss of weight, fatigue, anaemia, nutritional oedema, lowered resistance to infection, and poor healing of wounds. Protein deficiency is more marked during periods when protein needs are more, e.g., during infancy, childhood, pregnancy, and lactation. The deficiency occurs when an individual does not eat enough proteins or obtains insufficient calories. Protein calorie malnutrition (PCM) is common in pre-school children in developing countries and manifests itself in the form of *kwashiorkor*, a deficiency of protein or *marasmus*, a deficiency of calories as well as proteins, which is equivalent to starvation in adults.

Protein deficiency is also seen in people who follow a crash diet for weight loss. It can be prevented by including correct mixture of inexpensive protein-rich foods in the diet.

An excessive intake of protein is not beneficial to health. When the diet provides more protein than what is necessary for body building, repair, and regulatory functions, the excess protein is used as energy or converted to fat and stored in the adipose tissue in the body.

A high protein intake has many disadvantages.

1. Once the body needs have been taken care of, the excess protein is deaminated by the liver and urea is synthesized. The kidneys have to work more to excrete the additional amount of urea. A high protein intake is an unnecessary burden on two vital organs, i.e., the liver and the kidneys. If these organs are diseased, toxic wastes tend to accumulate in the body.
2. When animal proteins, such as meat, poultry, and whole milk products, form a substantial part of the high-protein diet, there is a risk of high blood levels of cholesterol.
3. A high intake of protein increases the loss of calcium through the urine.
4. Protein-rich foods are much costlier, are in short supply, and are not an economical source

of energy.

SUMMARY

Proteins are important constituents of all living cells and are made up of units called amino acids. Proteins differ from one another because of the different kinds and amounts of amino acids of which they are composed. Amino acids are classified as essential and non-essential. Non-essential amino acids can be synthesized by the body in required amounts. Essential amino acids cannot be synthesized by the body and must be included in the diet. The quality of any protein depends upon the essential amino acids present. On the basis of quality, proteins are classified as complete, partially complete, and incomplete. Animal proteins except gelatin are complete proteins while plant proteins are partially complete proteins. The quality of plant proteins can be improved when several plant foods are combined together or small quantities of animal proteins are included in each meal. For tissue synthesis to take place all essential amino acids should be present at the same time.

Proteins perform three basic functions, namely the structural function of body building and repair, the regulatory and protective function, and as a source of energy when no other source is available.

The chemical digestion of protein begins in the stomach where protein is broken down to polypeptides. In the intestine, polypeptides are further broken down into dipeptides and amino acids, which are absorbed into the blood stream and sent to various tissue cells via the liver.

Proteins are present in abundance both in animal and plant foods such as eggs, milk, meat, pulses, especially soya beans, groundnuts, and textured vegetable proteins. Most vegetables and all fruits are poor sources of protein. How much protein an individual will require depends on many factors such as age, body weight, special physiological needs, adequacy of calorie intake, quality of protein, and previous state of nutrition.

An excessive intake of protein is not beneficial as it increases the burden on two vital organs, namely the liver and kidneys to metabolize and excrete the wastes arising from amino acid breakdown. Protein-rich foods are costlier than carbohydrates, which provide the same number of calories per gram. When the protein intake is inadequate, protein cannot perform the required functions in the body and a deficiency results. Deficiency symptoms are common in the vulnerable age group in developing countries. Protein deficiency can be prevented by proper menu planning and including low-cost plant proteins such as textured vegetable proteins in the diet.

KEY TERMS

Amino acids They are organic acids that contain an amino group (NH_2) and an acid or carboxyl group (COOH) attached to the same carbon atom. They are the basic units from which proteins are built.

Biological value The percentage of absorbed nitrogen retained by the body.

Collagen The intercellular cementing protein/ structural protein in bone, cartilage, connective tissue, etc.

Deamination The removal of the amino group from the amino acid by the liver.

Digestibility The percentage of protein that is absorbed by the body.

Essential amino acid An amino acid that cannot be synthesized by our body and needs to be supplied by our diet.

Non-essential amino acid An amino acid that can be synthesized in the body and need not be present in the diet.

Peptidases Enzymes that breakdown short polypeptides and dipeptides into amino acids.

Peptide linkage The linkage between the amino group of one amino acid and the carboxyl group of another amino acid.

Proteolytic enzymes Protein-splitting enzymes that reduce proteins to shorter chain polypetides and dipeptides.

REVIEW EXERCISES

1. List five cereal pulse combinations, which are popular items in a fast food restaurant.
2. How can the protein quality of a vegetarian diet be improved?
3. List the names of amino acids essential for children. What is the difference between essential and non-essential amino acids?
4. Classify proteins on the basis of their quality.
5. Define the following terms
   (a) Essential amino acid

Fill in the blanks

1. The basic building blocks of proteins are called _____.
2. Cereals are deficient in amino acid _____ and pulses are deficient in amino acid _____.
3. In a protein, the amino acids are linked together by _____ linkages.
4. The essential amino acid _____ is converted to niacin in the human body.
5. The quality of protein depends upon the _____ and _____ of amino acids present in them.

(b) Biological value
6. List and briefly explain the functions performed by proteins.
7. List the symptoms of protein deficiency in adults.
8. Why are proteins called an uneconomical source of energy?
9. Recollect and list the sources of animal and vegetable proteins, which you have consumed in your diet the day before.

Give scientific reasons for the following

1. *Rajma*, *kabuli channa*, and *urad dal* are partially complete proteins.
2. The biological value of dal and rice increases when it is consumed together.
3. An excessive intake of protein is not beneficial to health.
4. Even though gelatin is an animal protein, it does not promote growth.
5. An additional intake of protein is required during pregnancy.

CHAPTER 17

Lipids

LEARNING OBJECTIVES

After reading this chapter, you should be able to
- identify the fats and other lipids which are essential in the diet
- describe their chemical nature and functions in the human body
- list the food sources of various lipids and essential fatty acids
- determine how much and what type of fats should be included in our daily diet
- know how the body digests, absorbs, and metabolizes fat
- understand the consequences of a deficient or excessive consumption of lipids

INTRODUCTION

Fats and oils belong to a group of compounds called lipids, which are insoluble in water but soluble in fat solvents. Like carbohydrates, they are mainly made up of carbon, hydrogen, and oxygen. They contain much smaller proportions of oxygen than carbohydrates and larger proportions of carbon and hydrogen. Hence, they are a more concentrated source of energy, providing two and a quarter times more energy than carbohydrates and proteins.

The lipids of importance to our health are fatty acids, fats, oils, phospholipids, lipoproteins, and sterols.

CLASSIFICATION OF LIPIDS

Classification Based on Structure

Based on their structure lipids are classified into simple lipids, compound lipids, derived lipids, and sterols (Fig. 17.1).

Simple lipids They constitute more than 98 per cent of food and body fats. Simple lipids are made up of three fatty acids attached to glycerol. They are mixed triglycerides

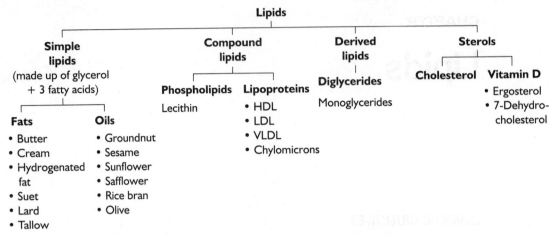

Fig. 17.1 Classification of lipids based on structure

which means that more than one type of fatty acid is present in the fat, e.g., cooking oils and butter.

Compound lipids They are fats in which at least one fatty acid is replaced by carbohydrate, protein, or phosphorous, i.e., they are fats + non-fat molecule, e.g., phospholipids, glycolipids, and lipoprotein.

Derived lipids They are the breakdown products of fats and include diglycerides, monoglycerides, glycerol, and fatty acids.

Sterols They are not made up of fatty acids and glycerol but have a benzene ring structure. These fat-like substances include cholesterol and fat-soluble vitamins A, D, E, and K.

As mentioned in Chapter 7, the basic chemical structure of fats and oils (Fig. 17.2) is a molecule of glycerol to which three fatty acids are attached. Such a fat is called a simple triglyceride. Triglycerides constitute 90 per cent of all food fats.

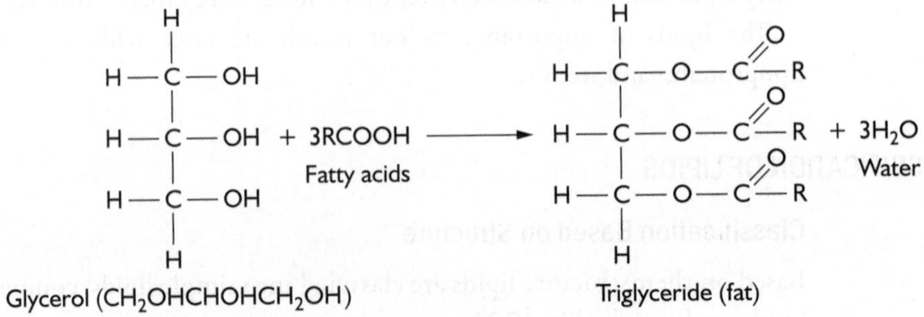

Glycerol ($CH_2OHCHOHCH_2OH$) + 3RCOOH (Fatty acids) → Triglyceride (fat) + $3H_2O$ (Water)

Fig. 17.2 Basic chemical structure of fats and oils

R is the carbon chain of varying length ending with methyl group (CH_3) and COOH is the acid group and is a double bond.

FATTY ACIDS

Fatty acids consist of chains of carbon atoms with a methyl (CH_3) group at one end and a carboxyl (COOH) group at the other end. Fatty acids may have short chains or they may have long chains (12–22 carbon chains). They may be saturated or unsaturated (Fig. 17.3). Saturated fats have single bonds between carbon atoms, while unsaturated fats have one or more double bonds between the carbon atoms. Fatty acids with two or more double bonds are called polyunsaturated.

Unsaturated fatty acids are highly reactive to oxygen at the point of unsaturation and turn rancid. Hydrogen is added at the double bond during hydrogenation of oils. The more the number of double bonds, the more unstable is the fat.

Food fats are generally a mixture of both types of fatty acids. Natural fats contain more than one kind of triglyceride molecules. Fats are mixtures of triglyceride molecules differing in length and in degree of unsaturation of the fatty acid chain. For example, butter contains 13 different fatty acids esterified to glycerol.

Both fats and oils are triglycerides but fats have a higher proportion of saturated fatty acids and are solid at room temperature, while oils have more unsaturated fatty acids and are liquid at room temperature.

The type of fatty acids present in fat determines the nature of the fat, its flavour, and other properties such as smoke point and melting point. The chemical structure of fatty acids is shown in Fig. 17.4.

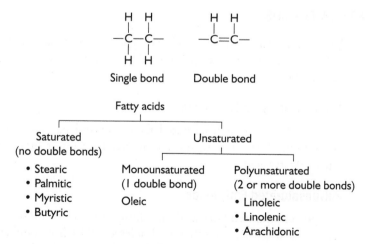

Fig. 17.3 Classification of fatty acids

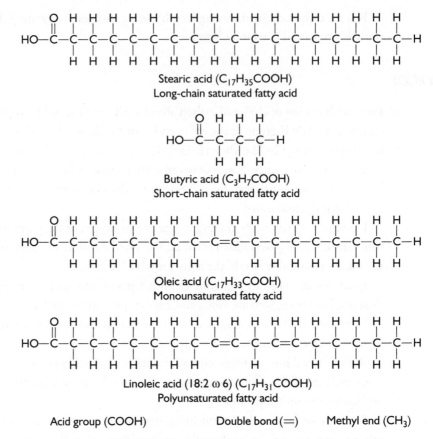

Fig. 17.4 Chemical structure of fatty acids

UNSATURATED FATTY ACIDS

Unsaturated fatty acids are of two types: monounsaturated fatty acids (MUFA) and polyunsaturated fatty acids (PUFA). Table 17.1 lists some of the common unsaturated fatty acids and their sources.

Monounsaturated Fatty Acids

Oleic acid is a monounsaturated fatty acid and has one double bond. It is found in groundnut, olive oil, corn oil, etc. It may help lower blood cholesterol levels. It is an omega-9 fatty acid.

Polyunsaturated Fatty Acids

The polyunsaturated fatty acids are those with two or more double bonds. They include linoleic acid (two double bonds) linolenic acid (three double bonds), and arachidonic acid (four double bonds). They help in lowering blood cholesterol levels and prevent atherosclerosis and coronary heart disease.

TABLE 17.1 Some unsaturated fatty acids present in food

Fatty acid	No. of carbon atoms	No. of double bonds	Food source
Oleic acid	18	1	Groundnuts, sesame, olives, butter, cocoa butter, cashew nuts, avocado
Linoleic acid	18	2	Safflower, sunflower, cottonseed, corn, soya bean, groundnut, salmon, tuna
Linolenic acid	18	3	Soya bean, rapeseed, sesame, butter
Arachidonic acid	20	4	Animal fats, groundnut
Eicosapentaenoic acid	20	5	Fish oils
Erucic acid	22	1	Rapeseed oil/mustard oil

Essential fatty acids

Two of the PUFA cannot be synthesized by the body. They have to be provided in the required amount by our diet and are called essential fatty acids.

They are linoleic acid, an omega-6 fatty acid, and linolenic acid, an omega-3 fatty acid.

Omega-3 and omega-6 fatty acids Omega-3 fatty acids are polyunsaturated fatty acids with the end most double bond on the third carbon from the methyl end. Omega (ω) is the last letter of the Greek alphabet used by scientists for naming fatty acids.

18:3 ω 3 is the abbreviation for linolenic acid which is a long chain fatty acid made up of 18 carbons with three double bonds with the last double bond between carbons 3 and 4 from the methyl/omega end.

Fish oils are especially rich in eicosapentaenoic acid (EPA) which is abbreviated as 20:5 ω 3, i.e., a 20-carbon fatty acid with five double bonds, and the last double bond is on carbon 3 from the omega end.

Omega-6 fatty acids have the last double bond located on the sixth carbon from the methyl or omega end. Essential fatty acid linoleic acid (18:2 ω 6) and arachidonic acid (20:4 ω 6) are omega-6 fatty acids. They are present in a number of foods.

Omega-6 rich oils include safflower, sunflower, cottonseed, corn, sesame, and groundnut.

Omega-3 rich foods include olive oil, fish oils, mustard oil, soya bean, flax seed, fenugreek seeds, mackerel, black gram, *rajma*, and green leafy vegetables.

When consumption of omega-6 goes up, need for omega-3 increases. Omega-3 and omega-6 in the correct ratio helps in reducing blood cholesterol levels.

Eating 200–300 g of fish/shellfish per week or 15–20 g of flax seeds daily meets the RDA (0.5–1.0 g/day of omega-3 fats).

To ensure that the body gets the required amounts of essential fatty acid, a blend of different oils should be used for cooking.

Oil recommended for cooking

1. Sesame + mustard
2. Groundnut + mustard
3. Soya bean + olive
4. Corn + rice bran

Omega-3 fatty acid is an essential part of each and every cell membrane. It helps in maintaining the cells membrane and prevents free radicals from attacking dioxyribonucleic acid (DNA) in the cell.

Free radicals are O, OH, CO, NO, and NOO. The percentage of free radicals increase because of the following:

1. High protein diet
2. High fat diet
3. Stress
4. Smoking
5. Alcohol

An optimum balance between omega-3 and omega-6 fatty acids is essential for maintaining good health. They are beneficial for the cardiovascular system, for inflammatory reactions, and immune response.

In the body, linoleic acid is converted to arachidonic acid which is required for normal growth, healthy skin, and metabolism of cholesterol. Hence, arachidonic acid is not an essential fatty acid.

ANTIOXIDANTS

Antioxidants are substances that prevent or delay oxidation by chemically protecting other substances in food from getting oxidized. They prevent changes in colour or flavour caused by oxygen in the air. They also prevent rancid taste and odour from developing in fats and oils during storage and in the fatty phases of foods such as *farsan*, pickles, and commercial cake mixes. Oxidation leads to degenerative changes in our body, i.e., it contributes to the breakdown of body cells as we age.

Free radicals are highly unstable and cause damage to DNA, carbohydrates, and lipids and proteins in the body that leads to the development of heart diseases and aging. Antioxidants are capable of neutralizing these highly reactive molecules in the body.

Antioxidants, such as vitamin C, vitamin E, beta-carotene, and selenium, help protect against free radical damage. They scavenge free radicals and protect body cells against cancer. They prevent atherosclerosis and coronary artery diseases (CAD).

The sources of antioxidants are listed below.

1. *Vitamin E* Soya oil, sunflower oil, almonds, spinach, and mint
2. *Vitamin C* Amla, guava, green leafy vegetables, all citrus fruit, papaya, tomato, cabbage, and capsicum

3. *Beta-carotene* All green leafy vegetables, and all yellow, orange, and red fruits and vegetables
4. *Selenium* Whole grains, whole pulses, green leafy vegetables, and cauliflower
5. *Non-nutrient antioxidants* Phenolic compounds, flavonoids, and isoflavones present in beans, cloves, oats, tea, coffee, grapes, turmeric, mustard, red wine, etc.

We need to consume much more than the recommended daily allowances (RDA) for antioxidant effect.

SATURATED FATTY ACIDS

These are found in animal foods such as meat, butter, cheese, and egg yolk and in plant foods such as coconut oil, palm oil, and cocoa butter. Hydrogenated fats used in bakery products and confections have a high percentage of saturated fatty acids. Stearic acid, palmitic acid, myristic acid, and butyric acid are some of the saturated fatty acids. A maximum of 10 per cent of our total calories should come from saturated fats. Table 17.2 shows some saturated fatty acids present in food.

TABLE 17.2 Some saturated fatty acids present in food

Fatty acid	No. of carbon atoms	Food source
Acetic acid	2	Vinegar
Butyric acid	4	Butter
Caproic acid	6	Butter
Caprylic acid	8	Coconut, palm kernel
Lauric acid	12	Palm kernel, coconut
Myristic acid	14	Coconut, butter
Palmitic acid	16	Palm, soya, sesame, butter, lard, cotton seed
Stearic acid	18	Beef tallow, cocoa butter, lard

PHOSPHOLIPIDS

They are composed of fats, phosphoric acid, and a nitrogenous base, e.g., lecithins and cephalins. They are required for cell permeability and for the formation of brain and nervous tissue. They help in transporting fats throughout the body as they form a part of the lipoproteins.

LIPOPROTEINS

They include chylomicrons, very low-density lipoproteins (VLDL), low-density lipoproteins (LDL), and high-density lipoproteins (HDL). They are composed of lipids (triglycerides, cholesterol, and phospholipids) and proteins in varying proportions with percentage of proteins being least in chylomicrons and most in HDL. Lipoproteins are required for transporting triglycerides to various tissues in the body via blood circulation. Triglycerides are encased by a covering of water-soluble proteins which helps them to circulate in water-based blood. These lipid–protein complexes are called lipoproteins.

Since LDL are the main carriers of cholesterol, an increase in LDL increases the risk of heart disease. High-density lipoproteins help in lowering cholesterol levels. An LDL/HDL ratio of less than 3 is desirable.

GLYCOLIPIDS

They contain glucose or galactose in place of one of the fatty acids in the triglyceride molecule.

CHOLESTEROL

It is a fat-like substance present in food. It is different in structure from triglycerides, as it has a ring structure. It is present in all cells of the body and in large amounts in brain and nerve tissue. Cholesterol if consumed in excess is responsible for diseases of the cardiovascular system. The normal blood cholesterol level for adults should be below 200 mg/100 ml blood.

The human body gets cholesterol from two sources:

1. Synthesis in the liver
2. Food rich in cholesterol

If the diet is deficient in cholesterol, the body can synthesize the required cholesterol. The functions of cholesterol are listed below.

1. Cholesterol is a precursor of all steroid hormones, e.g., sex hormones.
2. A precursor of vitamin D, 7-dehydrocholesterol is present in the skin which is irradiated by ultra violet (UV) rays of sunlight to form vitamin D.
3. It is required for formation of bile.
4. It is an essential constituent of cell membranes.

Sources

Cholesterol is present in animal foods only. Whole milk, butter, ghee, cream, egg yolk, organ meat, and shellfish are rich sources. The approximate cholesterol content of some common foods are given in Table 17.3.

Cholesterol is also synthesized by the body independent of the dietary intake.

TABLE 17.3 Approximate cholesterol content of some common foods (per 100 g edible portion)

Food	Cholesterol (mg)	Food	Cholesterol (mg)
Beef tallow	109	Mutton	70
Lard	95	Beef	70
Butter	250	Pork	70
Processed cheese	150	Chicken with skin	80
Paneer	19	Liver	300
Ice cream	40	Brain	2,000
Whole milk	14	Fish	60
Skimmed milk	2	Shellfish	150
Mawa-based sweets	65	*Vanaspati*	0
Egg white (1 egg)	0	Margarine (veg fat)	0
Egg yolk (1 egg)	252	All plant foods	0

FUNCTIONS OF FATS

Energy Fats are a concentrated source of energy in our diet. One gram of fat/oil gives 9 kcal when it is oxidized in the body. All tissues, except those of the central nervous system and brain, can utilize fat as a source of energy.

Protein sparing action The kilocalories from fat spare dietary proteins from being oxidized for energy. An adequate intake of fat in the diet allows proteins to perform their main functions of growth and maintenance.

Thermal insulation Subcutaneous fat acts as an insulation and helps in retaining body heat.

Protection of vital organs Fat provides a protective padding to vital organs from mechanical shock and keeps them in place.

Absorption of fat-soluble vitamins Fat is necessary for the absorption of fat-soluble vitamins A, D, E, and K.

Essential fatty acids An adequate intake of fats/oils is necessary to meet the body's requirements for linoleic and linolenic acids.

Satiety value Fats slow down the secretion of gastric juice and speed of digestion.

Food is more flavoursome because of volatile essential oils naturally present and fats used for cooking. A well-cooked meal containing fats is more satisfying than a meal devoid of fats.

Synthesis of cell membranes Fats are an important constituent of all cell membranes.

Synthesis of hormones   The lipid cholesterol is necessary for the synthesis of some hormones, e.g., sex hormones.

DIGESTION, ABSORPTION, AND METABOLISM OF FATS

The fats and oils consumed in the diet need to be broken down into their constituent components, namely glycerol and fatty acids, before they can be utilized by the body.

Digestion

No chemical digestion of fat takes place in the mouth. Fat is broken into smaller particles by chewing and is mixed with saliva.

In the stomach, peristaltic movements churn the food along with the gastric juice. Two enzymes help in digesting fats, namely gastric lipase in the gastric juice and pancreatic lipase from the pancreas which acts in the small intestine. For fats to be digested, they first need to be emulsified. Gastric lipase acts on emulsified butterfat, and the main digestion of fats begins in the small intestine.

The presence of fats in the duodenum stimulates the secretion of bile from the gall bladder. Bile acts as an emulsifier and breaks down large fat globules into smaller particles. This increases the total surface area of fat and increases the efficiency of enzyme action. The alkaline nature of bile helps pancreatic lipase to remove fatty acids from the triglyceride, converting them to diglycerides and monoglycerides and finally to fatty acids and glycerol.

The final products of fat digestion to be absorbed are fatty acids, glycerol, monoglycerides, and diglycerides. Some remaining fat which is undigested may be excreted through the faeces. Figure 17.5 shows the digestion and absorption of fat in the body.

Absorption

Since fats are insoluble in water, they cannot be directly absorbed into the intestines and blood stream without making them absorbable. Bile helps in absorption of fat by forming a complex with fatty acids and glycerides which is absorbed by the intestinal wall. Once absorbed, bile separates and returns to the intestine to recombine with fatty acids and glycerides and the process continues.

Metabolism

In the intestinal wall two important reactions take place:

1. The enzyme enteric lipase breaks down the remaining mono- and diglycerides into fatty acids and glycerol.
2. The fatty acids and glycerol recombine to form new body fats or newly formed triglycerides which need to be absorbed and transported via the blood circulation. The newly formed triglycerides and fats are covered with small amounts of protein to form lipoproteins called chylomicrons. Chylomicrons enter the lymphatic circulation

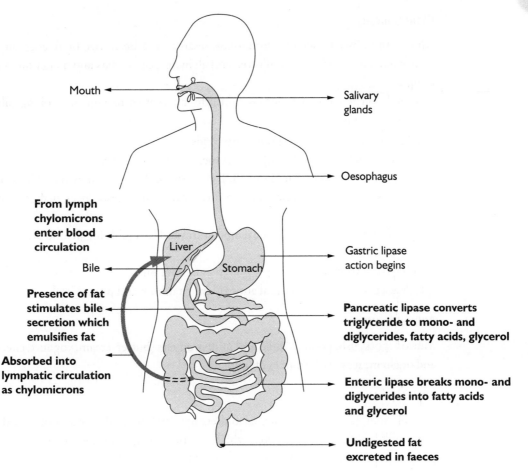

Mouth

Salivary
glands

Oesophagus

**From lymph
chylomicrons
enter blood
circulation**

Liver

Bile

Stomach

Gastric lipase
action begins

**Presence of fat
stimulates bile
secretion which
emulsifies fat**

**Pancreatic lipase converts
triglyceride to mono- and
diglycerides, fatty acids, glycerol**

**Absorbed into
lymphatic circulation
as chylomicrons**

**Enteric lipase breaks mono- and
diglycerides into fatty acids
and glycerol**

**Undigested fat
excreted in faeces**

Fig. 17.5   Digestion and absorption of lipids

from lymph vessels in the small intestine. From the lymphatic system, they enter into the portal circulation and are converted into other lipoproteins in the liver. These lipoproteins are circulated to all body cells for energy and other structural functions, or stored in the adipose tissue as a reserve source of energy.

FOOD SOURCES

Most foods, except the bread cereal group and the vegetable fruit group (except olives and avocado), contain varying percentages of lipids. Some fats are visible such as fats and oils added to food or used for frying. Many sources are hidden or invisible such as the fats and oils naturally present in the food, e.g., milk, egg yolk, oily fish, and meat (see Plate 2). Both visible and invisible sources must be taken into account while calculating the fat content of a meal.

Plant Sources

All oils and oilseeds, such as groundnut, sesame, soya bean, rice bran, coconut, almond, cashewnut, corn, safflower, sunflower, and all hydrogenated fats and margarine, are sources of lipids.

Canola oil is recommended as a healthy alternative to regular cooking oils for the following reasons.

1. It is low in saturated and trans fatty acids
2. It has a higher ratio of omega-3 to omega-6 fatty acids, i.e., 1:2
3. It is believed to lower levels of LDL cholesterol (bad cholesterol) and in turn reduces the risk of high blood prersure, coronary heart problems, cancer, diabetes, and loss of memory
4. It can withstand high cooking temperatures and is suitable for all food products because of its mild flavour.
5. Its MUFA(omega-9) content is high as in olive oil.
6. It is a good source of natural antioxidant vitamin E and phytosterols.

Animal Sources

Mutton, pork, fish, poultry, milk, and milk products (butter, cream, yoghurt, cheese), eggs, and organ meat are rich sources of lipids.

Invisible Sources

Invisible sources of fats are nuts, salad dressings, flesh food, desserts, cookies, cakes, milk, eggs, milk-based sweetmeats, etc., which are rich in fat, but the fat is not visible. The percentage of fat in some foods is given in Table 17.4.

TABLE 17.4   Percentage of fat in some Indian foods

Foodstuff	% fat	Foodstuff	% fat	Foodstuff	% fat
Bajra	5	Coconut (dry)	62	Turmeric	5
Rice bran	16.2	Coconut (fresh)	42	Fruits	0.3–1.5
Dals	1.4–5.6	Sesame seeds	43	Mackarel	1.7
Wheat germ	7.4	Groundnuts	40	Black pomfret	2.6
Wheat flour	1.7	Oil/*vanaspati*	100	Prawns	1
Soya beans	19.5	Niger seeds	24	*Surmai*	1.4
Butter	86	Walnuts	64	Egg	13.3
Fenugreek leaves	0.9	Cloves	9	Mutton	13.3
Potato, beetroot	0.1	Mace	24	Liver	3
Peas, beans, gourds	0.1–0.3	Nutmeg	36	Margarine	86
Almonds	59	*Omum*	22		
Cashew nut	47	Pepper	4		

TABLE 17.5 Fatty acid composition of some commonly used oils

Cooking oil	Saturated fatty acids	Unsaturated fatty acids		
		Omega-3 Alpha linolenic acid (ALA)	Omega-6 EFA linoleic acid (LA)	Omega-9 MUFA
Canola oil	7%	10%	19%	64%
Safflower oil	10%	Traces	76%	14%
Sunflower oil	12%	1%	71%	16%
Olive oil	15%	1%	9%	75%
Soya bean oil	15%	8%	54%	23%
Groundnut oil	19%	Traces	33%	48%
Palm oil	51%	Traces	10%	39%
Coconut oil	91%	2%	–	7%

The fatty acid composition of some commonly used oils are shown in Table 17.5.

DEFICIENCY OF FATS

A deficiency of fat causes a deficiency of essential fatty acids, linoleic and linolenic acids, and subsequently a deficiency of arachidonic acid. These (PUFA) are required for healthy cell membranes and their permeability. A deficiency results in characteristic eczema and skin lesions. It is seen in infants as dry scaly lesions on the skin. Toad skin or dry papules are seen on upper limbs.

A deficiency of fat may result in a deficiency of fat-soluble vitamins, and growth and weight may be affected in children.

Since fat is present in minute quantities in almost all foods including cereals and pulses, a deficiency in adults is unlikely because these foods are consumed in large quantities. What is of greater concern today is the problems related to excessive intake.

SYMPTOMS OF EXCESSIVE INTAKE

The percentage consumption of fat varies widely in different regions and in different income groups. In oriental diets the percentage of fat is 10 per cent, while in the United States approximately 40 per cent of the total calories come from fat. The percentage consumption increases directly with incomes, and today it is a major problem faced in urban areas and changing lifestyles.

Excess intake of fat causes obesity because more kilocalories are consumed than required by the body. Excess fat is stored in the adipose tissue. Excessive consumption of saturated fats can elevate blood cholesterol levels. A high intake of saturated fats and cholesterol are predisposing factors for cardiovascular diseases, while foods rich in omega-3 fatty acids have a protective effect.

RECOMMENDED DIETARY ALLOWANCES

Fats should contribute not more than 30 per cent of the total kilocalories. Kilocalories from saturated fat should not exceed 10 per cent of total calories and at least 10 per cent calories should be provided by PUFA to ensure an adequate intake of essential fatty acids. The correct ratio of omega-3 to omega-6 fatty acids should be maintained.

The cholesterol intake should not exceed 200 mg/day. A variety of cooking oils should be used everyday to ensure consumption of all essential fatty acids. Non-vegetarians should eat groundnut, corn, soya, and olive oil throughout the year, while for fish eaters a mixture of safflower and sunflower oil is adequate. Rice bran oil and corn oil is recommended for vegetarians.

The fat content of the diet can be reduced by following simple measures, such as

1. Use skimmed cow's milk and its products.
2. Select lean meat and trim off visible fat.
3. Steam, boil, or poach food instead of frying.
4. Avoid salad dressing or use low-fat dressing.
5. Select fruit for dessert instead of baked puddings and pastries.
6. For flavour add herbs, spices, and lime juice instead of fats.
7. Dry powdered chutneys of flax and niger seeds are rich in essential fatty acids, and are a good substitute for oil-based pickles.

 ## SUMMARY

Fats, oils, and fat-like substances belong to a group collectively known as lipids. Lipids of importance in human nutrition include simple fats and oils such as butter, cooking oils, phospholipids, lipoproteins, and cholesterol. Simple fats which constitute 98 per cent of dietary fats are made up of glycerol and three fatty acid molecules. Food fats or triglycerides are mixed triglycerides with saturated, monounsaturated, or polyunsaturated fatty acids. Two fatty acids which are polyunsaturated, namely linoleic and linolenic acid, are essential as they cannot be synthesized by the body and must be present in the diet. They belong to omega-3 and omega-6 fatty acids which are essential for maintaining the integrity of cell membranes and lowering blood cholesterol levels.

Depending on whether saturated or unsaturated fatty acids are present, the fat is solid or liquid at room temperature. Different foods contain different percentages of fat. Cereals, pulses, fruits, and vegetables are low in fat, but yet make a significant contribution because they are consumed in fairly large quantities in the Indian diet. Fats are a major source of calories providing 9 kcal per gram of fat/oil. They help in absorption of fat-soluble vitamins and provide thermal insulation and protection to vital organs. A deficiency of fat leads to a deficiency of essential fatty acids which manifests itself as eczema in children. Polyunsaturated fatty acids help lower blood cholesterol levels. Hence, a mixture of oils is preferable to using only one type of oil.

An excessive consumption of saturated fats leads to raised levels of blood cholesterol, atherosclerosis, and cardiovascular diseases. Excess fats are converted to adipose tissue and stored as body fat which is a reserve source of energy for the body. A 20 per cent or more rise in ideal body weight leads to obesity. The diet should not exceed more than 30 per cent of total calories from fat of which less than 10 per cent should be saturated and at least 10 per cent should be polyunsaturated.

 ## KEY TERMS

Adipose tissue It is a fatty tissue.
Arachidonic acid A 20-carbon polyunsaturated fatty acid with four double bonds. In the body it is synthesized from essential fatty acid linoleic acid.

Atherosclerosis A condition of narrowing of the lumen of the arteries due to deposition of cholesterol and other material and hardening of arterial walls.
Bile Greenish yellow brown alkaline secretion of

the liver which is stored in the gall bladder and is needed for digestion of fat. It is composed of bile salts, cholesterol, etc.

Chylomicrons Lipoprotein complexes of very fine droplets of fat covered with a protein casing so that they can be transported through the intestinal wall into lymphatic circulation, giving lymph a milky white appearance.

Cocoa butter A yellowish white fat prepared from cacao seeds (cocoa beans).

Coronary heart disease A disease resulting in a reduction or stoppage of blood supply to part of the heart muscles due to narrowing or blockages in a blood vessel.

Eczema A skin disorder with inflammation and dry scaly lesions seen in essential fatty acid deficiency.

Erucic acid Monounsaturated fatty acid present in rape seed/mustard seed. Amount used in hydrogenated fat is limited as it is known to damage heart muscle in experimental animals. Low erucic acid varieties are being developed.

Essential fatty acid The fatty acid linoleic acid and linolenic acid which cannot be synthesized by the body and should be supplied by the diet. It serves as a precursor for arachidonic acid.

Ester Compound formed when an acid reacts with an alcohol. Fats and oils are esters of glycerol and fatty acids.

Glycerides Group name given to mono-, di-, and triglycerides meaning fats and oils found in adipose tissue and plant and animal foods.

Lipoproteins Compound lipids made up of lipid and protein present in four forms, namely, chylomicrons, very low density lipoproteins, low density lipoproteins, and high density lipoproteins. Form in which triglycerides, cholesterol, and other fats are transported in water-based blood.

Lymphatic system All vessels and structures that carry lymph from the tissues to the blood.

Mixed triglycerides Triglycerides in which all three fatty acids attached to glycerol are different.

Obesity A condition of overweight in which weight exceeds more than 20 per cent of desirable body weight.

Omega-3 fatty acids Long-chain polyunsaturated fatty acids with the first double bond between carbons 3 and 4 from the omega or methyl end (omega means last).

Portal vein The vein carrying blood from the wall of the intestine to the liver.

REVIEW EXERCISES

1. Differentiate between
   (a) Fats and oils
   (b) Monounsaturated and poyunsaturated fats
   (c) Omega-3 and omega-6 fats
   (d) Visible and hidden fats
2. How do saturated fats differ from unsaturated fats?
3. List five important functions of fat in the body.
4. Which of the following are rich sources of cholesterol?
   (a) Hydrogenated fat   (e) Mutton
   (b) Prawns   (f) Coconut oil
   (c) Egg white   (g) Processed cheese
   (d) Organ meat   (h) Palm oil
5. Explain the following:
   (a) Role of compound lipids in the body
   (b) Consequences of excessive consumption of fat
   (c) Digestion of fats
   (d) Role of antioxidants
6. Why is a mixture of oils recommended for daily consumption? Explain giving suitable examples.
7. Suggest five simple measures to reduce the fat intake in your daily diet.

Fill in the blanks

1. Simple fats are made up of _____ and _____.
2. Fats supply _____ times the energy as compared to carbohydrates.
3. Cholesterol is present in foods of _____ origin only.
4. The body obtains cholesterol from _____ sources and from _____ in the body.
5. The secretion of the liver _____ is essential for digestion and absorption of fats.

CHAPTER 18

Water

LEARNING OBJECTIVES

After reading this chapter, you should be able to
- describe the main functions of water in our body
- understand how the body maintains water balance
- identify the various ways of water intake and loss from the body
- describe the treatment of dehydration

INTRODUCTION

Water is so familiar and so large a constituent of the body that its fundamental importance in both structure and functioning of all tissues tends to be overlooked.

Water is the most essential constituent of our body. It accounts for 55–70 per cent of our total body weight. Men have a higher proportion of water in their body as compared to women. Lean individuals have more water than the obese, and infants and children have a greater proportion of water than adults.

The total body fluid is distributed among two major compartments:

1. The extracellular fluid or water present outside the cells in the interstitial spaces and blood plasma
2. The intracellular fluid or the water present inside the cells

Considering an average of 60 per cent of body weight contributed by water, an adult weighing 70 kg has a total body water of 42 litres of which 28 litres is intracellular and 14 litres is extracellular. Of the 14 litres, 11 litres is present as interstitial fluid and 3 litres as plasma. Water present in the body is never plain water but has electrolytes dissolved in it. Similarly, when the body loses water, it loses electrolytes as well.

Sodium is the principal electrolyte of the extracellular fluid while potassium is predominant in the intracellular spaces. The normal concentration of ions in the intracellular and extracellular fluids needs to be maintained at all times. This concentration of ions is preserved by a balance between the intake of water and the output or loss of body water.

FUNCTIONS

1. Water quenches thirst and is the most refreshing and cooling of all liquids.
2. It is a structural component of all cells. In the bone, water is tightly bound, but in most tissues, a constant interchange takes place between the body compartments of water.
3. Water is the medium in which all chemical reactions take place.
4. It is an essential component of all body fluids such as blood, lymph, cerebrospinal fluid, bile, digestive juices, and urine.
5. It acts as a lubricant and helps food to be swallowed and digested food to pass through the gastro-intestinal tract.
6. It acts as a solvent for the products of digestion and helps in transporting these products to different tissues.
7. Water regulates body temperature by taking up and distributing heat produced in cells when metabolic reactions take place.
8. It helps in excreting waste products of metabolic reactions.
9. Water is essential to maintain the turgidity of cells.

DAILY INTAKE OF WATER

Apart from the water we drink during the day to relieve thirst between and during meals, there are three major sources of water.

Beverages and liquid foods   Hot and cold beverages such as tea, coffee, milk shakes, fruit juices, and soups are largely made up of water. Both stimulating beverages and refreshing beverages are important sources of water and nutrients (refer the section on beverages in this chapter).

Water content of solid foods   Another important source of water is fruits, vegetables, and the water used for cooking food. Solid foods contain varying percentages of water. The water consumed from beverages and solid food amounts to 2,100 ml/day approximately.

Metabolic water   It is synthesized in the body as a result of oxidation of fat, proteins, and carbohydrates, adding to about 200 ml/day.

$$\text{Oxidation of 100 g fat} \longrightarrow 107 \text{ ml water}$$
$$100 \text{ g protein} \longrightarrow 41 \text{ ml water}$$
$$100 \text{ g carbohydrate} \longrightarrow 56 \text{ ml water}$$

The intake of fluid varies among different people and also varies according to the climate, habits, and physical activity on a day-to-day basis.

DAILY LOSS OF BODY WATER

Insensible water loss   It is the loss of water we are not consciously aware of even though it occurs continuously in all living beings. It includes,

1. Continuous loss of fluid by evaporation from the skin, which occurs independently of sweating. This loss by diffusion through the skin is about 300–400 ml/day.
2. Insensible water loss through the respiratory tract, which is about 300–400 ml/day. This loss of water is greater in cold weather.

Water loss through sweat   The extent of water loss through perspiration or sweat largely depends on physical activity and environmental temperature. The volume of sweat secreted is normally about 100 ml/day but could increase to a few litres in very hot weather or during heavy exercise.

Water loss in urine   This is the most important mechanism by which the body maintains a balance between fluid intake and output as well as electrolyte homeostasis. Urine volume can be as low as 0.5 litre/day in a dehydrated person or as high as 20 litres/day in a person who has been drinking tremendous amount of fluid.

The rate of filtration of water in the normal kidney is about 125 ml/minute or approximately 180 litres daily for an adult. About 99 per cent of the water filtered is re-absorbed into the blood while 500–2,000 ml is excreted as urine.

Water loss in faeces   Only a small amount of water (100 ml/day) is normally lost in faeces. The saliva, gastrointestinal secretion, and bile may together add to 8 litres or more fluid per day. All but a small proportion of this is re-absorbed in the gut (large intestine). If there is diarrhoea or vomiting, fluid losses may be large and cause dehydration.

Table 18.1 provides details of daily intake and output of water.

TABLE 18.1   Daily intake and output of water (in ml/day)

Intake		Output	
Fluids ingested	2,200	Insensible—skin	350
From metabolism	200	Insensible—lungs	350
		Sweat	100
		Faeces	100
		Urine	1,500
Total	2,400		2,400

Note: Prolonged heavy workout may result in sweat losses as great as 1–5 litres/day, accompanied by a reduction in urine output.

WATER BALANCE

Deficiency of Water

Excessive loss of water could take place due to diarrhoea, vomiting, fever, excessive perspiration, strenuous exercise, and uncontrolled diabetes mellitus. It can result in dehydration. Dehydration can be classified as

- Mild   –   <5 per cent fluid loss
- Moderate   –   5–15 per cent fluid loss
- Severe   –   15–20 per cent fluid loss

TABLE 18.2 Oral rehydration salts

ORS Formula	
Ingredients	Amount in grams
Sodium chloride (NaCl)	3.5
Trisodium citrate dehydrate	2.9
Potassium chloride	1.5
Glucose anhydrous	20
Water	1 litre

A 20 per cent loss of fluid from the body can be fatal.

A dehydrated person feels thirsty, has a dry mouth, sunken and dry eyes, and may feel restless, irritable, or even lethargic or unconscious in severe cases. The skin when pinched does not go back quickly. A dehydrated person is usually managed by oral rehydration therapy (ORT). The Would Health Organization (WHO) recommends oral rehydration salts (ORS) that are to be dissolved in 1 litre of water (see Table 18.2). This is to be sipped till hydration returns to normal.

Oral rehydration salts are most often prescribed in cases of diarrhoea. Glucose present in ORS enhances the absorption of salt.

Apart from ORS, ORT also includes any of the following:

1. Sugar and salt solution
   40 g sucrose + 4 g NaCl in 1 litre of water
2. Rice water with salt
   50 g rice + 4 g salt in 1 litre water
3. Dilute salted *lassi*
4. Plain water, lemon water, coconut water, thin soups, or dal water may also be given along with ORT.

If vomiting is severe, intravenous fluids such as normal saline (0.9 per cent NaCl) and dextrose need to be administered. When the body loses fluids, it loses both water and electrolytes, hence ORS or dextrose normal saline (DNS) is given. Dehydration cannot be treated by giving pure water only.

Retention of Water

Oedema is the retention of salt and water in the interstitial fluid giving rise to swelling of the skin. A pit or depression is formed when pressure is applied with the finger to the swollen skin and this is how oedema is distinguished from swelling. Water and salt may need to be restricted.

Daily Requirement

A minimum of six to eight glasses of water is recommended to enable the body to perform optimally and keep one active and refreshed throughout the day. It should be consumed at regular intervals so that the body is always well hydrated. This quantity is independent of other fluids consumed.

BEVERAGES

Water is the simplest and cheapest of all beverages and the main constituent of all beverages. Beverages are consumed mainly for their thirst quenching properties or for their stimulating effect. They can be classified on the basis of serving temperature, i.e., hot and cold beverages, on the basis of aeration as carbonated and non-carbonated or on the basis of their stimulating effect or alcohol content or as nourishing beverages.

Non-alcoholic stimulating beverages include tea, coffee and cocoa. They are refreshing and stimulating and contain the stimulants caffeine (in tea) and coffee and theobromine in (cocoa). Carbonated non-alcoholic beverages or soft drinks may contain artificial flavour, fruit flavour or fruit juice or plain sparkling soda water. Popular soft drinks are based on cola. They contain water, sugar or sweeteners, and a variety of additives such as flavouring agents, food colours, acids, preservatives, carbon dioxide, etc.

Alcoholic beverages include malted beverages such as beer and ale, fermented fruit juices such as wine and cider, and distilled liquors such as brandy, whiskey, rum, and vodka.

Cocktails, mocktails, fortified wines, liqueurs, cider, and perry are other popular alcoholic beverages, the exception being mocktails.

Nutritious beverages include fruit juices, milk-based beverages such as milkshakes, milk chocolate, health drinks, probiotic beverages, eggnog, and soups.

Nutritive Value of Beverages

Carbonated beverages are generally purely synthetic with the exception of fizzy fruit juices. They are sweetened with sugar or artificial sweeteners along with other additives and are empty or hollow calorie foods because they provide only calories from sugar. The diet versions provide zero calories while normal colas provide approximately 70 calories per glass and 40 mg caffeine.

Alcoholic beverages provide 7 kcal/g alcohol or 5.6 kcal/ml alcohol. Alcoholic beverages contribute significant amounts of calories which vary from one beverage to another. Refer Table 15.5 in Chapter 15 for calorie content of alcoholic beverages. Red wine contains antioxidant resveratrol.

Tea and coffee have no nutritive value as such. The nutritive value depends on the quantity of milk and sugar added to the beverage. Tea and beverages are popular because of their refreshing and stimulating effect. They can contribute significantly towards the calorie intake if consumed in excess.

Cocoa and chocolate are milk-based stimulating beverages. The primary stimulant is the alkaloid theobromine. These beverages provide carbohydrates, fats, and proteins. Cocoa powder is prepared after removing cocoa butter from the cocoa beans and is used in preparing cocoa beverage.

Fruit juices, smoothies, milkshakes, eggnog, and soups are nourishing beverages ideal for all age groups. Soups, milk-based beverages, and juices are recommended for patients and during convalescence as they are light and nourishing. Fresh juices contain both fruit, and vegetables that are rich in vitamin C.

SUMMARY

Water is a vital constituent of our body necessary for the structure and functioning of all cells and tissues in the body. It accounts for 55–70 per cent of our body weight. Body fluid is distributed as extracellular and intracellular fluids. Intracellular fluid is present inside the cell while extracellular fluid is present between cells in tissues and in blood plasma. The concentration of electrolytes in both extracellular and intracellular compartments needs to be maintained at all times.

Apart from the water which we drink, the body gets water from beverages, liquid and solid foods, and from the oxidation of proteins, carbohydrates, and fats in the body. The body loses water by evaporation through the skin, perspiration, urine, and faeces. The major loss is through the kidneys in the form of urine, by which toxic metabolites are excreted from the blood.

Water performs many functions in the body and is the medium for all chemical reactions. It acts as a lubricant, solvent, temperature regulator, and a means of excreting waste products. It is present in all cells and body fluids and maintains the turgidity of cells.

Excessive loss of water results in dehydration while accumulation of water in the extracellular spaces is called oedema. Both cases need to be treated because a loss of 20 per cent fluid from the body could be fatal. Dehydration is treated by ORT in which ORS are given gradually.

For optimum health, a minimum intake of six to eight glasses of water is recommended.

KEY TERMS

DNS   Dextrose normal saline is an intravenous fluid containing 5 per cent dextrose and 0.9 per cent normal saline.

Electrolyte   A chemical element or compound that dissociates into ions when in solution.

Homeostasis   A state of equilibrium in the body between body parts and functions.

Interstitial fluid   Fluid present in the spaces or interstices between the cells and tissues in an organ.

Ion   A charged particle.

Oedema   The accumulation of large amount of fluid in extracellular spaces.

ORS   Oral rehydration salts are a mixture of electrolytes and glucose used for ORT.

ORT   Oral rehydration therapy is used for treatment of dehydration by orally feeding fluids to which sugar and salt are added.

REVIEW EXERCISES

1. Why is water an essential nutrient? Discuss the functions of water.
2. List the various ways of water loss from the body.
3. What are the major sources of water to our body? Explain, giving suitable examples.
4. List the various conditions which lead to excessive loss of body water.
5. Explain briefly:
   (a) Oedema
   (b) ORT
   (c) Water balance
6. Discuss the nutritive value of beverages.

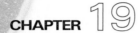

Vitamins

LEARNING OBJECTIVES

After reading this chapter, you should be able to
- define the term vitamin and classify different vitamins
- understand the role of different vitamins in the body
- identify the food sources of vitamins
- relate each vitamin's functions to a state of deficiency or excess
- retain maximum vitamins while cooking and storing food
- appreciate various processes which increase the vitamin content of food

INTRODUCTION

The term vitamin was coined from the words *vital amine,* as early scientists felt these chemicals, which are vital for life, were amines. Vitamins were discovered one at a time from 1900 to 1950, some as a cure for classic diseases such as beriberi, pellagra, and scurvy, while others were discovered after research on various body functions.

Vitamins like carbohydrates, proteins, and fats are organic compounds. Unlike these nutrients, vitamins are required in minute quantities and are also called micronutrients. They do not provide energy and are present in very small quantities in food, but nonetheless are vital for life processes. All vitamins can be synthesized on a commercial scale, though fresh foods are always preferred.

Definition   Vitamins is the term used for a group of potent organic compounds other than proteins, carbohydrates, and fats which occur in minute quantities in food and which are essential for some specific body functions such as regulation, maintenance, growth, and protection. Many of them cannot be synthesized, at least in adequate amounts, by the body and must be obtained from the diet.

CLASSIFICATION

Vitamins are grouped according to their solubility in either fat or water (see Table 19.1).

Fat-soluble vitamins   The fat-soluble vitamins are vitamins A, D, E, and K. They require fat for their absorption and can be stored in the body. If their intake is poor, but body stores are ample, deficiency symptoms will not be seen immediately.

Water-soluble vitamins   The water-soluble vitamins are B-complex vitamins and vitamin C. Being water soluble, they are easily absorbed and the excess consumed is excreted in the urine. They are not stored in the body.

TABLE 19.1   Classification of vitamins

Fat soluble	Water soluble
1. Vitamin A (retinol, retinal, retinoic acid) Precursor—carotenes such as α-, β-, and γ-carotene and cryptoxanthin	1. B-complex (a) Vitamin B_1 (thiamine) (b) Vitamin B_2 (riboflavin)
2. Vitamin D (a) D_2—activated ergosterol or calciferol (b) D_3—activated 7-dehydrocholesterol or cholecalciferol	(c) Niacin (i) Nicotinic acid (ii) Nicotinamide (d) Vitamin B_6 (i) Pyridoxine (ii) Pyridoxal (iii) Pyridoxamine
3. Vitamin E (tocopherols) (a) α-Tocopherol (b) Tocotrienols	(e) Vitamin B_{12} (i) Cyanocobalamin or cobalamin
4. Vitamin K (quinones) (a) K_1—phylloquinones (b) K_2—synthesized by intestinal bacteria (c) K_3—menadione (the water soluble synthetic form)	(f) Folic acid or folacin (g) Pantothenic acid (h) Biotin 2. Vitamin C (ascorbic acid)

FAT-SOLUBLE VITAMINS

Vitamin A

Vitamin A is the generic name given to a group of compounds having vitamin A activity. These compounds are retinol, retinal, and retinoic acid. They are found only in the fatty phases of foods of animal origin. Plant foods contain yellow, orange, and/or red coloured pigments called carotene which give colour to vegetables and fruits. Carotene pigments

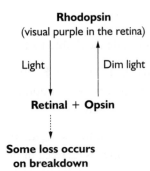

Rhodopsin
(visual purple in the retina)

Light | Dim light

Retinal + Opsin

Some loss occurs on breakdown

Fig. 19.1   Role of vitamin A in vision

are converted to vitamin A in the body, i.e., carotene is a provitamin or precursor of vitamin A. Carotene is synthesized by plants and is the ultimate source of all vitamin A.

Pure vitamin A is a pale yellow crystalline compound occuring naturally in the animal kingdom. It is soluble in fat, insoluble in water, and relatively stable to heat, acids, and alkalis. It is easily oxidized and rapidly destroyed by ultraviolet (UV) rays.

Functions   Vitamin A performs the following functions.

1. Vitamin A maintains normal vision in dim light. Rhodopsin or visual purple is present in the retina of the eye. It is required for vision in dim light. It is formed when vitamin A combines with protein opsin. In bright light, rhodopsin absorbs light and breaks down into protein opsin and retinal. Every time rhodopsin breaks down, some retinal is lost. Figure 19.1 shows the role of vitamin A in vision.

   In dim light or darkness, retinal and opsin re-combine rapidly to form rhodopsin provided there is an adequate supply of vitamin A. If there is a deficiency of vitamin A, the regeneration is slow and the person's eyes fail to adapt to changes in light quickly.

2. It helps in synthesis and maintenance of healthy epithelium—outermost lining of skin and innermost lining of mucous membranes of respiratory, gastrointestinal, and genitourinary tract. Epithelial glands secrete mucous that lubricates the lining of the eyes, respiratory and gastrointestinal tract, etc.

3. Vitamin A is required for normal bone and tooth development, and proper growth.

4. It helps the body to fight against infections by keeping mucous membranes in a healthy condition which act as a barrier to infection.

Deficiency   If the body has sufficient stores, deficiency does not develop at once.

Night blindness or nyctalopia   It is one of the earliest signs of vitamin A deficiency. In this condition, an individual is unable to see well in dim light, especially after coming from a brightly lit area. This happens because there is insufficient vitamin A to bring about quick formation of rhodopsin.

Epithelial changes   The epithelium becomes dry, scaly, and rough. Goose pimples are seen on upper forearms and thighs.

Changes in the eyes

(a) Secretion of tears decreases
(b) Eye ball becomes dry and lustreless
(c) Bitot spots (pigmented spots) are seen on conjunctiva
(d) Photophobia or sensitivity to bright light is observed

(e) Xeropthalmia: Cornea becomes dry and inflamed. If not treated it leads to keratomalacia.

(f) Keratomalacia or softening of the cornea and permanent blindness results.

Bone development   Growth failure and stunted bones are seen in children.

Hypervitaminosis A   High doses of vitamin A is not recommended as excess is stored in the liver. This excessive accumulation of vitamin A in the body is toxic. Symptoms of toxicity are nausea, vomiting, abdominal pain, loss of hair, thickening of long bones, and joint pain.

Sources   Animal foods, such as whole milk and milk products, eggs yolk, oily fish, fish-liver oils, organ meat, butter, cream, and clarified butter or pure ghee, are rich sources.

Sources of carotene   All yellow, orange, and red fruits and vegetables such as carrots, pumpkin, mango, papaya, peaches, and apricots, and all green leafy vegetables such as fenugreek leaves, spinach, colocasia leaves, amaranth, curry leaves, and turnip greens are rich sources of provitamin A.

Requirement   An adult requires 600 μg of retinol or 2,400 μg of β-carotene per day; 4 μg of β-carotene is converted to 1 μg of retinol in the intestinal wall and liver.

Vitamin D

It is a fat-soluble vitamin. The two important forms are vitamin D_2 (activated ergosterol or calciferol) and vitamin D_3 (activated 7-dehydrocholesterol or cholecalciferol). Vitamin D_3 is produced when 7-dehydrocholesterol in the skin is exposed to the UV rays in the Sun. Vitamin D differs from other fat-soluble vitamins because it is synthesized in the body, and we do not depend on our diet for it. Being fat soluble, it requires fat for its absorption.

Functions
1. Absorption of calcium and phosphorus from the small intestine requires the presence of vitamin D and the hormones of the parathyroid and thyroid gland.
2. Mineralization of bones and teeth: After calcium and phosphorus is absorbed, vitamin D is required to ensure that these minerals are deposited in bones and teeth to strengthen them.
3. Regulation of calcium and phosphorus levels in blood.

Sources   Sunlight is the main source of vitamin D. The precursor in skin is converted to active vitamin D_3. Barriers such as clothing, soot, fog, window glass, and melanin (pigment in the skin) interfere with synthesis of vitamin D. Sunscreen lotions with high SPF also prevent vitamin D formation.

It is found in fish liver oils, fortified milk, *vanaspati*, and margarine. Natural foods such as butter, milk, and fish have it in small amounts.

Deficiency   Vitamin D deficiency leads to lowered absorption of calcium, low serum levels of calcium, and reduced bone mineralization. Bones cannot withstand the weight and bend into deformities.

Rickets is seen in infants and children especially dark-skinned children. Bones are soft and yield to pressure. Joints are enlarged and there is delayed closing of the skull bones. Symptoms of rickets include enlarged skull, pigeon chest, poor muscle development, pot belly, and bowed legs or knocked knees.

Osteomalacia or adult rickets is more common in women who consume a diet deficient in calcium, phosphorus, and vitamin D, and have had several pregnancies. The softening of bones leads to a deformed spine, rheumatic pain in the legs and lower back, a waddling gait, and spontaneous fractures.

Hypervitaminosis D   Large doses of vitamin D can be toxic. Excessive use of fortified foods lead to loss of appetite, vomiting, diarrhoea, growth failure, and calcification of soft tissues and kidney stones.

Vitamin E

Vitamin E or tocopherol is a fat-soluble vitamin. It is stable to heat and acids. It is rapidly oxidized in rancid fats.

Many claims are being made that supplements of this vitamin can prevent or cure a wide variety of diseases, from reproductive function to skin problems such as psoriasis and acne, but there is no proof.

Functions   Vitamin E is the most potent natural antioxidant found in food. Polyunsaturated fatty acids (PUFA) form a structural part of all cell membranes. They are prone to oxidative breakdown by free radicals in the cell. The main function of vitamin E is to act as an antioxidant. Vitamin E itself gets oxidized and protects cell membranes from oxidative damage. It performs the following functions:

1. Prevents oxidation of vitamin A in the intestine
2. Protects normal cell membranes by preventing their breakdown
3. Prevents hemolysis of red blood cells
4. Prevents oxidation of PUFAs.

Sources   Vitamin E is widely distributed in foods, particularly vegetable oils (corn, soya, sunflower, safflower), wheat germ, whole grains, legumes, nuts, and dark green leafy vegetables.

Deficiency   In severe deficiency, although uncommon, increased haemolysis of red blood cells is seen in premature infants.

Vitamin K

Vitamin K is essential in the diet because it is needed for synthesis of prothrombin and other blood clotting factors. It exists as K_1 (found in plants), K_2 (synthesized by bacteria in the intestinal tract), and K$_3$ (synthetic form). Being fat soluble, it requires fat and bile salts for efficient absorption.

Functions Vitamin K is required for the formation of prothrombin and several other proteins involved in clotting of blood. The ability of blood to clot is dependent upon a high blood level of prothrombin.

Deficiency A deficiency of vitamin K is uncommon in adults. New born infants have a sterile intestinal tract, hence they are given a single dose of vitamin K to prevent haemorrhagic disease.

A deficiency interferes with formation of prothrombinogen and, thus, reduces clotting tendency of blood. It may occur during diseases of malabsorption, oral use of sulfa drugs and antibiotics, or certain drugs which are vitamin K antagonists and can cause haemorrhages.

Sources Bacterial synthesis in the intestinal tract supplies at least half of the daily needs. Green leafy vegetables, cabbage, cauliflower, and pork liver are excellent sources. Cheese, egg yolk, and tomato also supply vitamin K.

Table 19.2 provides the details of the recommended dietary allowances (RDAs) and main sources of fat-soluble vitamins.

TABLE 19.2 Recommended dietary allowances and main sources of fat-soluble vitamins

Vitamin	RDA for adults	Main source
Vitamin A (retinol) or	600 µg	Whole milk, butter, egg yolk
Provitamin carotene	2,400 µg	Yellow, orange, and red fruits and vegetables, green leafy vegetables
Vitamin D	200 IU	Sunlight, fish-liver oils, fortified *vanaspati*
Vitamin E	8–10 mg	Vegetable oils, wheat germ, green leafy vegetables
Vitamin K	60–80 µg	Green leafy vegetables, liver, cheese, egg yolk, intestinal flora

WATER-SOLUBLE VITAMINS

B-Complex Vitamins

Scientists discovered eleven water-soluble B-complex vitamins of which eight are considered essential for humans.

They differ from each other in their structure, distribution in foods, stability, and symptoms that result from their deficiency. They are

1. Thiamine (vitamin B_1)
2. Riboflavin (vitamin B_2)
3. Niacin
4. Pyridoxine (vitamin B_6)
5. Pantothenic acid
6. Biotin
7. Folic acid
8. Cyanocobalamin (vitamin B_{12})

They are all water soluble.

These eight vitamins are grouped together because their functions are closely related. The remaining three B-complex vitamins, namely para-aminobenzoic acid (PABA), choline, and inositol play an active role in cell metabolism but the diet and intestinal synthesis can make good this requirement.

The B-complex vitamins which are essential in human nutrition are broadly grouped into the following categories:

1. Classic deficiency disease vitamins

   (a) Thiamine   –   Beriberi
   (b) Riboflavin   –   Ariboflavinosis
   (c) Niacin   –   Pellagra

2. Anaemia preventing vitamins

   (a) Pyridoxine   –   Hypochromic anaemia
   (b) Folic acid   –   Macrocytic anaemia
   (c) Cyanocobalamin   –   Pernicious anaemia

3. Recently discovered coenzyme factors

   (a) Pantothenic acid
   (b) Biotin

Thiamine (vitamin B_1)

Thiamine performs the following functions.

1. Thiamine functions mainly as a co-enzyme, thiamine pyrophosphate (TPP), which is required in the breakdown of glucose to yield energy.
2. It helps to maintain a healthy nervous system.
3. It is required for normal appetite and digestion.

Daily requirement of thiamine is 0.5 mg/1,000 kcal. Thus, an adult who needs 3,000 calories would require 1.5 mg of vitamin B_1 per day.

Sources   Foods rich in protein such as pork, liver, pulses, groundnut, and eggs are good sources. Wholegrain and enriched cereals, parboiled rice, unpolished rice, and sprouted pulses contribute B_1. Soya bean is a rich source.

Effect of cooking and processing B_1 is easily destroyed by cooking food in neutral or alkaline medium. Losses are greater when food is cooked at high temperatures, overcooked, and cooking water discarded.

Deficiency The symptoms of deficiency occur because the tissue cells are unable to receive sufficient energy from glucose. Therefore, they cannot carry out their normal functions. The gastrointestinal, nervous, and cardiovascular systems are specially affected.

Early symptoms of deficiency include fatigue, irritability, depression, poor appetite, tingling, and numbness of the legs. A severe deficiency causes beriberi. Beriberi is of two types.

1. *Dry beriberi* Polyneuritis or inflammation of the nerves, numbness of extremities, muscle weakness, and cramps are the main symptoms.
2. *Wet beriberi* Severe oedema, enlargement of the heart, palpitation, and increase in rate of heart beat are seen in wet beriberi.

A person may suffer from either type of beriberi. Beriberi is also known as rice-eaters' disease because it is seen in people whose chief diet consists of polished rice.

Prevention Parboiling rice to retain B_1.

Riboflavin (vitamin B_2)

Riboflavin performs the following functions.

1. As a co-enzyme, just like B_1 is a vital factor in carbohydrate metabolism, B_2 is vital is protein metabolism.
2. As a co-enzyme in carbohydrate metabolism, B_2 is a constituent of co-enzymes flavin mono nucleotide (FMN) and flavin adenine dinucleotide (FAD).

Daily requirement is 0.55 mg/1,000 kcal.

Sources Milk and cheese are rich in B_2. Organ meat, eggs, dark green leafy vegetables, and enriched cereal foods.

Effect of cooking and processing B_2 is sensitive to light. If milk is kept in clear glass bottles, three-fourths of B_2 is lost in a short time. Cooking in open containers and in excess water is harmful.

Deficiency

1. Swelling of lips with cheilosis
2. Cracks in the skin at the corners of the lip, i.e., angular stomatitis
3. Redness and swelling of the tongue or glossitis
4. Eyes look bloodshot, eye fatigue, itching, burning, watering, and sensitivity to bright light, i.e., photophobia.

Niacin

Niacin or nicotinic acid is a vitamin intimately connected with several metabolic reactions it takes part in as a component.

Functions   Like B_1 and B_2, niacin is also required for enzymes that bring about breakdown of glucose, amino acids, and fatty acids to yield energy, i.e., for release of energy from food.

1. As a constituent of two co-enzymes, nicotinamide adenine dinucleotide (NAD) and nicotinamide adenine dinucleotide phosphate (NADP), to release energy from carbohydrates, proteins, and fats.
2. For a healthy skin, normal gastrointestinal tract, and maintenance of the nervous system.

Because this vitamin takes part in many reactions of energy metabolism in the breakdown of proteins, carbohydrates, and fats, its requirement is related to calorie intake (6.6 mg/1,000 kcal). Although milk is not a good source of niacin, it contains essential amino acid tryptophan which is converted to niacin in the body.

$$60 \text{ mg tryptophan} \xrightarrow{\frac{B_2}{B_6}} 1 \text{ mg niacin}$$

Sources   Protein rich foods such as poultry, fish, meat, groundnut, beans, and peas are good sources. Grains are fair sources except maize and rice; green leafy vegetables, potatoes, milk, eggs, and cheese are poor sources of preformed niacin but rich sources of tryptophan.

Effect of cooking and processing   It is most stable of all B-complex vitamins. Fairly stable to heat, acid, alkali, light, oxidation, and autoclaving.

Deficiency   It is seen in low-protein or maize-based diets. Pellagra, which means rough skin, is characterized by four Ds—diarrhoea, dermatitis, dementia, and death. Deficiency begins with weakness, headache, loss of appetite and weight, and a sore and swollen tongue. Dermatitis is symmetrical and on exposed parts of the body (forearms, legs, and hands) and is aggravated by sunlight.

Dementia or depression, confusion, poor memory, delirium, and hallucinations occur in severe deficiency. Without treatment, it results in death.

Anaemia-preventing Vitamins

Folic acid, vitamin B_{12}, and vitamin B_6 help in the formation of either red blood corpuscles (RBCs) or haemoglobin and help in preventing anaemia.

Folic acid or folacin

It derives its name from the Latin word *folium*, which means leaf.

Sources   Liver, kidney, green leafy vegetables, whole pulses, and yeast, and in fermented food such as idli, *dhokla*, and dosa. Some bacteria present in the intestinal tract are capable of synthesizing the vitamin.

Functions   In order to perform its functions, folic acid needs to be converted into its active form. Vitamin C is needed for this conversion.

$$\text{Inactive folic acid} \xrightarrow{\text{Vitamin C}} \text{Active folic acid}$$

It is a component of specific enzymes required for formation of DNA and haeme in the RBCs. B_{12} is required along with folic acid for maturation of RBCs.

Deficiency Deficiency results in megaloblastic anaemia which is common in underdeveloped countries, among the vulnerable age group. In folic acid deficiency, the bone marrow releases large nucleated cells into the circulation. The anaemia is a macrocytic, megaloblastic anaemia. Megaloblasts are large nucleated cells or immature RBCs. Other symptoms are weakness, loss of weight, pallor, and glossitis. Haemoglobin level may fall as low as 2–4 g/100 ml and blood transfusion may be needed. Normal Hb level is 11.5–14.5 g for women and 12.5–16.5 g/100 ml blood for adult men.

Cyanocobalamin (vitamin B₁₂)

It is found only in foods of animal origin. Liver, kidney, milk, eggs, and cheese are good sources. Small amounts of animal protein in the diet take care of B_{12} requirement.

Functions
1. It helps folic acid in the synthesis and maturation of RBCs.
2. It is essential for formation of myelin sheath around nerve fibres.

Absorption Vitamin B_{12} is absorbed only if a glycoprotein known as 'intrinsic factor' is present in gastric juice.

Deficiency Vitamin B_{12} deficiency results either in megaloblastic aneamia or in pernicious anaemia. The latter is more common and is serious. Megaloblastic anaemia is seen in strict vegetarians who do not consume milk. It is because of a dietary deficiency of B_{12}.

Pernicious anaemia occurs due to absence of intrinsic factor in the person's gastric juice. So, even if diet provides enough B_{12}, it will not be absorbed and deficiency will result.

Symptoms The person appears well nourished with respect to body weight. Skin and eyes are pale, tongue is raw and red, and mouth ulcers are present. There is numbness, tingling sensation, and a feeling of pins and needles in the fingers, as nervous system is affected. Haemoglobin level is low and megaloblasts appear in blood. Treatment of pernicious anaemia involves injections of B_{12} throughout life as oral doses cannot be absorbed due to lack of intrinsic factor.

Pyridoxine (vitamin B₆)

Liver, kidney, meat, wholegrain cereals, soya beans, and groundnuts are sources of pyridoxine.

Functions
1. Essential for synthesis and breakdown of amino acids
2. Helps in conversion of tryptophan to niacin

3. Conversion of linoleic acid to arachidonic acid
4. Needed for synthesis of haeme
5. Production of antibodies.

The requirement increases with an increase in protein content of diet.

Deficiency   Anaemia is hypochromic anaemia because Hb is not synthesized for the red colour of RBCs. Red blood cells are pale in colour. Soreness of tongue, depression, and sleepiness are other symptoms. Deficiency occurs along with other nutrient deficiencies, e.g., PCM and B-complex deficiency.

Pantothenic acid and biotin   They are both co-enzymes required for release of energy from carbohydrates, fats, and proteins. Biotin is synthesized in the intestinal tract. Both vitamins are widely present in foods and deficiency is rare in normal circumstances.

Egg white contains a protein 'avidin' that interferes with absorption of biotin from the intestinal tract. Only raw egg whites can cause a deficiency as avidin is inactivated when eggs are cooked. Having a few raw egg whites in a week is not harmful and do not cause a deficiency.

Vitamin C

Vitamin C, also known as the fresh fruit and vegetable vitamin, was discovered as an acid in lime juice which prevented scurvy among British sailors on long voyages at sea. It was named ascorbic acid because of its antiscorbutic or antiscurvy properties.

It is highly soluble in water and most easily destroyed as compared to all other vitamins. It is readily oxidized and destroyed by heat and presence of alkali. It is lost when food is dehydrated.

Functions
1. Synthesis of collagen which is the intercellular cementing substance that keeps cells in bone and muscle tissue together
2. Making haemoglobin by helping in absorption of iron from food
3. Healing of wounds and fractures
4. Increasing resistance to infections and fevers
5. Proper growth during periods of increased need or during rapid growth
6. As an antioxidant, like vitamin E, it prevents the oxidation of vitamin A and unsaturated fatty acids.

Deficiency   Deprivation of vitamin C results in defective formation of the intercellular cementing substance.

Symptoms
1. Poor wound healing because collagen is not synthesized
2. Increased susceptibility to infections
3. Painful joints and bleeding gums

4. Skin bruises by slightest injury
5. Severe deficiency causes scurvy. The symptoms are swelling, infection and bleeding of gums, and anaemia.

Excessive intake   The benefits of consuming megadoses of vitamin C to prevent common cold and cancer is still controversial. An increased intake beyond the RDA is advised in certain cases such as surgical cases, infections, and drug therapies, but benefits of megadoses of 1–5 g daily is still under study.

Sources   Fresh citrus fruits such as orange, sweet lime, grape fruit, lemon; other fruits and vegetables such as guava, *amla*, cabbage, capsicum, green chillies, green leafy vegetables, and tomatoes are excellent sources of vitamin C (see Plate 2). Cereals and pulses are poor in vitamin C, but when dry pulses are sprouted ascorbic acid is formed in them. 85 per cent of the vitamin is formed in the grain and 15 per cent in the sprout. Green gram contains thrice as much vitamin C as compared to bengal gram. Sprouted pulses are a good alternative to fresh fruits and vegetables during periods of scarcity. Sprouts can be lightly steamed or consumed raw.

Berries such as zizyphus, strawberries, gooseberries, and cashewfruit are seasonal rich sources. *Amla* is the richest source providing 600 mg/100 g as compared to oranges which provide 30 mg/100 g, i.e., *amla* contains 20 times as much vitamin C as compared to orange. Heating and dehydration reduces the vitamin C content of all fresh fruits except amla, which retains some vitamin C in the preserve.

Table 19.3 presents the RDA and the main sources of water-soluble vitamins.

TABLE 19.3   RDA and the main sources of water-soluble vitamins

Vitamin	RDA for adults	Main source
• Thiamine (B$_1$)	0.5 mg/1,000 kcal	• Whole grains, pulses, wheat, groundnuts
• Riboflavin (B$_2$)	0.55 mg/1,000 kcal	• Milk, eggs, organ meat
• Niacin	6.6 mg/1,000 kcal	• All protein rich foods—groundnuts, beans, peas, meat, fish
• Provitamin — tryptophan		
• Pyridoxine (B$_6$)	0.6–2.5 mg	• Wheat, *jowar*, red gram, meat, liver, fish, parboiled rice
• Pantothenic acid	4–7 mg	• Milk, egg, intestinal flora
• Biotin	30–100 μg	• Intestinal flora, egg yolk, liver
• Folic acid	100 μg	• Green leafy vegetables, lentils, intestinal synthesis
• Cyanocobalamin (B$_{12}$)	1 μg	• Milk and milk products, egg, meat
• Ascorbic acid (vitamin C)	40 mg	• Fresh fruits and vegetables eaten uncooked, citrus fruits, guava, *amla*

EFFECT OF COOKING ON VITAMINS

Water-soluble vitamins are more easily lost during cooking and storing food. Losses occur due to oxidation or exposure to air which is catalysed by enzymes. Blanching fruits and vegetables, which need to be refrigerated or frozen, destroys the enzymes and preserves vitamin C. High temperature, prolonged heating, and alkaline medium favour destruction of vitamins. To retain maximum vitamins in food, observe the following rules.

1. Select good quality, fresh fruits and vegetables. Stale, wilted, and poor-quality produce may be cheaper, but has lower vitamin content.
2. Always wash fruits and vegetable before peeling or cutting and not afterwards, as water-soluble vitamins get leached into water and are lost.
3. Cut fruits and vegetables for salads just before they are to be served and store in a cool place. Keep food covered. This prevents oxidative losses.
4. Avoid cutting into small pieces as more surface area is exposed.
5. Avoid soaking in water as water-soluble vitamins leach out.
6. Cook in minimum quantity water so that extra cooking is not required to dry up the excess liquid. Use shortest cooking time.
7. Cook in a covered pan, except while cooking greens—cook uncovered for a few minutes to allow volatile acids to escape which helps in preserving green colour.
8. Do not overcook. Refresh greens and use pot liquor or cooking liquid in soups, gravies, or for kneading dough.
9. Do not add alkali (soda bicarbonate) to enhance green colour or hasten the cooking of pulses such as *kabuli channa* as B-complex and vitamin C are readily destroyed in an alkaline medium.
10. Store food in a refrigerator, covered with a lid, aluminium foil, or cling film to retain nutrients.
11. Reheat only what is required.
12. Pressure cooking helps in retaining vitamins as food is cooked in a covered container for a shorter time.
13. Fat-soluble vitamins are lost during deep fat frying, if the food to be fried is not coated prior to frying.
14. Vitamin A and carotene are lost due to oxidation and dehydration, so keep food covered to prevent oxidative and moisture loss.

SUMMARY

Vitamins are vital organic compounds required by the body to perform specific functions such as the release of energy from food and other growth related, protective and regulatory functions. They are required in minute amounts and hence are categorized as micronutrients.

They are broadly classified as fat soluble (vitamin A, D, E, and K) and water soluble (B-complex and vitamin C) vitamins. Each vitamin has a specific role to perform and cannot be replaced by another vitamin. Fat-soluble vitamins require fat for their absorption and can be stored in the body. Water-soluble vitamins are readily absorbed but are not stored in the body. Excessive intake of fat-soluble vitamins leads to toxicity or hypervitaminosis.

Vitamin A is present in animal foods only. Carotene, a precursor of vitamin A, is present in yellow, orange, and red fruits and vegetables, and in green leafy vegetables. We get our requirement of vitamin D from sunlight. The precursor in the skin '7-dehydrocholesterol' is activated by UV rays from sunlight. A deficiency of vitamins E and K is rarely seen in adults as both vitamins are wide-spread in nature.

The B-complex vitamins are water soluble and include eight vitamins, namely thiamine or B_1, riboflavin or B_2, niacin, pyridoxine or B_6, folic acid, cyanocobalamine or B_{12}, pantothenic acid, and biotin. They mainly function as co-enzymes in the release of energy from carbohydrates, fats, and proteins. Three B-complex vitamins are designated 'anaemia preventing vitamins' as they are needed for synthesis of haeme and for the maturation of red blood cells. Apart from the food sources, the bacterial flora in the intestine are capable of synthesizing vitamins, namely vitamin K and B-complex vitamins.

Vitamin C is the most susceptible of all vitamins. It is present in fresh fruits and vegetables and in sprouted grain. It is destroyed by oxidation, heat, and an alkaline medium. Proper cooking practices need to be followed if vitamin content of food has to be retained.

 KEY TERMS

Anaemia A condition in which number of RBCs or haemoglobin content of blood is reduced.

Antagonist A substance that interferes with the action of another substance.

Antioxidant A substance naturally present or added to a product to prevent its breakdown by oxygen.

Carotene Reddish orange colour pigment in yellow/ orange/red fruits and vegetables and green leafy vegetables which include α-, β-, and γ-carotenes and cryptoxanthin.

β-carotene A fat-soluble carotenoid pigment which is present in plants and is a precursor of vitamin A.

Cheilosis Swollen, cracked, and red lips.

Co-enzyme A substance that must be present along with an enzyme for a specific reaction to occur.

Collagen Intercellular cementing substances which is protein matrix of cartilage, connective tissue, and bone.

Glossitis Inflammation of the tongue.

Hypochromic anaemia Hypo means less and chroma means colour. A type of anaemia in which RBCs are pale in colour. It is seen in iron and B_6 deficiency.

Intrinsic factor A mucoprotein in gastric juice which helps in absorption of vitamin B_{12}.

Macrocytic anaemia Macro means large and cytes means cells. A type of anaemia in which large, immature RBCs or megaloblasts are released in blood. Also called megaloblastic anaemia, caused by deficiency of folic acid and B_{12}.

Neuritis Inflammation of the nerves.

Oedema Retention of fluid in extracellular spaces. Sodium, the electrolyte in the extracellular fluid, is also retained along with water resulting in swelling.

Parboiling Steaming of rice in the husk before milling so that B-complex vitamins diffuse from the husk and bran into the grain.

Pernicious anaemia Chronic macrocytic anaemia caused by absence of intrinsic factor needed for absorption of B_{12} accompanied by nervous disturbances.

Photophobia Abnormal sensitivity to light.

Precursor Another term used to describe provitamin.

Preformed vitamin Active form of the vitamin.

Provitamin A provitamin is a substance which can be converted into the active vitamin in the human body.

Rhodopsin or visual purple A light sensitive pigment in the rods of the retina needed for vision in dim light or for dark adaptation.

Vulnerable age group   The ages when nutrient needs are high because of synthesis of new tissues, e.g., infancy, preschool children, adolescents, and pregnant and lactating women. They are more susceptible to deficiency diseases.

REVIEW EXERCISES

1. Define vitamins and classify them.
2. Differentiate between water-soluble and fat-soluble vitamins.
3. Explain the following briefly:
   (a) Role of vitamin A in vision
   (b) Role of vitamin E in maintaining the integrity of cell membranes
   (c) Role of vitamin K in coagulation
   (d) B-complex vitamins and energy metabolism
4. List the anaemia preventing vitamins and their functions.
5. List five rich sources of each of the following vitamins:
   (a) Carotene
   (b) Niacin
   (c) Vitamin B_{12}
   (d) Ascorbic acid
   (e) Vitamin E
6. List any 10 measures which will help in retaining vitamins while cooking.
7. What are the symptoms of the following deficiency diseases
   (a) Beriberi
   (b) Pellagra
   (c) Scurvy
8. Match the following items in column I with a suitable answer from column II.

I	II
(i) Niacin	(a) Rice-eaters' disease
(ii) Vitamin D	(b) Lost on exposure to light
(iii) Beriberi	(c) Precursor tryptophan
(iv) Riboflavin	(d) *Amla*
(v) Ascorbic acid	(e) Sunlight
	(f) Night blindness
	(g) 9 kcal/g

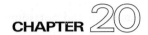

Minerals

LEARNING OBJECTIVES

After reading this chapter, you should be able to
- define the term mineral and identify the different minerals required by the body
- know the approximate amount of minerals required and the form in which they are present
- describe the function of each mineral in the body
- co-relate the functions with the deficiency symptoms
- understand the factors that affect their absorption
- list the rich sources of minerals in our daily diet

INTRODUCTION

Mineral elements are inorganic substances found in body tissues and fluids. They occur in foods as salts, e.g., sodium chloride, calcium phosphate, and ferrous sulphate. They constitute 4 per cent of our body weight.

Unlike carbohydrates, fats, and proteins, they do not furnish energy. They have many functions in our body such as tissue building and regulation of body fluids. Like vitamins, they are required in small quantities and are vital to the body. They should be supplied daily as they are excreted through the kidney, the bowel, and the skin.

Minerals are present in the body

1. As components of organic compounds, e.g., haemoglobin contains iron and thyroxine contains iodine
2. As inorganic compounds, e.g., calcium phosphate in the bones
3. As free ions in every cell in the body
4. In all body fluids

Sodium is the main electrolyte in the extracellular fluid, and potassium is the main electrolyte in the intracellular fluid.

The mineral elements are not destroyed by heat, oxidation, acid, or alkali. Since they are soluble in water, some loss occurs due to leaching when cooking water is discarded.

Definition   Minerals are inorganic elements required by the body in varying amounts to carry out various body functions. They remain largely as ash when plant and animal tissues are ignited.

CLASSIFICATION

Minerals may be classified into three groups.

Major minerals or macrominerals   Seven minerals are required in large amounts of over 100 mg/day, e.g., calcium, phosphorus, sodium, chlorine, potassium, magnesium, and sulphur.

Minor minerals   These are required in small quantities, less than 100 mg/day, e.g., iron and manganese.

Trace elements   A few micrograms to a few milligrams are required per day, e.g., iodine, fluorine, zinc, and molybdenum.

GENERAL FUNCTIONS OF MINERALS

1. Minerals form the structural components of bones, teeth, soft tissues, blood, and muscles, e.g., calcium, phosphorus, and magnesium in bones.
2. They regulate activity of nerves with regard to stimuli and contraction of muscles, e.g., calcium.
3. Maintain acid–base balance of body fluids, e.g., sodium and chlorine.
4. They control water balance by means of osmotic pressure and permeability of cell membranes, e.g., sodium and potassium.
5. They are constituents of vitamins, e.g., thiamine contains sulphur and cyanocobalamin contains cobalt.
6. They form part of molecules of hormones and enzymes, e.g., iodine in thyroxine and zinc in insulin.
7. They activate enzymes, e.g., calcium activates enzyme lipase.
8. They regulate cellular oxidation, e.g., iron and manganese.
9. Necessary for clotting of blood, e.g., calcium.

Minerals which are often deficient in the diet are shown in Table 20.1.

TABLE 20.1 Mineral elements

Mineral	Functions	Factors favouring absorption	Deficiency symptoms	Sources
1. *Calcium* Most abundant mineral in the skeletal tissues and bones (1,200 g)	1. 99% calcium is in the form of $Ca_3 PO_4$ to give hardness to bones to hold body weight 2. Catalyzes clotting of blood 3. For contraction and relaxation of muscles 4. For cell permeability	1. Body needs 2. Gastric acidity 3. Vitamin D 4. Lactose 5. Ascorbic acid	1. Rickets in children 2. Osteomalacia in adults (refer vitamin D) 3. Osteoporosis 4. Tetany	Milk and milk products such as curds, butter milk, and cheese; green leafy vegetables; small fish; ragi; *paan*; (betel leaf with lime)
2. *Phosphorus* vital as it forms DNA and RNA	1. 85% is found along with calcium in the bones and teeth 2. Constituent of DNA and RNA 3. Regulates many metabolic processes in the energy chain	Phytic and oxalic acid inhibit absorption	Deficiency is rare	Widely distributed in foods
3. *Iron* Generally deficient in Indian diet; 70% is in haemoglobin	1. Component of haemoglobin necessary for carrying O_2 2. Part of enzyme structure	1. Acid medium, vitamin C, HCl favour 2. Phytates and oxalates inhibit absorption. 3. Iron in foods is present in two forms: (a) Haeme iron associated with haemoglobin (b) Non-haeme iron. 23% haeme iron is absorbed and only 3–8% non-haeme iron is absorbed	1. Hypochromic anaemia, cells are pale 2. General fatigue 3. Breathlessness on exertion 4. Headache 5. Oedema 6. Pallor 7. Haemoglobin 5–9 g/100 ml 8. Spoon-shaped nails	Liver, organ meat, shellfish, lean meat, egg yolk, peaches, apricots, green leafy vegetables, wholegrain and enriched cereals, jaggery, legumes, *poha*, iron cooking utensils

Contd

Table 20.1 Contd

Mineral	Functions	Factors favouring absorption	Deficiency symptoms	Sources
4. *Iodine* Affects growth and metabolism in very minute amounts	1. As a constituent of thyroid hormone thyroxine it regulates rate of oxidation in the cell and determines rate of metabolism	1. Prevalence seen in hilly areas, far away from the sea 2. Iodine content of food depends on iodine content of soil on which they are grown 3. Goitrogens interfere with thyroxine activity—seen in cabbage, peanuts, etc.	1. Goitre—an enlargement of the thyroid gland in an attempt to secrete more thyroxine 2. Cretinism in infants born to thyroxine deficient women 3. Low BMR, muscular flabbiness, dry skin, thick lips, mental and skeletal retardation. Deficiency is more in females	Saltwater fish, shellfish, iodine content of eggs, meat, dairy products depend on iodine content of diet of animal. Fortification of salt with potassium iodate
5. *Fluorine* Exists in bones and teeth along with calcium	1. Fluoride along with calcium forms tooth enamel which is more resistant to decay 2. Maintains bone structure		Deficiency causes (a) tooth decay (b) osteoporosis Excess (more than 1.5 ppm) causes (a) mottled teeth, teeth are discoloured, have a chalky white appearance (dental fluorosis) (b) skeletal fluorosis	Food, water, milk, eggs, fish, fluoridated water, topical applications of stannous fluoride by dentists; 1 ppm or 1 mg per litre is the ideal level of fluoride in drinking water

Calcium

The adult body contains 1.2 kg of calcium of which 99 per cent is present in bones and teeth. The bones provide

1. A rigid framework for the body and
2. Reserves of calcium

The remaining 1 per cent is distributed in extracellular and intracellular fluids and has the following functions.

1. Calcium acts as a catalyst in clotting of blood.
2. It increases permeability of cell membranes thus helping in absorption.
3. It regulates contraction and relaxation of muscles including the heart beat.
4. It activates a number of enzymes such as pancreatic lipase and acts as a co-factor.

Factors affecting calcium absorption   The amount of calcium absorbed by humans depends on the body's need. Approximately 40 per cent of calcium ingested is absorbed.

1. Phosphate and phytic acid is present in cereals and form insoluble calcium salts if present in excess.
2. An alkaline intestinal pH (above 7) reduces absorption by forming insoluble salts.
3. Excess fibre decreases absorption of calcium.
4. Oxalic acid in green leafy vegetables forms insoluble calcium oxalate, which is excreted.
5. Faulty absorption of fats and fatty acids form insoluble calcium salts, which are excreted.
6. Lactose increases calcium absorption.
7. High protein intake increases absorption.

The parathyroids regulate the calcium level in blood and calcium metabolism in bone. The calcium to phosphorus ratio should always be 1:1.

Sources   Various sources of calcium are

1. Milk and milk products excluding butter, ghee, and cream
2. Ragi, green leafy vegetables especially drumstick leaves, cabbage, curry leaves, carrot, and cauliflower tops, and amaranth
3. Small dried fish, nuts, and oilseeds such as gingelly seeds
4. Betel leaf with slaked lime is a rich source of calcium.

Deficiency   A severe deficiency of calcium leads to rickets in children and osteomalacia and osteoporosis in adults (refer vitamin D deficiency for symptoms of rickets and osteomalacia in Chapter 19).

1. *Osteoporosis*   In osteoporosis, the bones become porous because of bone mineral loss. This causes compression of the vertebrae that results in loss of height, back and hip pain, and increased susceptibility to fractures. It is seen in post-menopausal women and can be controlled by weight bearing exercises such as walking, calcium supplements, and hormone therapy.
2. *Tetany*   A decrease in serum calcium levels gives rise to a condition called tetany. The symptoms of tetany are severe intermittent spasms of the muscles of hands and feet, accompanied by muscular pain. Twitching of facial muscles occurs.

Phosphorus

Phosphorus comprises 1 per cent of total body weight. It occurs along with calcium in human nutrition and also has many other functions in the body.

1. Building bones and teeth along with calcium and magnesium.
2. Deoxyribonucleic acid (DNA) and ribonucleic acid (RNA), the nucleic acids needed for genetic coding contain phosphorus.
3. As phospholipids, they regulate the absorption and transport of fats.
4. Adenosine triphosphate (ATP) and adenosine diphosphate (ADP)are necessary for storing and releasing energy according to body needs.
5. As part of enzymes needed for the metabolism of carbohydrates, fats, and proteins.

Sources   Phosphorus is widely distributed in foods. Milk and meat are rich in phosphorus. Wholegrain cereals, legumes, nuts, carrots, and fish are also rich sources of phosphorus.

Deficiency   Phosphorus deficiency is rare since a diet that contains adequate protein and calcium will be rich in phosphorus. Deficiency symptoms are similar to calcium deficiency.

Iron

The human body contains 3–5 g of iron of which 70 per cent is in the circulating haemoglobin.

Functions

1. Essential for carrying O_2 to the lungs where O_2 is released and CO_2 is picked up to be exhaled by haemoglobin in the red blood cells.
2. It is an essential part of several oxidative enzymes.
3. It helps in specific brain functions such as a good attention span and capacity to learn and memorize.
4. It facilitates the complete oxidation of carbohydrates, proteins, and fats within the cell and release of energy for performing physical work.

Diet provides iron in two forms:

1. Haeme iron, i.e., iron associated to the protein, globin, to form haemoglobin. Haeme iron is found in flesh food only.
2. Non-haeme iron is the form present in all plant sources plus 60 per cent of animal sources.

Haeme iron is present in small quantities in food. About 40 per cent iron in flesh food is haeme iron while 60 per cent is non-haeme iron. It is rapidly absorbed and transported. About 23 per cent is absorbed.

Non-haeme iron is the larger portion of iron in food. It is tightly bound to organic molecules in the form of ferric iron (Fe^{+++}). In the acidic medium of the stomach, it is dissociated and reduced to its more soluble ferrous form (Fe^{++}). The absorption rate of non-haeme iron is slow and approximately 8 per cent is absorbed.

Vitamin C from the diet and hydrochloric acid in gastric juice help in converting ferric iron to ferrous iron.

Factors affecting iron absorption   The following factors enhance absorption.

Body need   In periods of extra demand or in a deficiency, more iron is absorbed.

Acidic medium   Gastric acidity and ascorbic acid in the meal favour absorption.

Form of iron   Haeme iron and ferrous form are better absorbed.

Complete proteins   Complete proteins, such as meat, favour absorption.

The following factors decrease absorption.

1. Ferric iron or non-haeme iron in the absence of protein and ascorbic acid are poorly absorbed.
2. Achlorhydria or lack of hydrochloric acid in gastric juice and use of antacids with meals interfere with absorption.
3. Tea and coffee with meals.
4. Excessive intake of phytates and oxalates interferes with absorption.
5. Malabsorption due to intestinal disorders.

Iron is required for replacement of daily losses through excretion in urine, sweat, hair, and worn-out cells. It is also needed for replacement of blood losses and an expanding blood volume in all stages of growth.

Sources   Various sources of iron are

1. Liver, organ meats, shellfish, lean meat, egg yolk are all good sources
2. Green leafy vegetables, wholegrain and enriched cereals, legumes, and jaggery

3. Garden cress seeds and niger seeds are excellent sources
4. Peaches, apricots, *manukas* (black raisins), and figs
5. Use of iron cooking utensils contributes significantly to the iron content of the diet

Non-haeme iron is present in plant foods such as green vegetables, and cereals. 40 per cent iron in meat, poultry, and fish is haeme iron and 60 per cent is non-haeme iron.

Deficiency   Iron deficiency or anaemia is very common in the vulnerable age groups in all developing countries. Haemoglobin level may be as low as 5–9 g per cent. Normal haemo-globin levels for females are 11.5–14.5 g per cent and for males 12.5–16.5 g per cent.

Symptoms   General fatigue, breathlessness on exertion, giddiness and pallor of skin (paleness), oedema of ankles and spoon shaped nails are the common symptoms of iron deficiency.

Iron deficiency causes microcytic and hypochromic anaemia. Red blood cell's appear pale and smaller in size. Iron deficiency may also be seen if excessive blood loss occurs or because of faulty absorption, intestinal disease, or parasites especially hookworm and roundworm infestations.

Iodine

Most of the iodine in an adult body is found in the thyroid gland. The only known function of iodine is as a constituent of thyroxine. The thyroid hormone regulates the rate of oxidation within the cells. The iodine absorbed is incorporated into the amino acid tyrosine to form the hormone thyroxine.

$$\text{Iodine + Tyrosine} \longrightarrow \text{Thyroxine}$$

If intake of iodine is inadequate, the stores of thyroxine are gradually depleted and the thyroid gland enlarges in an attempt to produce the necessary thyroxine.

Sources   Seafood contains maximum iodine and fruits contain the least. Wide variations are seen because food content of iodine depends upon the soil where they are grown. To provide sufficient iodine, salt is being iodized. Salt is a universally used dietary item. It is cheap and addition of iodine does not affect its flavour. It is added in the form of sodium or potassium iodide in the proportion of 1 mg for every 10 g of salt.

Deficiency   Deficiency occurs when iodine content of the soil is so low that insufficient iodine is obtained through food, e.g., the soil in the Kangra valley in the Himalayan belt is deficient in iodine. Deficiency of iodine results in goitre.

Symptoms
1. Enlargement of the thyroid gland.
2. Cretinism in children (stunted growth). Cretinism is characterized by a low basal metabolism rate (BMR), flabby and weak muscles, dry skin. Skeletal development stops and mental retardation is seen.

Goitrogens are substances in food known to interfere with the use of thyroxine and can produce goitre. They are present in the red skin of peanuts and in vegetables such as cabbage and cauliflower, turnips and mustard.

Fluorine

Fluorine is the normal constituent of the body, found mainly in bones and teeth. Small amounts of fluorine bring about striking reductions in tooth decay probably because the tooth enamel is made more resistant to the action of acids produced by bacteria in the mouth.

Sources   Milk, eggs, and fish are important sources. Fluoridation of water to ensure a concentration of 1 ppm is a safe and economical way to reduce the incidence of dental caries.

Deficiency   A deficiency results in dental caries and is seen in areas where drinking water contains less than 0.5 ppm of fluorine. Adding fluorine at a level of 1 ppm reduces the incidence of dental caries by 50 per cent. Foods as well as water contain varying amounts of fluorine.

Fluorosis   Fluorosis or mottling of teeth occurs in parts of the world where drinking water contains excessive amounts of fluorine, i.e., 3–5 ppm. Teeth lose their lustrous appearance. Enamel becomes dull and unglazed and chalky white patches are seen. Sometimes enamel is pitted giving the tooth surface a corroded appearance. Skeletal fluorosis may also be seen. There is hypercalcification of the bones. Mottled areas may get yellow brown stains or discoloured.

Sodium

Sodium chloride or common salt is a daily ingredient in our diet. The adult body contains 180 g of sodium most of which is present in the extracellular fluid of the body.

The functions of sodium are listed below:
1. Maintaining fluid balance and normal osmotic pressure between intracellular and extracellular compartments.
2. It maintains normal irritability of nerves and helps in muscle contraction.
3. Regulates the alkalinity and acidity of body fluids along with the mineral chloride.
4. Regulates cell permeability or passage of substances into and out of the cell.

Sources   Milk, egg white, meat, poultry, green leafy vegetables, bengal gram dal, beetroot, and knolkhol are good sources.

The sodium from additives should also be included in the sodium content of a meal.

Deficiency   A deficiency is seen in people engaged in heavy physical activities such as farm and mine workers and in atheletes. It may also occur in cases of severe vomiting or diarrhoea.

It results in weakness, giddiness, nausea, and muscle cramps. It can be treated by adding salt to water or lime juice and if this is not retained, intravenous saline could be given.

Excess   An excessive intake of sodium should be avoided as it predisposes a person to hypertension. Salt is 40 per cent sodium, which means that a teaspoon of salt provides 2 g or 2,000 mg of sodium. Sodium is present in food as well as in many ingredients added to food such as sodium bicarbonate, monosodium glutamate, sodium benzoate, sodium propionate, and sodium nitrate. These need to be curtailed on a low-sodium diet.

Potassium

It is present as the major electrolyte in all body cells.

Functions

1. As a component of all cells in the intracellular fluid it helps in regulating the water balance along with sodium.
2. It regulates the acid–base balance like sodium.
3. It helps in transmitting nerve impulses and contraction of muscle tissues.

Sources   Fruits, vegetables, pulses, nuts, flesh food, and whole grains are rich in potassium.

Deficiency   Deficiency of potassium is unlikely in normal circumstances but may occur in severe malnutrition, chronic alcoholism, surgery, and prolonged infection.

Magnesium

About 60 per cent is found along with calcium and phosphorus in the bones and teeth. The remaining 40 per cent is present in tissues and body fluids and performs the following functions.

1. It is present mainly in the intracellular fluid and helps in maintaining fluid balance along with sodium, potassium, and calcium.
2. It helps in transmission of nerve impulses, muscle contractions, and regulation of the heart beat.
3. It acts as a co-factor in many metabolic reactions.

Sources   Milk, cheese, fish, meat, whole grains, pulses, and nuts contain magnesium.

Deficiency   Deficiency of magnesium is uncommon. It may occur in malnutrition and alcoholism. Symptoms of deficiency are similar to tetany and include muscle tremors, spasms, and convulsions.

Some more mineral elements are shown in Table 20.2.

TABLE 20.2 Other mineral elements

Mineral	Main function	Deficiency symptoms	Sources
Chloride	• Electrolyte in extracellular fluid • Water balance • Acid–base balance • Digestion—as part of gastric juice	• Seen in severe vomiting or diarrhoea resulting in alkalosis	• Common salt
Sulphur	• As a constituent of amino acids, vitamins, skin and hair, etc. • In cartilage, bones, and skin as chondroitin sulfate • Enzyme activity	• Uncommon	• All protein food rich in amino acid methionine and cystine such as milk, meat, eggs, poultry, pulses, nuts
Copper	• Haemoglobin synthesis • Part of several enzyme systems • Synthesis of melanin pigment and integrity of myelin sheath	• Uncommon • Anaemia • Excessive intake is toxic	• Liver, meat, seafood, whole grains, pulses, nuts, and copper utensils (see Plate 2)
Zinc	• Constituent of enzymes involved in metabolism • Functioning of insulin • Healing of wounds • Normal skin, bones, and hair • Normal taste acuity	• Loss of appetite • Stunted growth in children • Loss of taste sensitivity • Dull hair • Delayed wound healing	• Widely distributed in wheat bran, liver, peanuts, cheese, oysters, seafood, eggs, and whole grains (see Plate 2)
Cobalt	• As a component of vitamin B_{12} for proper formation of red blood cells	• Unknown	• Vitamin B_{12}
Manganese	• As a component of enzymes in glucose metabolism	• Unknown	• Wholegrain cereals, legumes, soya beans, and leafy vegetables
Molybdenum	• It acts as a catalyst for metalloenzymes and for several metabolic reactions	• Unknown	• Whole grains, pulses, milk, green leafy vegetables, organ meat

SUMMARY

Mineral elements are inorganic compounds present in body tissues and fluids in small amounts and are referred to as micronutrients. They constitute 4 per cent of body weight and do not provide any energy. They are classified into three groups based on the quantity required by the body. Major minerals or macrominerals are required in large amounts exceeding 100 mg/day. Minor minerals are required in amounts less than 100 mg/day and trace elements are those whose requirement is a few milligrams or in micrograms per day.

The minerals of importance to the body are calcium, phosphorus, sodium, chloride, magnesium potassium, sulphur, all of which are major minerals. Iron, manganese, fluorine, zinc, molybdenum, copper, cobalt, and iodine are required in much smaller quantities.

Minerals occur in the body as components of organic compounds, as components of inorganic compounds, and as free ions in all cells. They perform various functions related to growth and maintenance and regulation of body functions.

They are widely distributed in nature and a balanced diet with variety in choice of foods ensures an adequate intake and prevention of deficiency. However, many factors affect the absorption and utilization of minerals and these need to be known to enhance availability of minerals.

KEY TERMS

Betel leaf   Leaf of the creeper Piper betle, which is consumed along with slaked lime and betel nut for its digestive properties.

Co-factor   A mineral element which activates an enzyme.

Electrolyte   An element or compound which dissociates, when in solution, into ions.

Garden cress seeds   Maroon red seeds, which when soaked in water develop a mucilaginous covering.

Haeme iron   Iron associated with the haemoglobin molecule and is better absorbed than non-haeme iron.

Niger seeds   Also called black gingelly seeds or *karal*.

Non-haeme iron   Iron present in plant foods and partly in meat, fish, and poultry, which is not associated with haemoglobin.

Oxalic acid   An organic acid present in green leafy vegetables and cocoa.

Phytic acid   An organic acid present in outer layers of cereals which combines with calcium forming insoluble calcium phytate.

REVIEW EXERCISES

1. List the seven major minerals. Describe the functions of minerals in general.
2. Classify mineral elements, giving two examples for each.
3. State the factors which affect absorption of iron and calcium in the body.
4. Define the following terms:
   (a) Mineral elements
   (b) Co-factor
   (c) Trace elements
   (d) Goitrogens
5. List the various sources of sodium in our diet.
6. The iodine content of food depends on the iodine content of the soil on which it has grown. Explain this statement.
7. Match the following minerals in column I with a deficiency symptom in column II.

I	II
(i) Calcium	(a) Tooth decay
(ii) Iron	(b) Cretinism
(iii) Sodium	(c) Muscle cramps
(iv) Iodine	(d) Alkalosis
(v) Fluorine	(e) Spoon-shaped nails
(vi) Chloride	(f) Macrocytic anaemia
(vii) Phosphorus	(g) Osteoporosis
	(h) Glossitis
	(i) Tetany
	(j) Night blindness

CHAPTER 21

Energy Metabolism

LEARNING OBJECTIVES

After reading this chapter, you should be able to
- define the terms energy and basal metabolism
- identify and compare the basic units used in measuring energy
- understand the factors which influence our energy requirements
- describe the conditions resulting from energy imbalance
- modify the energy content of meals and know rich sources of high- and low-calorie foods
- determine individual energy needs

INTRODUCTION

Next to air and water, the body requires food as a continuous source of energy to stay alive and keep all organs and systems functioning efficiently. Just as every engine requires fuel to keep going, the human body too requires fuel in the form of food as a source of power to work continuously.

The human body is far more complex than any machine invented and as long as there is life, its energy supply cannot be turned off.

The first and foremost function of food is to supply energy to the body. This takes priority over building of new tissues, repair of wear and tear, and regulation of body functions. For example, if a diet contains adequate protein but is deficient in carbohydrate and/or fat, the protein will be oxidized to meet the energy needs first and balance used for other functions.

When food is digested, the complex nutrients carbohydrates, fats, and proteins are broken down into monosaccharides, fatty acids, glycerol, and amino acids, respectively. These simple forms are absorbed into the bloodstream and supplied to the millions of cells in the body to be oxidized by a series of complex steps to release energy (see Fig. 21.1).

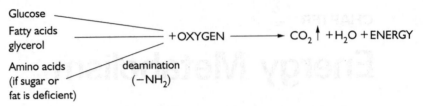

Fig. 21.1   Oxidation of nutrients to release energy

FORMS OF ENERGY

Energy is defined as the ability to do work. Energy exists in several forms (see Fig. 21.2). The forms of energy important in nutrition are

1. Chemical energy in food
2. Light or solar energy for synthesis of vitamin D in the skin and for photosynthesis in plants
3. Mechanical energy for movement of muscles
4. Electrical energy for functioning of the brain and nerve cells
5. Heat energy, generally produced when energy is converted from one form to another. The energy from food is finally converted into heat energy.

The various forms of energy are interconvertible.

Living cells are capable of releasing the energy stored in certain nutrients. This energy is used to perform various activities in the cell such as synthesis of proteins, maintaining warmth, and contraction of muscle.

The energy from the breakdown of food is stored in the body in the form of a high-energy compound, adenosine triphosphate (ATP). Adenosine triphosphate acts as a store

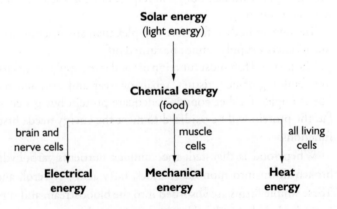

Fig. 21.2   Forms of energy

ATP ⟶ ADP + 8 kcal
adenosine triphosphate ⟵ adenosine
+ phosphate diphosphate
ion

Fig. 21.3   Release and transfer of energy

of energy-rich phosphate bonds. Living cells can use energy only in the form of energy-rich phosphate bonds.

When energy is required for cellular activity, living cells release energy from ATP which gets converted to adenosine diphosphate (ADP). One mole (molecular weight in gram) of ATP provides 8 kcal/33 kJ of energy. Adenosine diphosphate is reconverted to ATP by addition of phosphate ions. Phosphate ions help in release and transfer of energy (see Fig. 21.3).

UNITS OF MEASUREMENT

The energy present in food or the energy needed by the body is measured in units called joules or calories. The calorie in nutrition is the large calorie or kilocalorie. The kilocalorie is defined as the amount of heat required to raise the temperature of 1 kg (1,000 g) of water by 1°C. This calorie is 1,000 times bigger than the calorie used in physics.

The international unit for energy is the joule (J) and it is the energy expended when 1 kilogram (kg) is moved 1 metre (m) by a force of 1 newton (N).

Scientists and nutritionists are concerned with large amounts of energy, so they use the units kilocalorie, kilojoule (kJ = 10^3J), or megajoule (MJ = 10^6 J) to express energy.

1 kilocalorie = 4.184 kilojoules
1 megajoule = 239 kilocalories

ENERGY VALUE OF FOOD

The energy content of various foods can be measured in two ways: by calorimetry or by proximate composition.

Calorimetry

The bomb calorimeter is based on the principle of calorimetry. It measures the heat produced when the food sample is ignited by an electric spark in the presence of oxygen and platinum which acts as a catalyst. The bomb calorimeter is made up of two main parts—an inner part in which a measured quantity of food sample to be tested is placed and an outer portion which contains a known volume of water. When the food sample is electrically ignited, the surrounding water absorbs the heat produced. The energy value of the food is calculated by measuring the rise in temperature of water, based on the definition of the term calorie (see Fig. 21.4).

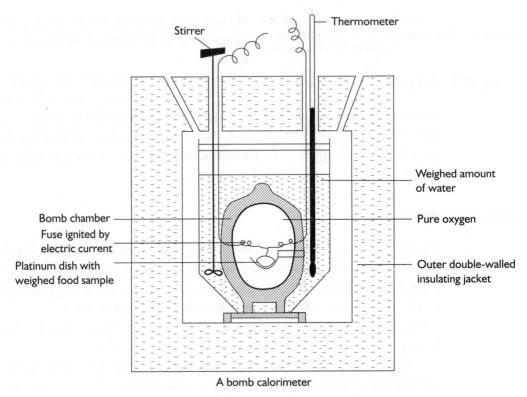

A bomb calorimeter

Fig. 21.4 Measuring the potential energy of food

Proximate Composition

This is a simpler and faster way of determining the calorie content of food. The approximate carbohydrate, fat, and protein content of a food given in the food composition tables is multiplied by their fuel factor, i.e., calories provided by 1 g of the nutrient and this total gives the energy value of a food.

The energy content of food given in the food composition tables are derived values. The carbohydrate content is calculated by difference, subtracting water, minerals, proteins, fats, and crude fibre content. However, foods contain undigestible carbohydrates which do not provide any energy and these values need some correction.

The energy value of food obtained by igniting it in the bomb calorimeter is the potential energy value of food.

The potential energy present in food when measured in a bomb calorimeter is higher than the energy released in the body. This is because some losses occur during digestion, absorption, and metabolism. The potential energy value must be corrected to allow for the losses that occur during digestion, absorption, and metabolism of nutrients (see Table 21.1).

The physiological fuel factors are based upon the corrections for losses of unabsorbed nutrients in the faeces and nitrogenous products excreted in the urine. On a mixed diet

TABLE 21.1 Energy value of food

	Potential energy in food (kcal/g)	Physiological fuel value (kcal/g)
Carbohydrates	4.15	4.0
Proteins	5.65	4.0
Fats	9.4	9.0

containing high-quality protein, 85–90 per cent carbohydrate, 95 per cent fat, and 92 per cent proteins are digested and absorbed.

The carbohydrates and proteins which are absorbed are fully oxidized.

However, when proteins are oxidized as a source of energy, they first need to be deaminated (removal of amino group). The amino group is converted to urea and is excreted in the urine. Hence, the body loses a part of the protein that is digested and absorbed. This loss of protein is about 25 per cent.

The net energy value obtained from food by the body is lesser than that measured in a bomb calorimeter.

ENERGY NEEDS OF THE BODY

The energy requirement for an average healthy person is based on the energy required to carry out basal processes as well as the energy cost of activities one indulges in. The average requirements for both the sexes belonging to different age categories is given in Table 14.1 on recommended dietary allowances (RDAs) in Chapter 14.

These allowances are suggested for a reference man weighing 60 kg and a reference woman weighing 50 kg in the 20–39 year age group.

Reference man The reference man is between 20–39 years of age and weighs 60 kg. He is in a state of good health, free from disease, and physically fit for active work. He is moderately active and is employed for 8 hours in moderate work. He spends 8 hours in bed, 4–6 hours sitting or engaged in light work, and 2 hours in walking, active recreation, or household chores. On an average his energy requirement is 2,875 kcal.

Reference woman The reference woman is between 20–39 years of age, healthy, and weighs 50 kg. She is moderately active and spends 8 hours in routine household work or in light work. She spends 8 hours in bed, 4–6 hours sitting or moving around and performing light activity, and 2 hours in walking or active recreation or household chores. On an average her energy requirement is 2,225 kcal.

Carbohydrates, fats, and proteins provide us with energy. About 60–65 per cent of the total calorie requirement should be from carbohydrates. The energy from fat should not exceed 30 per cent, preferably 15 per cent calories from fat of which 15 g should be polyunsaturated vegetable oils to meet the requirement for essential fatty acids; and 10–15 per cent calories from proteins.

TOTAL ENERGY REQUIREMENT

The total energy required by a person is the sum total of basal energy needs, the energy effect of food intake or the specific dynamic action and energy cost of physical activity (see Fig. 21.5). Energy is needed for growth, for maintenance, for the innumerable processes continuously taking place, for regulating body temperature, and for physical and mental activity. Activities that need energy are broadly classified into the following:

1. Voluntary activities, e.g., activities under the control of our will such as walking, sitting, cycling, and dish washing.
2. Involuntary activities that go on irrespective of whether we want them to. They are not under the control of our will and are vital activities on which our survival depends such as beating of the heart, respiration, and maintaing body temperature. Energy is first provided for these activities and is referred to as basal metabolism.

$$\text{Total energy needed by the body} = \text{Basal metabolic rate} + \text{Specific dynamic action} + \text{Activity}$$

Fig. 21.5 Total energy

BASAL METABOLIC RATE

The amount of energy required by the body for carrying out involuntary work and maintaining the body temperature is known as the basal metabolic rate (BMR). The involuntary work includes the functioning of various organs and systems which work continuously to keep the body processes going such as the heart and blood circulation, the kidneys and excretion. Approximately one-third of this energy is needed for these processes, while the remaining two-thirds is utilized for maintenance of muscle tone.

Test for Basal Metabolism

To measure the BMR, the following conditions need to be observed.

1. The test is conducted before breakfast 12–16 hours after the last meal, i.e., in a post-absorptive state, to eliminate the influence of food.
2. The subject should be relaxed and lying down but awake because sleep reduces BMR and activity or exercise increases the rate of oxidation in the cells.
3. The subject should have a normal pulse rate and be free from tension or fear of the test.
4. The ambient temperature should be comfortable as perspiration or shivering may affect the rate of oxidation.
5. The subject should be afebrile as fever increases the BMR by 7 per cent for every degree Fahrenheit rise in temperature.

The test is conducted by measuring the amount of oxygen consumed and/or carbon dioxide exhaled in a predetermined time, usually 6–8 minutes.

A deviation of 10–15 per cent from the accepted standards may be considered normal.

The adult BMR is 1 kcal/kg body weight/hour for men and 0.9 kcal/kg body weight/hour for women, or approximately 1,440 kcal for men and 1,080 kcal for women, respectively.

Factors Affecting the BMR

Many factors influence the BMR.

Body size Heat is continuously lost through the skin. A tall well-built person has a greater skin surface area than a shorter or smaller person and loses more heat through the skin and hence has a higher BMR.

Body composition The amount of muscle tissue and adipose or fatty tissue in the body affects the BMR. An athlete with well-built muscles and little body fat has a higher BMR than a non-athlete with more body fat of the same weight. The metabolic activity in muscle tissue or lean tissue is much more as compared to adipose or fatty tissue.

Age During periods of rapid growth, the BMR increases by 15–20 per cent because the growth hormone stimulates cell metabolism and new cells are formed. It is high during infancy, pre-school years, and puberty. During pregnancy and lactation it rapidly increases once again. The BMR gradually declines with age at the rate of 2 per cent for each decade after the age of 21 years.

Sex The BMR is 10 per cent higher in men as compared to women. The difference in BMR is attributed to a higher proportion of adipose tissue in females and hormonal variations between the sexes.

Fever Fever increases the BMR by 7 per cent for each degree Fahrenheit rise in body temperature. This is one of the reasons for loss of weight during fever.

State of health The BMR is low during starvation and malnutrition because of reduction in muscle tissue. In diseases and conditions where catabolic processes are high, such as cancers, tuberculosis, and burns, BMR is high.

Hormones Disorders of the thyroid gland markedly influence the BMR. Hyperthyroidism, a condition of excessive production of thyroid hormone, increases BMR and hypothyroidism or decreased production of thyroid hormone decreases BMR.

Climate The BMR rises when the climate is cold in order to maintain normal body temperature. In very warm climates leading to profuse sweating, BMR may increase by trying to reduce body temperature.

Psychological tension Worry and anxiety increase BMR.

SPECIFIC DYNAMIC ACTION

Specific dynamic action (SDA) is a term used to describe the effect food has in increasing the metabolic rate above the level found when fasting. Energy is needed to digest, absorb, and metabolize the food we eat. Food intake stimulates the metabolism process leading to an increase in energy expenditure. This is known as the thermogenic effect of food or the specific dynamic effect. Proteins have maximum effect on SDA, increasing the BMR by about 30 per cent when eaten alone, while carbohydrates and fats show smaller increases. When eaten together in a normal mixed diet, the increase is about 5–10 per cent of basal metabolism.

PHYSICAL ACTIVITY

Physical activity increases the energy requirement above the basal metabolism.

There is a wide variation in the energy required for physical activity among individuals. Physical activity includes energy needed for work, recreation, and mental activity, i.e., all voluntary activities. Some people use up more energy for physical activity than for basal metabolism.

On the basis of occupation, activities are grouped under three heads.

1. Sedentary/light work
2. Moderate work
3. Heavy work

Sedentary work   Teaching, office work, executive, housewife, tailoring

Moderate work   Farming, industrial labour, driver, maidservant

Heavy work   Stone cutter, miner, wood cutter

The energy requirement varies with the type of activity and the speed and efficiency with which it is performed (refer Table 14.1 on RDA in Chapter 14). For example, swimming uses up twice the energy of bicycling, and walking briskly uses up thrice the energy of walking at a moderate pace. The body size of the person also affects energy expended for a task. The larger the body size, the more energy would be needed just as more energy is needed to move a heavy sack of potatoes compared to a lighter one.

The energy expended for physical activities is measured indirectly by strapping a light-weight respirometer, collecting the expired air and analyzing the carbon dioxide and oxygen content to calculate the energy expended.

ENERGY BALANCE

The human body is constantly using energy which needs to be replaced. For this, a constant supply of energy is required. Energy is used for basal metabolism, specific dynamic action, and physical activity. The energy from the food we eat, mainly carbohydrates and fats, is used to meet the energy demands of the body. When food is not available during fasting or starvation, the body draws upon its own stores to meet the energy needs of the body. The body has three types of energy store.

Glycogen   The form in which carbohydrate is stored in the muscles and liver is adequate to last for 12–48 hours. Approximately 300 g glycogen is stored in the muscle and 100 g in the liver.

Muscle   Protein is stored in limited amounts in the muscle.

Adipose tissue   Fat is stored in the adipose tissue and the amount stored varies vastly from one person to another.

A person in energy balance neither gains weight nor loses weight. Excessive consumption of calories as compared to the output or activity leads to a condition called overweight, which in severe cases is called obesity. A deficient intake of carbohydrates and fats in the diet leads to underweight or undernutrition. Both underweight and obesity are undesirable conditions which need timely correction.

Definition   Energy balance is a condition in which the energy provided by food is nearly equal to the total energy expended by the body resulting in a steady body weight.

$$\text{Energy balance : Energy output} = \text{Energy input}$$

Overweight

Overweight and obesity affect over 25 per cent adults in developed countries and can lead to serious health consequences if not treated early. When an individual's energy intake consistently exceeds energy expenditure, weight gain occurs initially, leading to obesity. Since energy can neither be created nor destroyed but can be changed from one form to another, the excess chemical energy from food is converted into fat and stored as potential energy in the adipose tissues.

Overweight   A person whose body weight is 10 per cent more than the prescribed height for weight standards for his age and sex.

Obese   A person whose body weight is 20 per cent or more than that of the prescribed standards.

Grossly obese   A person who weighs 45 kg or 100 per cent more than accepted standards.

Underweight   A person whose weight is 15–20 per cent below the accepted standards.

Body mass index   The concept of ideal or desirable body weight has been changing from time to time and ideal weight for different body frames was initially computed. Today the weight of an individual is assessed on a more scientific basis known as the body mass index (BMI).

$$\text{Body mass index} = \frac{\text{Weight in kilograms}}{(\text{Height in metres})^2} = \frac{W}{H^2}$$

Normal values

Men $\dfrac{W}{H^2} = 20 - 25$

Women $\dfrac{W}{H^2} = 19 - 24$

Values over 25 indicate obesity.

A woman weighing 65 kg having a height of 155 cm will have a BMI of 27.

$$\text{BMI} = \frac{65}{1.5^2} = \frac{65}{2.4} = 27$$

On the basis of BMI, obesity is graded as follows:

Obesity	BMI
Grade I	25–29
Grade II	30–40
Grade III	>40

Causes of obesity

- Family food habits—rich high-calorie foods
- Ignorant of calorific value of food
- Skips breakfast, nibbles high-calorie snacks
- Sedentary lifestyle
- Lower metabolism with increasing age but failure to reduce intake
- Emotional outlet—eats more to overcome worry, stress, etc.
- Attends many social events
- Distress eating (to avoid wastage)

An obese person should lose one to two pounds per week. A reduction of 500 kcal/day will lead to a weight loss of one pound per week. Physical activity should be increased for faster weight loss and better muscle tone.

If 1 lb weight is to be lost per week, then

1 lb of body fat = 455 g

1g of body fat provides 7.7 kcal/g as it has some water in it.

Caloric equivalent of

1 lb body fat = $455 \times 7.7 = 3{,}500$ kcal

3,500 kcal to be lost in 1 week or 7 days

$\therefore$ Weight loss in 1 day = $\dfrac{3{,}500}{7}$ = 500 kcal/day

Underweight

Underweight is caused due to undernutrition which is the result of ingesting insufficient quantity of food. An energy intake less than the need is the most common cause. Other causes for underweight are poor assimilation of food due to digestive disorders, faulty absorption, intestinal infestations, infections, poor food habits, stress and tension, poverty, and lack of nutrition knowledge.

Teenagers are weight conscious and skip meals or consume junk food to maintain their weight. Anorexia nervosa is a condition of self-induced severe weight loss seen in adolescents and has psychological origins.

Undernutrition affects one's growth, health, behaviour, and brain structure and function. Such individuals should be prescribed a high-calorie, high-protein, moderate-fat diet for gaining weight. An excess of 500 kcal/day will help in gaining 1 lb/week.

CALCULATING THE ENERGY VALUE BASED ON PROXIMATE PRINCIPLES

Problem

A non-vegetarian meal provides 20 g protein, 10 g fat, and 125 g carbohydrate of which 5 g is fibre. Calculate the calories provided by this meal (see Table 21.2).

1. Protein

   1 g protein provides 4 kcal

   ∴ 20 g protein will provide 20 × 4 = 80 kcal
2. Fat

   1 g fat provides 9 kcal

   ∴ 20 g fat will provide 20 × 9 = 180 kcal
3. Carbohydrate

   1 g carbohydrate provides 4 kcal

   1 g fibre provides 0 kcal

   Digestible carbohydrate = 125 – 5 = 120 g

   120 g carbohydrate will provide 120 × 4 = 480 kcal

   Total calories provided by the meal = 80 + 180 + 480

   = 740 kcal

The meal provides 740 kcal.

TABLE 21.2 Sources of energy in the diet

	kcal/g	kJ/g
Proteins	4	17
Carbohydrates	4	17
Fats	9	38
Alcohol	7	29

DIETARY SOURCES

All foods provide energy. While selecting food, one must consider the other nutrients such as proteins, vitamins, minerals, and fibre present in the food and make a wise choice.

The nutrients carbohydrates and fats are consumed mainly as a source of energy. All refined carbohydrates, i.e., sugars and starch and all foods rich in fats are rich sources of energy (refer Chapters 15 and 17 for sources).

The cereal group is another excellent source of energy and supplies the highest percentage of calories.

Hollow-calorie foods or empty calories are provided by food which is rich in energy but lack other vital nutrients. Sugars, fats, and alcoholic beverages are referred to as empty-calorie foods because they contain traces of vitamins and minerals. They are low in nutrient density.

Nutrient-dense foods are those food which are rich in one or more nutrients apart from calories. It is a measure of the quantity of these nutrients supplied by a food in relation to its calorie content. Nutrient-dense foods are of special importance to weight watchers and those leading a sedentary lifestyle. It helps them get all the nutrients they need without consuming unnecessary calorie-rich foods and gaining weight.

Table 21.3 lists some hollow-calorie foods and some nutrient-dense foods.

TABLE 21.3 Hollow-calorie and nutrient-dense foods

Hollow-calorie foods	Nutrient-dense foods
• Aerated soft drinks as	• Milk, cheese, yoghurt
• Synthetic syrups	• Green leafy vegetables
• Candy and candy floss	• Pulses, sprouts
• Chocolates	• Soya beans, peanuts
• Iced cakes and fresh cream pastries	• Guava, *amla*
	• Liver, fish, meat
• Ice lolly	• Eggs
• Puff pastry	• Flaxseeds

ESTIMATION OF ENERGY REQUIREMENTS

The total energy required in a day can be estimated by two methods: RDA tables and actual record of activities.

The RDA table gives us the approximate calories required on the basis of age, sex, and activity. A specific estimate of ones energy needs can be calculated by adding energy needed for performing different activities in a 24-hour period. The energy cost of various activities is mentioned in Table 21.4. If the time taken for each activity is known, the energy cost can be easily calculated (see examples given in Table 21.5). A sum total of energy required for BMR + SDA + physical activity could also give us the total energy requirement.

TABLE 21.4   Energy cost of various activities

No activity (50–65 kcal/hour)	Sedentary (80–100 kcal/hour)	Light (110–160 kcal/hour)	Moderate (170–240 kcal/hour)	Heavy (250–400 kcal/hour)	Strenuous (400–600 kcal/hour)
Sleeping	• Sitting activities	• Standing and walking slowly	• Sitting/standing with active arm movements	• Vigorous activities	• Aerobic activities
	• Attending lectures	• Having a shower	• Sweeping	• Drying clothes	• Swimming
	• Sitting, chatting	• Getting dressed	• Mopping	• Washing large pots and pans	• Walking uphill
	• Eating	• Handwashing small clothes	• Scrubbing	• Moving furniture	• Climbing stairs
	• Watching TV	• Riding a bike	• Polishing surfaces	• Stripping beds	• Chopping wood
	• Reading	• Driving a car	• Bed making	• Weeding and digging the garden	• Shovelling snow
	• Writing	• Attending practicals	• Washing clothes		• Jogging
	• Using the computer	• Walking	• Bicycling		
		• Ironing clothes	• Painting		
		• Sewing, cooking, dusting			
		• Clerical work			

Note: These are approximate values. The actual energy expenditure will depend on weight of the individual, lean body mass, and physical fitness. BMR and SDA are included. Lower value is for women and higher value is for men.

TABLE 21.5   Activity record for an 18-year-old college boy

Activity	Time (hours/minute)	Energy cost of activity (kcal/hour)	Energy expended
Sleeping	8 hours	65	520
Bathing and dressing	30 minutes	160	80
Handwashing small clothes/ironing	30 minutes	160	80
Tidying your room	10 minutes	240	40
Driving a bike	15 minutes	160	40
Climbing stairs	15 minutes	420	105
Attending lectures	4 hours	100	400
Sitting chatting	1 hour	100	100
Attending practicals	3 hours	160	480
Walking	50 minutes	160	130
Having meals	2 hours	100	200
Watching television	2 hours	100	200
Gym/aerobic exercises	30 minutes	500	250
Studying/writing journals	1 hour	100	100
Time	**24 hours**		
Total energy required			**2,725**
RDA			**2,640**

Note: These values include BMR + SDA.

Calculating Energy Requirements

Particulars—Adult woman, 25 years old, weight 50 kg, Height 155 cm
- Calculate energy required for basal metabolism. (BMR for females = 0.9 kcal/kg/hour)
  BMR for one day will be
  0.9×50 (weight in kg) $\times 24$ (hours in a day) = 1,080 kcal
- Estimate your level of physical activity as a percentage of BMR.

Activity	Energy cost as per cent of BMR
Sedentary	20 per cent
Moderate	35 per cent
Heavy	50 per cent

Energy cost of physical activity for a heavy worker will be

$$= (50 \text{ per cent} \times BMR) + BMR$$
$$= 50/100 \times 1{,}080 + 1{,}080$$
$$= 1{,}620 \text{ kcal}$$

Add energy cost of food intake (SDA) which is 6–10 per cent of total calories. On a vegetarian diet it is about 6 per cent and on a non-vegetarian diet it is about 10 per cent, approximately 100 kcal.

Total energy requirement = BMR + Physical activity + SDA

$$= 1{,}080 + 1{,}620 + 100 = 2{,}800$$
$$= 2{,}800 \text{ kcal}$$

MODIFYING ENERGY CONTENT OF MEALS

The energy content of the diet can be suitably modified to enable a person to gain or lose weight. It is essential to understand the causes of weight loss or weight gain before suggesting modifications. The weight gain or weight loss should be gradual.

Underweight

The cause of weight loss must be treated before a modified diet is prescribed.

To gain weight

- High-calorie diet, i.e., 500 kcal more per day for weight gain of 1 lb/week
- High-protein diet with good quality protein 1.2 g/kg desirable body weight
- Adequate vitamins and minerals. Sometimes supplements may be necessary
- Modify diet gradually
- Have six small meals a day
- Keep meal times pleasant and food should be appetizing and attractively served

Type of foods recommended

- Food which is easy to assimilate
- High-calorie, high-protein foods
- Salad dressings, cream soups
- Desserts
- Fresh fruits such as banana, mango, chikoo
- Whole milk, whole milk curd, and *paneer*
- Nutritious soups and stews
- Animal protein—baked fish, mutton stew, cheese sandwiches

Do not force the individual to eat, but serve meals which will whet one's appetite.

Overweight/Obesity

To reduce weight

- Low-calorie, high-fibre, high-protein diet
- Low fat, no salad dressings
- Low sugar and refined carbohydrate
- Avoid sugar in tea and coffee
- Use lean meat
- Have three meals a day

Type of foods recommended   Foods which give a feeling of fullness at the end of a meal, i.e., low energy density meals, lots of substance but lesser calories.

To create satiety, increase

1. Bulk or fibre content
2. Volume

Fats, butter, and oil should be used sparingly by an obese individual (see Plate 3).

Foods suggested

- *Soups* Large portion of liquid, rich in ingredients. The steamy aroma gives a sense of satisfaction.
- *Vegetable juices* Served before a meal reduces quantity of food consumed at mealtime.
- *Salads* A salad platter looks like a large portion of food served. It takes time to chew, has lots of fibre, and is low calorie. It is part of a low-energy-density meal recommended for all individuals. It is specially included in a weight reduction diet (see Plate 3).
- *High-fibre breakfast cereal* It requires time to eat and chew; keeps blood sugar levels steady.
- *Plain lassi* Made from skimmed milk and served diluted and unsweetened could be had before or between a meal.
- *Smoothies* Appetite suppressing fruit protein drinks. The volume is increased by whipping fruit and yoghurt/soya curd/protein powder in the blender with crushed ice for a longer time.

SUMMARY

The body requires a continuous source of energy to stay alive and to carry out all body functions, processes, and activities. This energy is derived from the oxidation of carbohydrates, proteins, and fats in the tissue cells, resulting in production of heat energy, and carbon dioxide and water which are excreted. The various forms of energy necessary for life are interconvertible.

Energy is stored in the form of high-energy phosphate bonds in ATP. Energy is measured in kilocalories or kilojoules. One kilocalorie = 4.184 or 4.2 kilojoules. The energy value of food can be measured in an instrument called a bomb calorimeter or by using food composition tables. This is the potential energy present in food. The energy available to the body is the physiological fuel factor that is lesser than the potential energy as some losses of carbohydrates, proteins, and fats occur during digestion and absorption.

The body needs energy to carry out the involuntary work of the body or for basal metabolism, for physical activity, and for releasing the nutrients or making them available to the body, i.e., the specific dynamic action. Many factors affect the BMR. The energy cost of different activities varies depending on the activity and the speed and efficiency with which it is carried out. The body is in energy balance if there is no weight loss or weight gain. Overweight and obesity result from an imbalance between energy intake, which is more, and energy output, which is less. Underweight results from deficient intake and more output. Both conditions can be cured by modifying the energy intake.

KEY TERMS

Adenosine triphosphate   A compound with three phosphate groups in which energy is stored.

Aerobic exercises   Exercises requiring oxygen.

Basal metabolism   The energy needed by the body to carry out involuntary activities while at rest.

Calorimeters   An instrument used to measure heat energy by noting the rise in temperature of a known volume of water.

Energy   The ability to do work. Energy from food is expressed in kilocalories and kilojoules.

Physiological fuel factor   The energy in proteins, carbohydrates, and fats which is available to the body. Physiological fuel factor for protein = 4 kcal/g, carbohydrates = 4 kcal/g, and fat = 9 kcal/g.

Proximate composition   The carbohydrate, fat, protein, water, minerals, and crude fibre content.

Specific dynamic action   Also known as post-prandial thermogenesis or calorigenic effect of food. It is the energy required to transform food into nutrients to be used by body cells and accounts for 6–10 per cent increase in energy expenditure.

REVIEW EXERCISES

1. Define the terms
   (a) Kilocalorie
   (b) Basal metabolism
   (c) Specific dynamic action
   (d) Potential energy in food
   (e) Physiological fuel factor
2. The basal metabolism is the rate of oxidation occurring in the body at rest. Why can the basal metabolism vary in two individuals of the same age?
3. On what factors does the total energy requirement depend on? Explain them briefly.
4. One serving of pudding provides 30 g carbohydrate, 10 g fat, and 2 g of protein. Calculate the calories provided by two such servings.
5. How are the fuel values of food estimated? Explain any two methods.

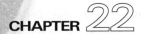

Balanced Diet

LEARNING OBJECTIVES

After reading this chapter, you should be able to
- define the term balanced diet
- understand the importance of consuming a balanced diet
- know the various factors which influence our RDA and the difference between requirement and RDA
- classify foods into appropriate groups
- explain the basis for dividing food into groups
- discuss the use of food groups and RDA in planning balanced diets

INTRODUCTION

Nutrients are needed by humans in specific amounts to ensure good health and well-being. These nutrient needs are met by eating the right kinds and amounts of food. But how does an individual know what the right kind and amount of food should be? If a diet is planned and given to an individual with the correct kinds and proportions of different nutrients, and he/she is asked to follow it every day, it will become monotonous. Also, a diet which is acceptable to one individual may not be acceptable to another individual for many different reasons such as food preferences, customs, food habits, age, economic reasons, and allergies.

RECOMMENDED DIETARY ALLOWANCE

While planning balanced diets, we need certain guidelines regarding the kinds and amounts of nutrients that we require for maintenance of good health. The recommended dietary allowance (RDA) is the guideline stating the amount of nutrients to be actually consumed in order to meet the requirements of the body. The RDA is based on requirements.

The requirement for a particular nutrient is the minimum level that needs to be consumed to perform specific functions in the body and to prevent deficiency symptoms. It should also maintain satisfactory stores of the nutrients in the body.

Recommended dietary allowances are based on a person's requirements for different nutrients. In other words,

Recommended dietary allowances = Requirement + Margin of safety

The margin of safety is added to take care of factors such as

1. Losses during cooking and processing
2. Short periods of deficient intake
3. Nature of the diet
4. Individual variations in requirements

For example, the requirement for iron in Western countries is 10 mg for adult men and 15 mg for adult women respectively, while Indian RDAs suggest an intake of 28 mg for adult men and 30 mg for adult women. This is because the form of iron consumed varies and the factors interfering with absorption of iron such as phytates in cereals and larger proportions of nonhaeme iron present in Indian diets. The requirement for vitamin C or ascorbic acid is actually 20 mg, but since the vitamin is easily destroyed during pre-preparation, cooking, and storage, the recommended intake is twice the requirement and is 40 mg/day.

The RDAs apply to healthy individuals and are set high enough to cover individual variation. They are based on gender, age, body size, activity level, and special physiological state. Disease and drugs prescribed for treatment can alter the requirement for one or more nutrients.

RDAs for specific nutrients

1. The RDAs are expressed in metric units such as kilocalorie (kcal), grams (g), milligrams (mg), and micrograms (μg).
2. They are based on gender and activity levels such as sedentary or light, moderate, and heavy.
3. The RDAs for B-complex vitamins B_1, B_2, and niacin are based on kilocalories or energy. The major role of these three vitamins is the release of energy from carbohydrates, proteins, and fats.
   The RDA for B_1 is 0.5 mg/1,000 kcal, B_2 is 0.55 mg/1,000 kcal, and niacin is 6.6 mg/1,000 kcal.
4. The RDAs for protein are based on body weight. Adults need 1 g/kg body weight while infants, children, adolescents, and pregnant and lactating mothers need more protein to meet the demands of growth and body building.
5. The RDAs, for practically all nutrients, increase during pregnancy and lactation to meet the needs of the growing foetus during pregnancy and for production of milk

during lactation. These additional needs depicted by a + sign in the RDA table take care of the physiological stress which results due to these conditions.

6. The RDAs for infants are expressed per kg body weight.
7. The RDAs for vitamin A are expressed in terms of retinol (preformed vitamin A) and β-carotene (precursor or provitamin A). β-carotene needs to be converted to vitamin A in the body. During this conversion certain losses occur and on an average only 25 per cent is converted to vitamin A. The total vitamin A or retinol could be calculated using the formula given below

$$\text{Total vitamin A in } \mu g = \mu g \text{ of retinol} + \frac{\mu g \text{ of } \beta\text{-carotene}}{4}$$

How much food each individual will need will depend on many factors which have been considered while computing the Recommended Dietary Allowances. Factors such as age, gender, and special physiological needs have been kept in mind. The RDA table gives us the quantity of different nutrients to be included in our daily diet. The second important factor we need to know to ensure the right selection of food is its nutritive value. Most foods contain more than a single nutrient. The nutritive value of different foods have been analysed in the laboratory and on the basis of this information, food composition tables have been formulated.

These tables give us the percentage of important nutrients in the edible portion of all foods we consume. If we know the weight of the food we have consumed, we can calculate its nutritive value with the help of the food composition tables. This can be compared with the RDAs which will tell us whether our diet is nutritionally adequate or not. The RDA is a goal to be achieved and food is selected so that we reach the goal.

However, this process is time consuming and not at all practical as lengthy calculations are necessary. What is needed is a practical guide which can help individuals to select foods of their choice according to their nutritional requirements. Since no single food provides all the nutrients in desirable amounts, and all foods differ in their nutrient content, it becomes necessary to divide food into groups to help us consume a balanced diet.

Definition

A balanced diet is one which includes a variety of foods in adequate amounts and correct proportions to meet the day's requirements of all essential nutrients such as proteins, carbohydrates, fats, vitamins, minerals, water, and fibre (see Plate 4). Such a diet helps to promote and preserve good health and also provides a safety margin or reserve of nutrients to withstand short durations of emergency.

The safety margin takes care of the days on which we fast, or on a certain day all nutrients may not be consumed. If the balanced diet meets the RDA for an individual, then the safety margin is already included as the RDA is formulated keeping extra allowances in mind.

A balanced diet takes care of the following aspects.

1. It includes a variety of food items.
2. It meets the RDA for all nutrients.
3. Nutrients are included in correct proportions.
4. Provides a safety margin for nutrients.
5. It promotes and preserves good health.
6. It helps maintain acceptable body weight for height.

BASIC FOOD GROUPS

One of the simplest ways to plan a balanced diet is to divide foods into groups. Foods are grouped on the basis of the predominant nutrients present in them. They may be classified into three, four, five, seven, or eleven food groups. This classification varies from one country to another depending on many factors. For example, in India we do not have milk and milk products or flesh foods as a separate food group because of religion, economic reasons, etc. The five food group classification is used in India as a guide to meal planning. Many factors have been considered while compiling these groups such as availability of food, cost, meal pattern, and deficiency diseases prevalent. Not all foods in each group are equal in their nutrient content. That is why a variety of foods from each group should be included in the diet (see Fig. 22.1).

A food group consists of a number of foods which have common characteristics. These common features may be the source of food, the physiological function performed, or the nutrients present.

On the basis of the source of food, at least 14 groups can be identified, e.g., cereals, pulses, milk and milk products, eggs, flesh foods, nuts and oilseeds, sugar and sweeteners, fats and oils, root vegetables, other vegetables, green leafy vegetables, fruits, condiments and spices, and miscellaneous foods. This does not simplify the planning of balanced meals.

A classification based on nutrients present will ensure that all nutrients are made available to the body and offer greater variety within the group.

There are five basic food groups:

1. Cereal and millets group
2. Protein or body building food group
3. Protective food group
4. Secondary protective food group
5. Fats and oils, sugar and jaggery group

Cereal and Millets Group

This group includes all cereals and millets which form the staple diet for a large majority of Indians. The major nutrients provided by this group are calories, protein, fibre, B-complex vitamins mainly thiamine, some minerals, and fibre. As the income decreases, the calories provided by this group increases.

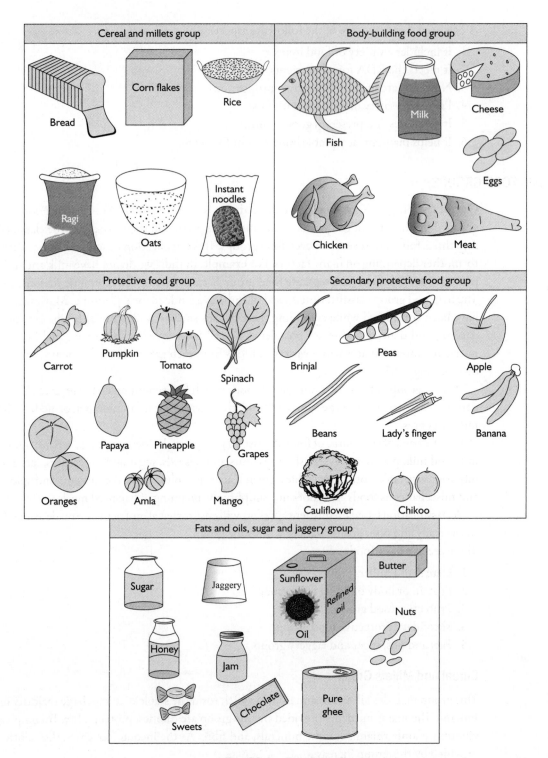

Fig. 22.1 Five basic food groups

The staple cereal consumed varies in different geographical areas and includes wheat, rice, maize, and millets such as *jowar*, *bajra*, *ragi*, and their products such as refined flour, semolina, broken wheat or dalia, parboiled rice, rice flakes or parched rice, puffed rice, popcorn, cornflakes, vermicelli, pastas, bread, and pizza. Other cereals are *triticale*, rye, oats, barley, etc. (see Table 22.1).

TABLE 22.1   Five basic food groups

Food group	Foods included	Serving size	Number of servings per day	Main nutrients provided
Cereal and millets	All cereals and their products such as wheat, rice, maize, millets such as *jowar*, *bajra*, *ragi*, semolina, *poha*, bread, noodles, pizza, puffed cereals	30 g	6–12 servings (1 serving is 1/2 cup cooked rice, 1 chappati, a slice of bread, 2 *poories*, a bowl of breakfast cereal)	Carbohydrates, partially complete proteins, fibre (except rice), B-complex vitamins, some are rich in iron or calcium
Protective foods	Yellow, orange, and red fruits and vegetables such as mango, papaya, carrots, pumpkin	50–75 g	1 or more servings (1 serving is 1/2 cup cooked vegetable or 1/2 cup cut fruit)	Rich source of carotene, iron, folic acid, fibre, other vitamins and minerals
	Green leafy vegetables such as spinach, fenugreek, colocasia	100 g		
	All citrus fruits, guava, tomato, pineapple, amla	50–75 g 10 g	1 or more servings (1 serving is 1 medium-sized fruit)	Rich source of ascorbic acid
Protein or body building foods	All pulses, nuts, and oilseeds such as Bengal gram, red gram, black gram, green gram, lentils, soya beans, sprouts, groundnuts, sesame, almonds	30 g	3–6 servings of any of the following (1 serving is 1 cup dal)	Partially complete proteins, carbohydrates, iron, B-complex vitamins B_1, B_2, niacin. Soya bean and oilseeds provide fat. Sprouts provide vitamin C
	Milk and milk products such as whole milk, skimmed milk, curds, *paneer*, cheese, ice cream, buttermilk	150 g	1 cup milk or curds 25 g cheese	Complete protein, calcium, phosphorous, fat, vitamins A, B_2, B_{12}, cholesterol
	Meat, fish, poultry Egg	40 g 40–50 g	1 medium size piece 1 egg	Protein, iron, fat, cholesterol, vitamins A, B_1, B_2, B_{12}, niacin
Secondary protective foods	All other fruits and vegetables not included in protective food group such as brinjal, beans, gourd vegetables, lady's finger, potato, onion, yam, colocasia, radish, beetroot, banana, apple, chikoo, grapes, melons, pears	50–75 g	2 or more servings (1 serving is 1/2 cup vegetable or fruit or 1 medium banana)	Carbohydrates, fibre, small amounts of vitamins and minerals
Fats and oils, sugar and jaggery	All fats such as *vanaspati*, margarine, shortenings, fresh cream, non-dairy cream, butter, clarified butter All oils such as groundnut, corn, soya, rice bran, sesame, salad oil, olive oil, fish oils	5 g	5 servings, of which 3 servings should be vegetable oil	Calories, Oils provide vitamin E and essential fatty acids Fats provide vitamins A and D
	Sugar, jaggery, honey, molasses, chocolates. Jam, jellies, marmalade	5 g	5 servings	Only calories; jaggery, honey, and preserves give very small amounts of minerals

One serving from this group is 30 g of cereal/by-product of cereal and includes

1. A slice of bread
2. A medium *phulka*
3. Half cup cooked rice
4. Two *poories*
5. A bowl of breakfast cereal.

It is preferable to use two or more different cereals everyday, of which some should be whole grain for maximum nutritional benefit. Ragi is the only cereal which is rich in calcium and wheat is rich in iron as compared to rice. When cereals and pulses are consumed together in the same meal, the quality of protein increases dramatically.

At least six or more servings should be selected from this group. Each serving provides 2–3 g of protein and 80–100 kcal.

Protein or Body-building Food Group

This group includes both plant and animal foods that are rich in protein, both quantitatively and qualitatively. All milk and milk products such as whole and skimmed milk, *paneer*, cheese, curds, buttermilk, milk powder, and *mawa* or *khoa* excluding butter, cream, and clarified butter or pure ghee which is included under fats and oils; pulses and their products such as roasted *channa*, bengal gram flour, soya products, such as soya flour, tofu, soya grits, and textured vegetable protein; meat, fish, poultry, game and organ meat, and eggs; and nuts and oilseeds such as groundnuts, sesame, and almonds.

Apart from proteins, this group also provides B-complex vitamins, vitamin A, iron, and calcium. Animal proteins supply B_{12} and cholesterol.

One serving from this group is equal to 30 g pulses, 1 egg, 40 g mutton, or 1 cup of milk or curd.

At least three servings should be included from this group daily.

The protein quality of a non-vegetarian diet is far superior to that of a vegetarian diet, except when cereals and pulses are consumed together, the protein quality improves. Those who depend on pulses for meeting their protein requirement can improve the protein content of the meal by one or all of the following ways:

1. Including at least one serving from this group in every meal
2. Adding a small amount of animal protein in every meal
3. Combining cereals and pulses or cereals and animal protein
4. Including a variety of pulses, especially whole grain or split pulses with the husk
5. Sprouting pulses to increase availability of nutrients and provide vitamin C and B-complex vitamins specially B_1, B_2, and niacin.

As a general rule, this group does not provide ascorbic acid or vitamin C to the diet. One serving from this group provides approximately 7 g protein and 70–100 kcal.

Protective Food Group

This group includes all vegetables and fruits that are rich in β-carotene and ascorbic acid. These nutrients increase the body's resistance to disease and protects the body against infection, hence the name protective. β-carotene is converted to vitamin A in the body.

The foods in this group are rich in carotenoid pigment which imparts a yellow, orange, or red colour to fruits and vegetables. In green leafy vegetables which are naturally rich in β-carotene, the orange colour of carotene pigment is masked by the green pigment of chlorophyll present in the leaf. Other rich sources are pumpkin, carrots, tomatoes, ripe jackfruit, mango, papaya, peaches, and apricots. This group also includes all citrus fruits such as oranges, sweet lime, grapefruit, lemon, guavas, *amla*, zizyphus, and pineapple which are rich in vitamin C.

Green leafy vegetables such as spinach, fenugreek leaves, radish leaves, amaranth, oniontops, colocasia leaves, drumstick leaves, mint, and cabbage are rich source of carotene. One serving from this group includes 50–75 g of vitamin C rich fruit or vegetable which is equal to half a cup or one whole fruit in the case of citrus fruits or 100 g of green leafy vegetable.

Choose at least two servings from this group, one in the form of a green leafy vegetable and the other in the form of a vitamin C rich fruit which is uncooked. Apart from carotene and vitamin C, this group provides negligible amounts of calories, protein, and fibre. Green leafy vegetables provide iron, calcium, and folic acid.

A serving from this group gives 25 kcal and 1 g protein.

Secondary Protective Group or Other Fruits and Vegetables

All fruits and vegetables which do not come under the protective food group are included in this category. This group provides some carbohydrates, minerals, vitamins, and fibres to the diet. The main role of this group is to add variety to the diet. Fruits such as banana, chikoo, pears, grapes, melons, custard apples, and apples are included in this group.

Vegetables such as brinjal, cucumber, and lady's finger; all gourds such as ash gourd, bottle gourd, bitter gourd, ridge gourd, and sponge gourd; tender peas and all beans; and roots and tubers such as potato, onion, radish, and yam and colocasia are also included in this group.

One serving from this group is equal to 50–75 g of vegetable or fruit which is half a cup of cut vegetables.

Two or more servings from this group should be included everyday. One serving provides 25–50 kcal and 1 g protein.

Fats and Oils, Sugar and Jaggery

The foods in this group are a concentrated source of energy and mainly provide calories only. Some foods such as animal fats provide vitamins A and D. Vegetable oils provide essential fatty acids. Sugar provides only calories while jaggery and honey provide small quantities of minerals as well.

This group includes sugar, jaggery, honey, molasses, and all forms of sugar such as icing sugar, castor sugar, Demerara sugar, glucose, corn syrup, and all natural sweeteners. All foods which are preserved with the help of sugar such as jams, jellies, and marmalades are included in this group. One gram of sugar provides 4 kcal, and this energy is available quickly.

Fats and oils are a concentrated source of energy since one gram of fat gives 9 kcal. Hydrogenated fat, margarine, butter, cream, and clarified butter are sources of fat. Groundnut, coconut, sunflower, safflower, gingelly, rice bran, corn, soya, mustard, etc. are sources of oil. Fats and oils should not exceed 30 per cent of the total calories. This includes the invisible fats in the diet. About 50 per cent of the fat intake should be from at least two to three vegetable oils to ensure consumption of essential fatty acids. 15–20 per cent of total calories from fat is recommended.

The diet should provide approximately 25–30 g of sugar and 25 g of fats and oils per day. This amount will vary depending on the total energy requirement. One serving is one teaspoon sugar or 5 g sugar providing 20 kcal and one teaspoon or 5 g fat providing 45 kcal.

This group does not contain any protein.

GUIDELINES FOR USING THE BASIC FOOD GROUP

1. Include at least one or a minimum number of servings from each food group in each meal.
2. Make choices within each group as foods within each group are similar but not identical in nutritive value.
3. If the meal is vegetarian, supplement vegetable proteins with suitable combinations to improve the overall protein quality of the diet. For example, serving cereal, pulse combinations or including small quantities of milk or curds in the meal.
4. Include uncooked vegetables and fruits in the meals.
5. Include at least one serving of milk to ensure a supply of calcium and other nutrients as milk contains all nutrients except iron, vitamin C, and fibre.
6. Cereals should not supply more than 75 per cent of total calories.

THE FOOD PYRAMID

The food pyramid is a carefully drawn up plan of exactly what the human body needs nutritionally. It is a guide prepared by the United States Department of Agriculture (USDA) which helps us plan our meals so that we get the correct amount of nutrients every day to keep us fit and healthy. The pyramid was designed to help us understand the concepts of

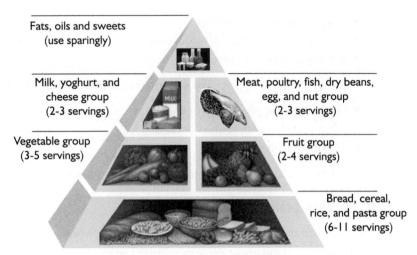

Fats, oils and sweets
(use sparingly)

Milk, yoghurt, and
cheese group
(2-3 servings)

Meat, poultry, fish, dry beans,
egg, and nut group
(2-3 servings)

Vegetable group
(3-5 servings)

Fruit group
(2-4 servings)

Bread, cereal,
rice, and pasta group
(6-11 servings)

Fig. 22.2   The food pyramid

variety, moderation and the inclusion of different types of foods in correct proportions in the daily diet. It does not have a set menu. In 2005 however, the food pyramid was updated and the two-dimensional food pyramid became three-dimensional. To show the added benefits of regular exercise, a figure running up a flight of stairs on the side of the food pyramid was added.

The earlier food pyramid had horizontal lines spanning the food pyramid with the food that we eat the most at the bottom and the food that we should eat the least at the top (see Fig. 22.2).

Like the basic food groups, the food pyramid tells us what foods are included in the group, nutrients provided, the number of servings to be consumed per day and the size of each serving. The aim of using the pyramid is the same as the basic food groups.

Bread, Grain, Cereal, and Pasta Form the Base

At the base of the food pyramid is the group that contains breads, grains, cereals and pastas. These foods provide complex carbohydrates, which are an important source of energy. 6 to 11 servings of these foods in a day. One serving of this group can be

- 1 slice of bread
- 1/2 cup of rice, cooked cereal or pasta
- 1 cup of ready-to-eat cereal
- 1 flat tortilla

Fruits and Vegetables

Fruits and vegetables are rich in nutrients. Many are excellent sources of vitamin A, vitamin C, folate or potassium. They are low in fat and sodium and high in fiber. The food pyramid suggests 3 to 5 servings of vegetables each day. One serving of vegetables can be

- 1 cup of raw leafy vegetables
- 1/2 cup of other vegetables, cooked or raw
- 3/4 cup of vegetable juice

The food pyramid suggests 2 to 4 servings of fruits each day. One serving of fruit can be

- One medium apple, orange or banana
- 1/2 cup of chopped, cooked or canned fruit
- 3/4 cup of fruit juice

Count only 100 per cent fruit juice as a fruit, and limit juice consumption.

Beans, Eggs, Lean Meat, and Fish

Meat, poultry and fish supply protein, iron and zinc. Non-meat foods such as dried peas and beans also provide many of these nutrients. The food pyramid suggests 2 to 3 servings of cooked meat, fish or poultry. Each serving should be between 2 and 3 ounces. The following foods count as one ounce of meat:

- One egg
- 2 tablespoons of peanut butter
- 1/2 cup cooked dry beans
- 1/3 cup of nuts

Dairy Products

Products made with milk provide protein and vitamins and minerals, especially calcium. The Food Pyramid suggests 2 to 3 servings each day. If you are breastfeeding, pregnant, a teenager or a young adult age 24 or under, try to have 3 servings. Most other people should have 2 servings daily.

- 1 cup of milk or yogurt
- $1^1/_2$ ounce of natural cheese
- 1 ounce of process cheese (remember that processed cheese usually contains a lot of sodium)

Fats and Sweets

A food pyramid's tip is the smallest part, so the fats and sweets in the top of the food pyramid should comprise the smallest percentage of your daily diet. The foods at the top of the food pyramid should be eaten sparingly because they provide calories but not much in the way of nutrition. These foods include salad dressings, oils, cream, butter, margarine, sugars, soft drinks, candies and sweet desserts.

The food guide pyramid can be extremely useful—whether you want to gain weight, lose weight or maintain your weight. Eating a healthy diet simpler easier if you base your choices on the food pyramid.

THE NEW FOOD PYRAMID

The new food pyramid however, is completely different. Apart from the fact that it has become three dimensional and has a figure climbing up the side of it, the horizontal lines have been replaced by vertical lines starting from the tip of the pyramid and radiating downward (see Fig. 22.3).

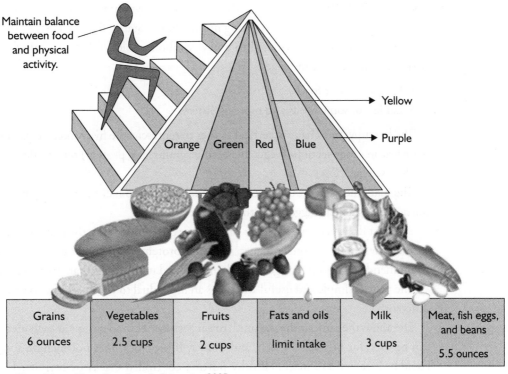

Maintain balance between food and physical activity.

Yellow

Purple

Orange Green Red Blue

Grains	Vegetables	Fruits	Fats and oils	Milk	Meat, fish eggs, and beans
6 ounces	2.5 cups	2 cups	limit intake	3 cups	5.5 ounces

Note: Adapted from Encyclopedia Britannica, 2005.

Fig. 22.3 The new food pyramid

The size of the section remains unchanged. Only in the new food pyramid, you now know that although you need to eat some food types more than others, even within those food groups there are some foods that you should only eat in moderation.

The new food pyramid is colour coded. The six coloured stripes denote the quantities of food you should consume. An orange stripe represents grains; a green stripe for

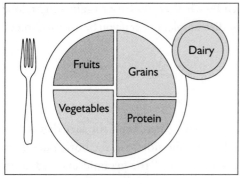

Source: www.choosemyplate.gov

Fig. 22. The food plate is now the new symbol for healthy eating

vegetables; a red stripe for fruits; a yellow stripe denotes how much fats and oils you should have; a blue stripe for the milk and dairy products that you are allowed; and a purple stripe shows the quantities of meat, fish, beans, and pulses that you should eat in a day. Like the basic food groups, foods are divided on the basis of their nutritive value in the pyramid. Today ,the food pyramid is being replaced by a plate which health care professionals feel will be easier to follow and have a more positive impact on the nutritional status of the population.

The food guide pyramid was the model for healthy eating in the United States. But the USDA, the agency in charge of nutrition, has switched to a new symbol, a colourful plate—called My Plate—with some of the same messages:

- Eat a variety of foods.
- Eat less of some foods and more of others.

The latest pyramid had six vertical stripes to represent the five food groups plus oils. The plate features four sections (vegetables, fruits, grains, and protein) plus a side order of dairy in blue (see Fig. 22.4).

The main message is that fruits and vegetables take up half the plate, with the vegetable portion being a little bigger than the fruit section.

And just like the pyramid where stripes were different widths, the plate has been divided so that the grain section is bigger than the protein section. Because nutrition experts recommend you eat more vegetables than fruit and more grains than protein foods.

The plate is simple and useful and helps an individual to view his or her own plate a little differently.

The aim is the same as the pyramid, to eat a variety of food groups at each meal .The plate can be used for breakfast, lunch, and dinner. If breakfast does not include a vegetable, it could be included as a snack. Healthy, portion-controlled snacks are permitted

The plate also shows how to balance your food groups. The protein section is smaller: You don't need as much from that group. Eating more fruits and vegetables will help one eat fewer calories overall, which helps you keep a healthy weight. Eating fruits and vegetables also gives lots of vitamins and minerals.

The divided plate also aims to discourage extra-large portions, which result in overeating and can cause weight gain. Nutrition experts are recommending different plates for healthy eating habits. Figure 22.5 shows us a food plate to maintain a healthy lifestyle.

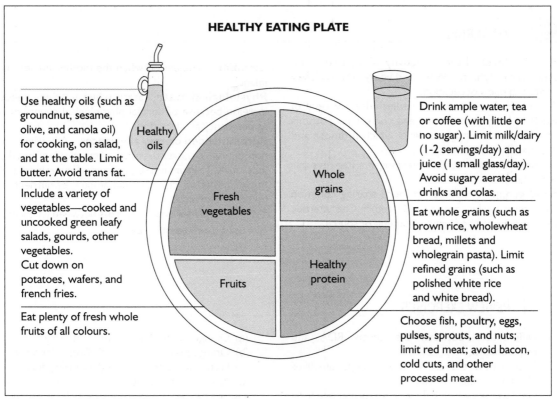

Source: www.health.havard.edu/plate/healthy-eating-plate

Fig. 22.5 A healthy eating plate

Both the food guide pyramid and the food plate are nutrition education tools that show dietary guidelines in an easy to understand graphic format.

 ## SUMMARY

Nutrients are needed in specific amounts to ensure good health and well-being. The nutrients needed by different age groups are mentioned in the RDA table. To enable us to consume these nutrients, food has been divided into five groups. These groups have been formulated on the basis of the nutrients present in them. If we select the number of servings recommended from each of the food groups, we can get a balanced meal.

A balanced diet has all nutrients in correct proportions and amounts to ensure good health and provide a margin of safety to take care of short periods of emergency. Food groups help us in getting a balanced diet. A choice must be made within each group since all foods in the group are not identical in nutrient content. The food pyramid and food plate have been designed to help us choose a healthy diet.

KEY TERMS

Activity level Level of activity of a person, i.e., sedentary or light, moderate, and heavy. This is closely related to one's occupation.

Balanced diet A diet which includes a variety of foods in adequate amounts and correct proportions to supply all essential nutrients which promote and preserve good health.

Demerara sugar Light brown sugar, a stage in sugar extraction.

Food group A number of foods sharing common characteristics which are grouped together. Characteristic for grouping may be function, nutrient, or source.

Lactation The period when the mother nurses her infant.

Physiological state State when nutrient needs increase because of normal physiological events such as pregnancy and lactation.

Recommended dietary allowances Allowances of nutrients which cover the needs of practically all healthy individuals. They are not requirements for any individual but guidelines which tell us the amount of nutrient to be consumed daily.

Triticale Cereal which is a cross between wheat and rye; used in breakfast cereals.

REVIEW EXERCISES

1. Differentiate between the terms RDA and requirement.
2. Explain how the use of food groups simplifies planning of balanced meals.
3. List 10 foods which belong to the protective food group, stating reasons for your choice.
4. In which food group would you include the following?

   (a) Orange marmalade
   (b) Orange juice
   (c) French dressing
   (d) Alcoholic beverages
   (e) Soft drinks
   (f) Coriander leaves
   (g) Nutrinuggets

5. List the five basic food groups giving four examples for each. State the main nutrients provided by each group.

CHAPTER 23

Menu Planning and Mass Food Production

LEARNING OBJECTIVES

After reading this chapter, you should be able to
- describe the concept and aim of meal planning
- understand the different factors which influence meal planning
- identify foods which must be included while planning nutritionally balanced meals for different age groups
- relate the RDA to nutritive value of meals served in catering establishments
- evaluate the nutritional adequacy of meals served to individuals
- understand the special requirements for nutrients at various stages in life and how these can be met

INTRODUCTION

In the past few decades, people ate in restaurants occassionally to celebrate a special event such as an anniversary, a birthday, or an achievement. It was an outing to look forward to, and if one indulged, it did not matter as these outings were rare.

Today, the scenario is different. Eating out has become a way of life. Education and employment has taken many of us away from home, and the mother's role now has an added responsibility of contributing to the family income. Modern day compulsions have made eating out a necessity. No longer does one find time for the traditional fare of yesteryears and depends on the caterer for the following:

1. Food for festivals and celebrations
2. Meals at the work place.
3. Ready-to-eat meals picked up on the way home from work
4. Snacks and sweetmeats for daily consumption

5. Preserves, pickles, papads, etc.
6. All meals served in institutions such as hospitals, school/college cafeteria, mess or dining hall, and boarding schools.

The number of reported cases of diabetes, hypertension, obesity, heart attacks, etc. is on the rise and so is the number of meals consumed away from home. This is not surprising because if one indulges practically everyday, it is bound to result in ill-health because of malnutrition. The caterer's role has become more significant as the responsibility now lies with the caterer for planning nutritionally adequate meals. Menu planning is the key to overcoming this problem.

Definition   Menu planning is defined as a simple process which involves application of the knowledge of food, nutrients, food habits, and likes and dislikes to plan wholesome and attractive meals.

The caterer who is responsible for providing meals has to decide on various aspects, such as

1. Menu
2. Serving size
3. Food cost
4. Suppliers and quantities to be purchased
5. Standardized recipes to be followed
6. Type of service
7. Meal timings
8. Clientele

The aim of menu planning are to

1. Meet the nutritional needs of the individuals who will be consuming the food
2. Plan meals within the food cost
3. Simplify purchase, preparation, and storage of meals
4. Provide attractive, appetizing meals with no monotony
5. Save time and money
6. Minimize overhead expenditure, i.e., fuel, electricity, water, labour.

Menu planning is the most important aspect of planning and organization in the food industry. It is an advance plan of a dietary pattern over a given period of time.

Menus are of the following types.

Table d'hôte or fixed price menu   It includes two or three courses at a set price. Each course may offer a choice of dishes.

A la carte   On this menu, dishes are individually priced and the customers can compile their own menu which may be one, two, or more courses.

Banquet menus   These are special menus for banquets or functions.

Institutional menus Hospital menus, boarding school menus, and industrial canteen menus.

Menus may be cyclic which means they are compiled to cover a specified period of time. The length of the cycle may vary and is decided upon by the management. A number of menus are set and repeated. They are often modified to take into account variations which may arise for a number of reasons.

FACTORS INFLUENCING MEAL PLANNING

Many factors influence the acceptability of a meal. Customers select what appeals most to them from a menu card based on individual likes and dislikes, budget, popularity of items, etc. However, while planning meals the following factors need to be considered.

Nutritional Adequacy

The most important consideration in menu planning is to ensure that the meal fulfils the nutrient needs of the individual consuming the meal. For example, if the meal is planned for an industrial worker, it must meet the recommended dietary allowances (RDAs) for that age group. Foods from all basic food groups should be included in each meal so that the meal is balanced and nutritionally adequate (see Plate 4). Nutrient needs may be modified for hospital diets (therapeutic diets).

Economic Considerations

The spending power of the clientele has to be kept in mind and meals have to be planned within the budget. Low cost nutritious substitutes should be included in the menu to keep the costs low. The food cost should be maintained, if the organization has to run profitably.

Type of Food Service

Menus should be planned in relation to the type of food service, whether it is cafeteria, seated service, buffet, etc.

Equipment and Work Space

The menu should be planned keeping the available equipment and work space in mind. Deep freezers, refrigerators, grinders, dough kneaders, deep fat fryers, boilers, etc. should be adequate.

Leftover Food

An effective manager should consider as to how leftovers could be rotated to obtain maximum profit. Adequate storage space and hygienic standards should be ensured to minimize the risk of contamination and spoilage of food.

Food Habits

Food habits of the customer is another important criteria which needs to be considered as food served has to be acceptable to the customer. Special attention should be paid when a particular type of community is catered to. Religious considerations should be known to the meal planner.

Availability

Some fruits and vegetables are seasonal. During the season the cost is reasonable and quality is better. Today, practically all fruits and vegetables are available throughout the year because of advanced preservation technology. However, seasonal fruits and vegetables should be given preference. Regional availability influences menu planning. For example, fish and sea food is fresh and cheaper in coastal areas.

Meal Frequency and Pattern

The meal timings and number of meals consumed in a day, whether meals are packed or served at the table, also influences the selection of food items on the menu. The age, activity level, physiological state, work schedule, and economic factors need to be known before planning meals for institutional catering.

Variety

This is one of the most important considerations while planning meals. A variety of foods from the different food groups should be included. The term variety means

1. Variety in food ingredients
2. Variety in recipe
3. Method of cooking
4. Colour, texture, and flavour
5. Variety in presentation and garnish.

A meal should look attractive and be appetizing. A judicious blend of flavours, attractive colour combinations, and different textures make food enjoyable and interesting. The method of cooking used for different items on the menu should vary. For example, two deep fried items would make the meal heavy. Simple processes such as fermentation and sprouting not only contribute to improved flavour and digestibility, but also enhance the nutritive value of the meal.

A well planned meal which is nutritionally adequate would have a good satiety value and prevent the occurence of hunger-pangs before it is time for the next meal. The nutritional adequacy of a meal in an a la carte service depends on the food choices made by the customer. It is the duty of the caterer to offer adequate, nutrient dense foods to the clients, to choose from.

PLANNING BALANCED MEALS

Meal planning involves proper selection of food to ensure balanced meals. In Chapter 22 on Balanced Diet we have studied how food is classified into five basic food groups to help us plan balanced diets. We have also read that food can be classified on the basis of its source, the nutrients present in it, or on the basis of its functions into 3–11 food groups. These food groups help us in planning balanced meals which supply all essential nutrients. In this chapter we will study the three basic food groups classified on the basis of functions performed by nutrients as this is the simplest way to ensure adequate nourishment to the body (see Fig. 23.1).

The three main functions performed by food are

1. Providing energy
2. Body building and maintenance
3. Regulation of body processes and protection against infection.

On the basis of functions performed, food is classified into the following three groups.

1. Protective/regulatory foods
2. Body-building foods
3. Energy-giving foods

Protective/Regulatory Foods

All fruits and vegetables including green leafy and other vegetables and all fruits, are protective/regulatory foods.

Green leafy vegetables; orange, yellow, and red fruits and vegetables; citrus fruits — Rich in carotene and ascorbic acid; also contain minerals, fibre, and carbohydrates

Body-building Foods

Foods rich in protein are included in this group. Nuts and oilseeds also provide fats.

1. All animal proteins — Protein vitamin, and mineral rich
2. Pulses, nuts, and oilseeds — Protein, vitamin, mineral, fibre, oils

Energy-giving Foods

This group provides mainly carbohydrates and fats, along with proteins, some vitamins and minerals, and essential fatty acids. Foods included in this group are:

1. Cereals and millets and roots and tubers — Carbohydrate rich with other nutrients
2. Sugars and jaggery — Only carbohydrates
3. Fats and oils — Mainly fats and oils

While planning meals one should ensure that foods from all three groups is included in each meal. This classification is simple and easy to use for menu planning.

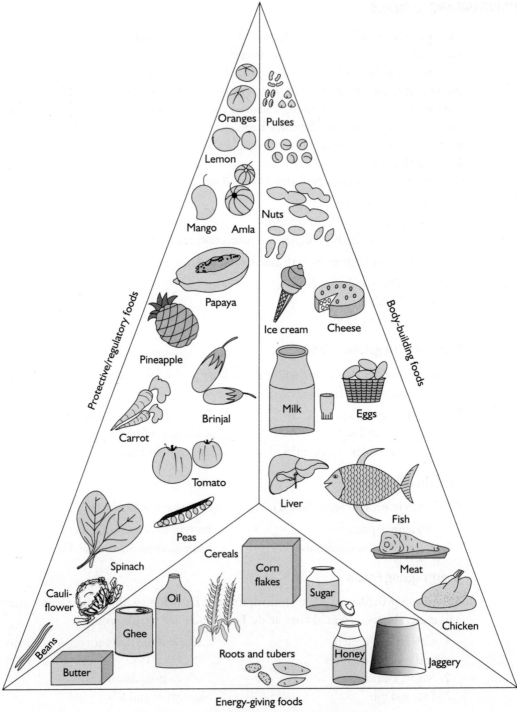

Fig. 23.1 The three food groups classification

STEPS IN PLANNING BALANCED MEALS

1. Collect information regarding the customer with respect to
   - Age
   - Gender
   - Activity level
   - Religion
   - Socio-economic background
   - Food habits
2. Check the RDAs for energy and proteins
3. Prepare a food plan, i.e., list number of servings from each food group to meet the RDA (see Table 23.1).
4. Decide on number of meals
5. Distribute servings for each meal
6. Select foods within each group and state their amount
7. Plan a menu
8. Cross-check to ensure that all food groups are included in requisite amounts.

Using the above steps, plan a balanced diet for a day.

TABLE 23.1   Serving size and nutritive value for food groups

Food group	Food	Size of serving (g)	Calories	Protein (g)
Energy-giving foods	• Cereals	20	70	2
	• Roots and tubers	60	70	2
	• Sugar	5	20	
	• Fat	5	45	
Body-building foods	• Milk	250 ml	170	8
	• Pulses	30	100	7
	• Meat/fish/ poultry	40	} 70	7
	• Egg	50		
Protective/ regulatory foods	• Green leafy vegetables	100	Negligible	Negligible
	• Other vegetables	100–150	40	2
	• Fruits	80–100	40	Negligible

Note: Two servings of green leafy vegetables = one serving of other vegetables.

Sample Balanced Diet

Planning balanced meals for college students residing in a hostel will have the following steps.
1. Basic information

Age	:	16–18 years
Gender	:	Male
Activity	:	Moderate
Religion	:	Hindu
Background	:	Urban, middle-income families
Food habits	:	Cosmopolitan

2. Recommended dietary allowances for

Calories	:	2,640
Protein	:	78 g

3. Food plan

Food group	No. of servings	Weight (g)	Calories (kcal)	Protein (g)
Energy-giving				
Cereals	16	320	1,120	32
Roots and tubers	3	180	210	06
Sugar	8	40	160	–
Fat	7	35	315	–
Body-building				
Milk	2	500	340	16
Pulses	2	60	200	14
Egg	1	50	70	7
Protective regulatory				
Green leafy veg.	1	100	–	–
Other veg.	3	300	120	3
Fruits	2	200	80	–
Total			2,640	81

4. Number of meals   :   04
5. Distribution of servings/meal

Food group	Food exchange	Number of servings	Serving per meal			
			Breakfast	Lunch	Tea	Dinner
Energ- giving foods	Cereals	16	4	5	2	5
	Roots and tubers	3	–	1	1	1
	Sugar	7	2	2	1½	1½
	Fat	8	2	2	2	2
Body-building foods	Milk	2	1	1/2	–	1/2
	Pulses	2	–	1	–	1
	Egg	1	1	–	–	–
Protective/regulatory foods	Green leafy veg.	1	–	1	–	–
	Other veg.	3	–	1	1	1
	Fruits	2	1	–	–	1

6. Select foods and plan the menu
7. Menu for the day

Menu for the day		
Bed tea	• 1 cup with milk	1 tsp sugar and 50 ml milk (from the day's allowance)
Breakfast	• Cornflakes	1 serving cereal
	• Milk	150 ml
	• Sugar	1 serving energy food
	• 3 slices of toast with butter	3 servings cereal 2 servings fat
	• 1 boiled egg	1 serving body building
	• 1 orange	1 serving protective
Lunch	• Palak aloo	1 serving green leafy vegetable
		1 serving roots and tubers
		1 serving fat for cooking
	• Dal	1 serving pulse
	• Rice	2 servings cereal
	• 3 *phulkas* and carrot *halwa*	3 servings cereals
		1 serving other vegetables
		1 serving fat
		2½ servings sugar
		1/2 serving milk
Tea	• Tea	1 serving sugar
		50 ml milk (from day's allowance)
	• 2 samosas	2 servings cereal
		1 serving roots and tubers
		1 serving other vegetable
		2 servings fat
	• Tamarind chutney	1/2 serving sugar
Dinner	• *Rajma*	1 serving pulses
		1/2 serving other vegetables
		1 serving fat
	• Colocasia (*dry arbi*)	1 serving roots and tubers
		1 serving fat
	• Green salad	1/2 serving other vegetables
	• 2 chappatis	3 servings cereals
	• Rice	2 servings cereals
	• Banana custard	1 serving fruit
		1/2 serving milk
		1½ servings sugar

8. Cross-check to ensure inclusion of all food groups in required amounts.

352 Food Science and Nutrition

CALCULATING THE NUTRITIVE VALUE OF A RECIPE

Using the food composition table, follow the steps given here to calculate nutritive value of a recipe. Refer Table 23.2 for food values.

1. List the ingredients used and their quantities in the recipe.
2. Prepare a table with the following blank columns, and fill up the ingredient and quantity column from the recipe.

S. no.	Ingredients	Quantity (g)	Protein (g)	Fat (g)	Carbohydrates (g)	Energy (kcal)
1						
2						
3						
4						
5						
6						
	Total value:					
	Value for 1 portion					

3. Refer to the food composition tables for the nutrients present in 100 g of edible portion of each ingredient.
4. Calculate the nutrients present for the quantities used in the recipe.
5. Weigh the finished product to know the total yeild.
6. Divide these values by the number of portions to know the nutritive value per portion.
7. For general calculations, do not include salt, spices, baking powder, stock, or ingredients which are used in very small quantities (less than 10 g) except for sugar and fat. Baking powder and salt are calculated for their sodium content, and not for their proximate principles, for sodium-restricted diets only.

Nutritive Value of Shrewsbury Biscuits

The nutritive value of one shrewsbury biscuit is described below (see Table 23.3).

Total yield from the recipe = 308 g

Number of biscuits = 14

Weight of one biscuit = 22 g

Nutritive value of one shrewsbury biscuit = Values for one recipe ÷ Number of biscuits

$$\text{Protein} = \frac{17}{14} = 1.2 \text{ g}$$

$$\text{Fats} = \frac{111}{14} = 8 \text{ g}$$

Recipe of shrewsbury biscuits

Ingredients	Quantity
Refined flour	150 g
Margarine	60 g
Amul butter	60 g
Castor sugar	75 g
Baking powder	1 g
Milk	15 ml

$$\text{Carbohydrate} = \frac{187}{14} = 13 \text{ g}$$

$$\text{Energy (kcal)} = \frac{1.817}{14} = 130 \text{ kcal}$$

Therefore, one shrewsbury biscuit (weight 22 g) provides

- 1.2 g protein
- 8 g fat
- 13 g carbohydrate
- 130 kcal energy

TABLE 23.2 Sample food composition table

Name of foodstuff	Protein (g)	Fat (g)	Fibre (g)	Carbohydrate (g)	Energy (kcal)	Calcium mg	Iron mg	Carotene µg	Vit. C mg
Cereals, grains, and products									
• Refined flour	11	0.9	0.3	74	348	23	2.7	25	0
• Whole wheat flour	12	1.7	1.9	69	341	48	4.9	29	0
• Rice	7	0.5	0.2	78	345	10	0.7	0	0
Pulses and legumes									
• Bengal gram whole	17	5	4	61	360	202	4.6	189	3
• Lentils	25	0.7	0.7	59	343	69	7.6	270	0
• Red gram dal	22	2	1.5	58	335	73	2.7	132	0
Green leafy vegetables									
• Spinach	2	0.7	0.6	3	26	73	1.1	5,580	28
• Fenugreek	4.4	1	1.1	6	49	395	2.0	2,340	52
Roots and tubers									
• Carrot	0.9	0.2	1.2	11	48	80	1	1,890	3
• Onion	1.2	0.1	0.6	11	50	47	0.6	0	11
• Potato	1.6	0.1	0.4	23	97	10	0.5	24	17
Other vegetables									
• Lady's fingers	2	0.2	1.2	6	35	66	0.4	52	1
• Cucumber	0.4	0.1	0.4	3	13	10	0.6	0	7
Nuts and oilseeds									
• Groundnuts	25	40	3.1	26	567	90	2.5	37	0
• Coconut (fresh)	4.5	42	3.6	13	444	10	1.7	0	1

Contd

Table 23.2 Contd

Name of foodstuff	Protein (g)	Fat (g)	Fibre (g)	Carbohydrate (g)	Energy (kcal)	Calcium mg	Iron mg	Carotene µg	Vit. C mg
Condiments and spices									
• Chillies (red)	16	6	30	32	246	160	2.3	345	50
• Coriander	14	16	33	22	288	630	7	942	0
• Cumin seeds	19	15	12	37	356	1,080	11.7	522	3
• Turmeric	6	5	3	70	349	150	67.8	30	0
Fruits									
• Banana	1	0.3	0.4	27	116	17	0.4	78	7
• Papaya	0.6	0.1	0.8	7	32	17	0.5	666	57
• Apple	0.2	0.5	1	13	59	10	0.7	0	1
• Orange	0.7	0.2	0.3	11	48	26	0.3	1,104	30
• *Amla*	0.5	0.1	3.4	14	58	50	1.2	9	600
Fish									
• Mackerel	19	1.7	–	0.5	93	429	4.5	–	
• Pomfret	17	1.3	–	1.8	87	200	0.9	–	–
• *Surmai*	20	1.4	–	–	92	92	2.0	–	
Meat and poultry									
• Egg	13.3	13.3	–	–	173	60	2.1	420*	0
• Mutton	18.5	13.3	–	–	194	150	2.5	9*	–
• Liver (sheep)	19	7.5	–	1.3	150	10	6.3	6690*	20
Milk and milk products									
• Milk (buffalo)	4.3	6.5	–	5	117	210	0.2	48*	1
• Milk (cow)	3.2	4.1	–	4.4	67	120	0.2	53*	2
• *Paneer*	18.3	20.8	–	1.2	265	208	–	110*	3
• Cream light	2.7	18	–	4	187	–	–	–	–
• Milk powder	26	27	–	38	496	950	0.6	420*	4
Fats and oils									
• Butter	–	81	–	–	729	–	–	960*	–
• Cooking oil	–	100	–	–	900	–	–	0	0
• Ghee (cow)	–	100	–	–	900	–	–	600*	0
Sugars									
• Sugar	–	–	–	99.4	398	12	0.1	–	–
• Honey	0.3	–	–	79.5	319	5	0.7	–	–
• Jaggery	0.4	0.1	–	95	383	80	2.6	–	–
• Jam	–	–		70	275	–	–		

Note: Values are for 100 g edible portion.

*These values represent vitamin A in µg.

TABLE 23.3   Nutritive value of shrewsbury biscuits

Ingredients	Quantity (g)	Protein (g)	Fat (g)	Carbohydrate (g)	Energy (kcal)
Refined flour	150	16.5	1.4	111	522
Margarine	60	—	60.00	—	540
Amul butter	60	—	48.60	—	437
Castor sugar	75	—	—	75	300
Baking powder	1	—	—	—	—
Milk	15 ml	0.6	1.00	1	18
Total		17	111	187	1,817

SPECIAL NUTRITIONAL REQUIREMENTS

Pregnancy

Every infant should have the right to begin life with a full-term healthy body and receive the advantage of mother's milk. For this to happen, every would-be mother should take special care of her nutritional needs. Pregnancy is a period of remarkable anabolic activity. A 3.2 kg infant develops in nine months of pregnancy from the nourishment received from the mother. If the diet is deficient during these months, the foetus draws upon the maternal reserves. A poor diet will ultimately affect both the infant and the mother, and may lead to complications of pregnancy such as premature birth and low birth weight.

Weight gain   A healthy woman is expected to gain 16–24 lbs in the three trimesters of pregnancy of which the full-term infant weighs 7 lbs. The remaining weight is due to increase in tissues, an expanding blood volume, and energy stored in the form of fat as a calorie reserve.

Energy   The energy needs increase during the second and third trimesters of pregnancy. An additional 300 kcal take care of the increased demands of pregnancy. Calorific value of food is adjusted according to the weight gained.

Protein   The protein requirement increases by 15 g for the synthesis of foetal and maternal tissues.

Minerals   The calcium requirement is 1,000 mg and iron is 38 mg for the formation of foetal bones and teeth, and formation of blood, respectively. The absorption of minerals improves because of the increased requirement. Iodine in the form of iodized salt, helps in protecting the mother and child against goitre and cretinism.

Vitamins With an increase in calories, the need for vitamins B_1, B_2, and niacin increases as they are needed for release of energy from carbohydrates, fats, and proteins. The need for folic acid and vitamin D also increases.

Nutrient dense foods should be selected to meet the extra demand for proteins, calcium, iron, vitamin D, and B-complex vitamins.

Lactation

Mother's milk is the most nutritious food designed for an infant. The nutritional needs during lactation are greater than the needs during pregnancy as the mother's body has to supply all nourishment to the rapidly growing infant. The conversion of dietary protein to milk protein is only 50 per cent which means 2 g of good quality protein is converted to 1 g of milk protein.

Energy Calorie requirements increase by 550 kcal during the first six months of lactation, followed by a marginal decrease during the next six months with 400 kcal being adequate to meet the additional demands.

Proteins An additional intake of 25 g in the first six months and 18 g in the next six months is adequate.

Minerals Calcium requirement is 1,000 mg which is necessary for synthesis of milk. Additional iron is not prescribed as milk is a poor source of iron.

Vitamins The requirement for vitamins A, D, B-complex, and vitamin C increases being

- Vitamin A – 950 µg
- Vitamin C – 80 mg
- Folic acid – 150 µg
- Vitamin B_{12} – 1.5 µg

Fluid The intake of fluid increases during lactation.

The diet should be nutritious, easy to digest with restrictions on strongly flavoured vegetables and spicy food.

Infancy

Human milk is the natural food for the infant. It is safe and convenient as it does not involve sterilizing bottles and preparing formulas throughout the day. At the same time, it is easy to assimilate, has the correct temperature, and gives a safe and secure feeling to the infant, and sense of satisfaction to the mother.

During the first few days after delivery, colostrum is secreted which is not mature milk but a substance richer in protein and vitamin A. Colostrum is secreted in small quantities but is valuable as it increases the resistance to certain infections during the first few months of life.

The intervals of feeding should be fairly flexible instead of following a rigid schedule or a self-demand schedule. For premature and low birth weight (weight less than 2.5 kg) babies a fixed schedule is preferable.

Milk is deficient in iron, vitamin C, and vitamin D. The baby is born with stores of these nutrients which suffice for 3 months. From the third month onwards, supplements should be gradually added to provide those nutrients which are not supplied by milk.

From the fifth to ninth month onwards, the infant should be weaned by substituting a cup feeding for a breastfeeding. This change should be gradual and at intervals till the infant is weaned from the breast to the cup before the age of one year.

Nutritional requirements   Human milk is the best food for infants. The next best substitute is cow's milk or modified buffalo milk. Buffalo milk is modified as it contains a larger percentage of protein, fat, calcium, and energy as compared to human milk and a lesser percentage of sugar. It is modified by partially skimming it, diluting it with water, and adding little sugar so that its composition resembles human milk.

Supplementary foods during the first year   The age at which supplementary foods should be included depends on a number of factors such as literacy of mother, economic factors, and time available. Supplements if not prepared, stored, and fed to the infant in hygienic conditions is one of the main causes for diarrhoea and gastro-intestinal upsets. While introducing a new food the following points should be borne in mind:

1. Introduce one food at a time till the infant's system is used to the new food. Season with salt
2. Give a teaspoonful in the beginning
3. Never force-feed an infant
4. Start with a thin smooth consistency initially
5. Once the infant is used to supplements, introduce variety
6. Follow hygienic practices and do not give any leftover food or drink to an infant.

Choice of food supplements for infants

1. Egg yolk
2. Strained cereals
3. Strained soup
4. Soft *khichdi*
5. Rice and dal
6. Pureed vegetables
7. Ready-to-eat cereals
8. Stewed fruit
9. Fruit juice

Childhood

During these stages rapid growth takes place. There is an increase in height and weight because of increase in the bone and muscle mass. Children use up a lot of energy in playing. They normally carry their lunch, which should be nutritious and interesting, or monotonous, in which case the packed lunch box comes back home unfinished or unopened. Special efforts should be made so that they do not meet their energy needs from junk food.

Energy   More energy per kg body weight is required for
1. Rapid growth which takes place in this age group
2. Enhanced physical activity
3. High basal metabolic rate (BMR) as compared to an adult.

Proteins   Good quality proteins should be included to take care of body building and maintenance of tissues. Milk proteins are complete proteins and provide calcium as well.

Carbohydrates and fats   They provide calories, and spare proteins from being oxidized for energy. Refined carbohydrates and poor dental hygiene are the reasons for dental caries in children. The consumption of fruits and vegetables, both cooked and uncooked, should be encouraged. Junk food and aerated beverages should be discouraged.

Vitamins and minerals   If the diet is well planned keeping the principles of menu planning in mind, supplements may not be necessary.

Fluid   Adequate fluid is necessary, specially in active children who play outdoor games and sweat a lot. Fluids should not kill the appetite, which is seen when children are thirsty and drink a lot of liquid just before a meal.

Points to be considered
1. Regular meal timings
2. No nibbling of low nutrient dense snacks between meals
3. Do not force-feed, let the normal appetite return
4. Meal timing should be pleasant
5. Food should be appetizing and attractively served. Finger foods should be preferred for children
6. Packed meals should not be messy to eat
7. Attractive colours and shapes appeal to children, and with a little imagination eating green vegetables and drinking milk could become more interesting.

Adolescence

Adolescence is a period of physiological stress for the body because of extremely rapid rate of growth. The appearance of sex characteristic is also accompanied by mental and emotional changes. The diet plays a crucial role in promoting growth, hence the RDAs for all nutrients are high during 13–18 years of age. Nutrients of particular importance are carbohydrates and fats for energy and proteins, iron and calcium for body building.

During adolescence the BMR accelerates once again because of the growth spurt and other hormonal changes which take place. The BMR of boys is higher than that of girls because of more muscle tissue.

Food habits change drastically because of peer pressure, maintaining one's figure and weight, skin problems, and the newly found independence.

Energy   Energy needs are high because of higher physical activity and BMR. Sports and aerobic exercises increase the energy requirements for sports people.

Proteins   A generous intake of high quality proteins is necessary for increase in muscles mass and skeletal development. A deficiency of calories and proteins can affect one's optimum height increase and resistance to infections.

Girls grow rapidly between 11–14 years and boys grow rapidly between 13–16 years. Initially, girls are taller than boys between 11–12 years. But later the growth rate is more in boys. Weight gain is a common problem in this age group which is tackled differently by both the sexes. Boys prefer exercise as a means of losing weight and body building while girls prefer going on a diet.

A deficiency of calcium/vitamin D during infancy or childhood results in rickets (deforming of bones). The weak bones cannot withstand the weight of the body and bend causing bow legs or knock knees (see Fig. 23.2). Once malformed, bones cannot be straightened. The effect of rickets is seen in adolescents and adults. Along with weight, emotional stress has an adverse effect on health and diet. Friction between parents and adolescents is another area of tension.

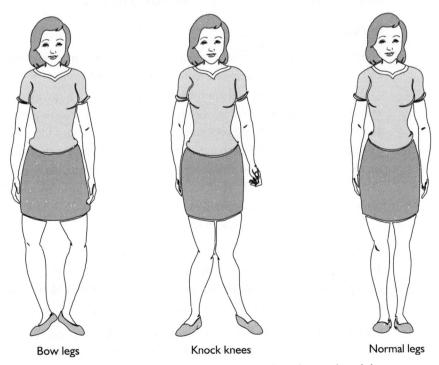

Bow legs   Knock knees   Normal legs

Fig. 23.2   Vitamin D deficiency can cause bow legs or knock knees

Snacks are the all-time favourite food, which often forms a large percentage of energy intake, favourite snacks being burgers, pizzas, pastries, ice creams, french fries, *pav wada*, *pav bhaji*, popcorn, and south Indian snacks. Milk is substituted by tea/coffee (which is more of a social need) or aerated beverages. This trend indicates a high consumption of refined flour, hydrogenated fats, and potato. South Indian snacks are a better option as they are made from a cereal–pulse combination.

In general, the diet is deficient in the protein food group and protective food group. Food such as milk, green leafy vegetables, yellow fruits and vegetables, citrus fruits, and whole grain cereals are deficient in the diet of adolescents. Deficiencies during infancy and childhood may leave their scar in adolescence.

Anorexia nervosa This is a disorder seen in adolescent girls concerning figure and weight control. The onset of puberty results in widening of the pelvis and deposition of subcutaneous fat creating a psychological problem in figure conscious young girls. They resort to crash diets for weight loss. This self-induced starvation to attain a slim figure leads to weight loss, loss of muscle tissue, a low BMR, and serious health problems.

Bulimia It is another disorder in which the appetite increases drastically followed by induced vomiting to throw out whatever has been consumed. Bulimia creates both emotional and physical problems and is also known as the gorging–purging syndrome. Both disorders are mainly seen in adolescent girls from affluent families.

Old Age

Nutrition in old age or geriatric nutrition is gaining importance as longevity has increased and 65 plus is the fastest growing segment of our population.

Aging is an individual phenomenon depending to a large extent on the health and nutrition status of an individual throughout his life span. People grow old at different rates and in different ways. Aging continues from birth throughout life.

Apart from the biological changes which occur with age, psychological and social changes are also seen. The body functions slow down, there is increasing social stress, and isolation. The elderly are often lonely, restless, and unhappy. They feel they are a burden and cannot contribute physically or monetarily to the family.

The following changes are seen in old age.

Body composition As age advance, adults lose muscle mass and gain fat. Since active muscle is lost, BMR reduces with age. Bone loss occurs leading to a reduction in height. Collagen content increases giving rise to loss of elasticity in blood vessels, joints, and skin, seen as easy bruises, painful joints, and a wrinkled skin.

Sensory changes The five senses of sight, hearing, taste, smell, and touch become dim with age. Old people cannot see without bright light, hearing is impaired affecting their social behaviour, and the other senses are less acute.

Digestive functions   Loss of teeth and ill-fitting dentures make it necessary to serve soft well-cooked food. Decreased secretion of saliva makes food difficult to swallow. Heartburn, diarrhoea, or constipation are other complaints.

Metabolic changes   Changes in metabolism, specially glucose tolerance and anaemias, are sometimes seen.

Osteopenia and osteoporosis are seen resulting in excessive bone loss, and fractures due to normal stress is another common finding. Because of age-related disabilities, the elderly should not live alone as they require assistance for all activities and company to overcome psychosocial changes in their life.

Nutritional requirements   The main features of the diet are as follows:

1. A low-calorie diet of 1,000–1,500 kcal is required, as there is a reduction in the BMR.
2. Good-quality protein, calcium, and iron; vitamin A, vitamin C, and folic acid should be consumed to prevent anaemia.
3. Food should be easy to chew, liquid preparations should be included in each meal as they are light and easy to digest.
4. Hot meals should be served attractively as appetite is low.
5. Five small meals should be preferred to a three meal pattern.
6. Gas forming foods and strongly flavoured vegetables such as bengal gram, cauliflower, cabbage, and onion should be avoided.
7. Fibre-rich foods, such as whole grains, green leafy vegetables, pulses, and fruits, are nutritious and provide fibre necessary for normal elimination. They should be incorporated into the diet gradually to prevent gastric irritation and gas.
8. Ample fluids are necessary to flush out toxic wastes. The kidneys function at a slower pace with age, but fluids help in excretion of toxins.
9. Low-calorie density and high-satiety value foods should be included.

EFFECT OF QUANTITY COOKING AND PROCESSING ON NUTRIENTS

Almost all foods consumed today need some form of cooking and processing before it is fit for service and consumption. Fruits and vegetables used in salads or for chutney are consumed uncooked. The nutrients we receive from the meals we consume depend to a large extent on cooking and processing practices which are being used. While some amount of nutrient loss is inevitable, cooking has many benefits which are listed below.

Benefits of Cooking Food

1. Cooking increases palatability.

2. Cooking makes food easier to digest by destroying anti-digestive factors such as trypsin inhibitor in soya beans.
3. Pathogenic microorganisms are destroyed.
4. Shelf life is increased by destruction of spoilage organisms and denaturation of enzymes.
5. The appearance of food improves, e.g., cooked meat versus raw meat.

Common Food Processing Techniques

1. Removal of unwanted outer layers, e.g., potato peels, inedible shells and scales of fish, and pea pods, and removal of inedible seeds, stone, etc.
2. Cutting, slicing, mincing, grinding, or reducing the size of vegetables, fruit, meat, etc.
3. Liquefaction and emulsification, milling, and blending
4. Heat treatment: Blanching, cooking by various methods such as boiling, frying, and roasting
5. Incorporation of air: Beating, whipping, aeration of soft drinks
6. Extrusion
7. Dehydration, freeze drying, deep freezing, etc.
8. Fermentation

Food prepared in large quantity in institutional kitchens or in food processing plants is more prone to loss of nutrients, if adequate care is not taken to retain or preserve the nutrient. This is because if food is cooked in bulk, the pre-preparation begins hours in advance, for example, vegetables have to be cut in advance and if these are not blanched and refrigerated to inactivate enzymes, oxidative losses of labile vitamins will continue at room temperature. Apart from nutritive value, the crisp texture of salads is also lost and phenol containing vegetables will discolour and turn brown, making the dish unattractive and unappetizing.

Effect of heat on nutrients   Cooking has beneficial effects on carbohydrates because of gelatinization of starch, favourable browning reactions such as Maillard reaction and caramelization of sugar which gives colour and flavour to food.

Proteins too take part in Maillard reaction along with sugar. Enzymes which catalyse undesirable enzymatic reactions in fruits such as apple and pears, and vegetables such as potato and brinjal are inactivated on blanching or cooking these foods. Enzymes which hasten oxidative destruction of vitamin C or ascorbic acid are denatured by blanching. Proteins get denatured by heat.

The chemical reactions that take place when oil is heated continuously during deep fat frying bring about hydrolysis, oxidation, and polymerization of the oil.

The moisture from the foods being fried hydrolyse fat into free fatty acids, mono- and diglycerides and glycerol.

$$\begin{array}{l} \mathrm{CH_2 \cdot O \cdot CO \cdot R_1} \\ | \\ \mathrm{CH \cdot O \cdot CO \cdot R_2 + H_2O} \\ | \\ \mathrm{CH_2 \cdot O \cdot CO \cdot R_3} \end{array} \longrightarrow \begin{array}{l} \mathrm{CH_2 \cdot O \cdot CO \cdot R_1} \\ | \\ \mathrm{CH \cdot O \cdot CO \cdot R_2 + HOOC \cdot R_3} \\ | \\ \mathrm{CH_2 \cdot OH} \end{array}$$

Triglyceride   Diglyceride   Fatty acid

The release of moisture, high frying temperatures of 160°–190°C, presence of carbonized crumbs in the oil, and oxygen from the atmosphere during frying brings about oxidation of the oil. Repeated use of the frying medium forms thermal and oxidative products which can cause gastro-intestinal irritation and destruction of vitamins. These products undergo polymerization and increase the viscosity of the oil. The oil darkens in colour, has a lower smoke point, and foams when used for frying. Such oil should be discarded. Fat-soluble vitamins dissolve in fat used for deep frying specially if food to be fried is not well coated.

Effect of alkali   Alkali is used during cooking and processing to soften vegetables, make pectin soluble, and dissolve hemicellulose. It is also used as lye (sodium hydroxide) to peel vegetables during processing. A pinch of sodium bicarbonate added to green vegetables helps in brightening the green colour. However, B-complex vitamins and ascorbic acid are destroyed in an alkaline medium. The use of alkali to hasten the cooking process for vegetables and pulses should be discouraged. Excessive cooking in an alkaline medium not only destroys vitamins, but makes the texture mushy and gives a soapy taste to the product.

Effect of acid   An acidic medium while cooking helps preserve water-soluble vitamins and retards enzymatic browning of certain fruits and vegetables. Vegetables and pulses take a longer time to cook in an acidic medium as acids precipitate pectin and hardens vegetables.

Effect of washing and soaking   While preparing food, water-soluble vitamins and minerals leach out into the cooking or washing water. These losses can be minimized by washing the uncut fruit or vegetables and not soaking the cut vegetable in water.

Soaking grains or pulses is beneficial as soaking increases digestibility and reduces cooking time. Figure 23.3 shows us simple measures which enhance nutrients.

Effect of sprouting and fermentation   Soaking whole grains overnight in water and tying them in a muslin cloth to allow them to germinate has many beneficial effects.

1. In sprouted grains, the dormant seed becomes active and synthesizes vitamin C.
2. Partial breakdown of carbohydrates, proteins, and fats begin, making it easier to digest.
3. The bioavailability of nutrients especially calcium and iron increases.

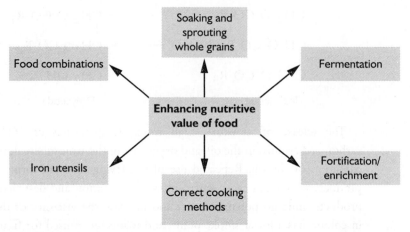

Fig. 23.3   Simple measures to enhance nutritive value of food

4. The active seeds synthesize vitamin C or ascorbic acid and thiamine, riboflavin, and niacin content increases. Table 23.4 shows processes which increase nutrient content of foodstuff.

TABLE 23.4   Enhancing nutritive value of food

Process	Foodstuff	Nutrient
Fortification/enrichment	Salt	Iodine
	Bread	Lysine (amino acid)
	Hydrogenated fat	Vitamin A and vitamin D
	Flour	Vitamin B$_1$, niacin, Fe, and Ca
	Fruit juice	Vitamin C
Sprouting	Wholegrain cereals and pulses	Vitamin C
		B-complex vitamin
		Bioavailability of iron increases
Fermentation	Cereal and pulse batters	Thiamine, riboflavin, and
	Bread dough	niacin
Food combinations	1. Cereal + pulse	Protein quality improves,
	2. Cereal + small quantity of animal protein	becomes complete protein
	3. Cereal + pulse + green leafy vegetable	
Iron utensils for cooking and tempering	Any food; preferably acidic food cooked or stirred or tempered with iron cooking utensils	Iron
Correct cooking methods	All foodstuffs; correct washing, pre-preparation, cooking, and storage procedures	Maximum retention of nutrients

Exposure to air or oxidation   Exposure of finely divided foods to oxygen of the air reduces the vitamin C content by oxidation. The enzyme ascorbic acid oxidase is released when fruits and vegetables are cut. The enzyme activity is temperature dependant and can be inactivated by blanching, or by storing cut fruits and vegetables at refrigeration temperatures or by adding acid.

Vitamin A is destroyed on exposure to air. The colour of cut carrots (carotene) fades due to oxidation and B-complex vitamins are also affected.

Milling   Whole meal flour contains all nutrients present in the grain. In flour with 100 per cent extraction no nutrients are lost. Low extraction flours (45 per cent extraction) are light in colour and are mainly starch with some protein and fat. Approximately 70 per cent of all B-complex vitamins, minerals, and dietary fibre present in the whole grain are lost during milling.

Polished rice (the form in which rice is consumed) loses 75 per cent vitamin B_1 or thiamine, while parboiling helps in retaining some of the vitamin.

Cooking and processing practices vary widely from one region to another, hence no authentic information on exact losses can be known. While cooking has both adverse and beneficial effects, proper practices can minimize the adverse effects and maximize the benefits so that food can become more wholesome and safe.

 ## SUMMARY

Meal planning and measures to retain nutrients in food cooked in large quantity is gaining greater significance because of the change in lifestyle since the past two to three decades. Eating out is no longer an occassional event but a way of life and the dependency on the caterer to provide the day's supply of nutrients has increased. Lifestyle diseases such as diabetes, obesity, hypertension, and heart attacks are on the rise because of lessened physical activity brought about by mechanization and increased intake of calorie and saturated fat-dense foods for the innumerable celebrations that are part of one's life.

The principle of menu planning is to provide wholesome and attractive meals at an affordable cost to individuals in all types of food service establishments, specially where the individual depends for all meals on the caterer. Meals are planned keeping all factors of menu planning in mind. The nutritive value and planning process can be simplified by following the three basic food group classification. This can be used to quickly check the adequacy of one's diet. The nutritive value of any recipe can be calculated using the food composition tables. This is a lengthy process.

Nutritional needs change during our lifetime because of physiological, psychological, and social changes which influence our meal consumption patterns. The changing needs should be kept in mind if optimum nutrition is to be maintained. Food cooked in bulk needs prior pre-preparation and remains hot for a longer time. It is reheated often over an extended lunch hour, which further reduces its nutritive value. The caterer should take all precautions to preserve and enhance the nutrient content of foods served.

KEY TERMS

Aging Process of gradual physiological changes which take place during life, specially visible in adulthood.

Anorexia nervosa Loss of appetite due to psychological disturbance resulting in loss of muscle tissue, weight loss, and low BMR. Self-imposed starvation.

Bulimia Gorging on food and throwing up to get rid of what is eaten.

Geriatrics The science dealing with disease and care of the elderly.

Osteopenia A disease characterized by very little bone mass.

Osteoporosis Reduction in bone tissue, weakening of the bones, making them prone to fractures.

Pathogens Microorganisms capable of causing disease.

Satiety value Feeling of satisfaction and fullness and not feeling hungry till the next meal.

Weaning Shifting the infant's feeding gradually from breast to bottle or cup.

REVIEW EXERCISES

1. What are the advantages of menu planning?
2. List any eight factors which influence menu planning.
3. Explain the three group classification of food. What is the basis for this classification?
4. Why should a pregnant woman be particular about her diet?
5. List any five advantages of breastfeeding.
6. What changes in old age affect menu planning for the elderly?
7. Explain the following:
    (a) Anorexia nervosa
    (b) Weaning foods
    (c) Food composition table
8. As a chef in a restaurant, what measures would you take to enhance the nutritive value of foods served?
9. Using the three basic food group classification, check the nutrient adequacy of the meals consumed by you in one day.
10. With the help of the food composition table, calculate the nutritive value of any four recipes you have prepared in the food production laboratory.

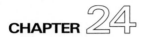

Modified Diets

LEARNING OBJECTIVES

After reading this chapter, you should be able to
- understand the need for modifying the diet
- know different kinds of modifications which can be made in the diet
- describe lifestyle-related and other common diseases and correlate the diet modifications to the symptoms of disease
- identify permitted and restricted foods in different diseases
- appreciate the role of food as a therapeutic agent in restoring and maintaining health

INTRODUCTION

In Chapter 22, we have read that a balanced diet is one which provides all the nutrients needed by a person to support life, maintain good health, to hasten recovery from illness, and take care of any short durations of emergency such as days on which one fasts, misses meals, or nutrients lacking in the diet. Very often illness or disease may alter the nutrient requirements of individuals.

Sometimes the patient's condition is such that he/she cannot tolerate or is not allowed to consume certain nutrients. For example, a diabetic cannot utilize glucose. Since the end-product of carbohydrate digestion is glucose, the carbohydrate content of the diet needs to be modified. In such cases, the diet is modified to bring down blood glucose levels, hasten recovery, and prevent complications arising due to diabetes mellitus.

The normal diet is used as the basis for all modified diets.

Diet therapy is defined as the use of food in the treatment of a disease. This is done by changing the normal diet in order to meet the altered requirements resulting from the illness or injury.

The aim of diet therapy is to maintain or restore good nutrition.

PURPOSE OF DIET THERAPY

- Maintain normal nutrition and health, e.g., modified diets are based on balanced diets
- Treat deficiency diseases, e.g., high-protein, high-calorie diet in protein calorie malnutrition
- Alter nutrient requirement according to body's ability to use the nutrient, e.g., modify carbohydrates in a diabetic diet
- Give rest to an organ or to the body, e.g., intravenous fluids in severe vomiting and diarrhoea
- Change body weight, e.g., low-calorie diet in obesity to lose weight.

The clinical dietitian in a hospital is responsible for planning therapeutic diets for patients as per the doctors diet prescription. The administrative dietitian manages food service establishments.

Dietetics   It is the science and art of feeding individuals or groups under different health and economic conditions according to the principles of nutrition and management.

CLASSIFICATION OF MODIFIED DIETS

The diet is normally altered or modified in the following ways (see Fig. 24.1)

1. Modification in consistency
2. Modification in nutrient content
3. Modification in quantity
4. Modification in method of feeding

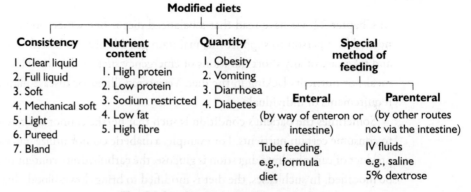

Fig. 24.1   Classification of modified diets

Modifications in Consistency

Clear fluid diet   The clear fluid or clear liquid diet is used for short periods when there is acute vomiting or diarrhoea, when minimal bowel residue is desired, and to test the individuals ability to tolerate oral food.

This diet is free from any solids, even those found in milk. The clear fluid diet is inadequate in all nutrients and should be used only for 1–2 days. The main purpose of this diet is to prevent dehydration and relieve thirst. It is high in simple sugars and needs to be modified for diabetic individuals. The amount of fluid given initially is 40–80 ml/hour, which is gradually increased to 100–120 ml/hour. Foods included:

1. Fruit juices: Apple, orange, grape juices
2. Cereal water: Barley water, arrowroot water, sago kanji, rice kanji
3. Soups: Clear consomme, fat-free broth
4. Beverages: Tea, coffee with lime and sugar (no milk), lime juice, coconut water, sugar cane juice, carbonated beverages
5. Flavoured gelatin and fruit ices

Full liquid diet This diet is prescribed for individuals who are unable to chew, swallow, or tolerate solid foods. It is given after the clear liquid diet and before starting solid foods.

It is composed of foods that are liquid at room temperature. If it is well planned it can meet most of the RDA's. However, due to difficulty in consuming adequate amounts of foods from the body building food and cereal food group, vitamin and mineral supplements should be given if the diet is to be used for longer durations.

It is prescribed during acute infections, gastritis, diarrhoea when milk is permitted, after surgery, and for people too ill to eat solid food.

Foods included:

1. Cream soups, dal soup, whipped potatoes
2. Eggnog, milkshakes, plain ice cream, China grass jelly, custard
3. Oatmeal, arrowroot, and *sago kanji* with milk
4. Soya milk, health drinks, *lassi*, cocoa

Soft diet This diet is given between the full liquid diet and light diet or the general hospital diet. It is given during convalescence, acute infections, gastrointestinal disorders, and after surgery.

The foods included in this diet are soft in texture and consistency, easy to chew and digest with very little fibre, spices, and condiments. Spicy, highly seasoned, and fried foods are avoided as they may cause heartburn, belching, and indigestion. Strongly flavoured vegetables and gassy foods can cause discomfort because of flatus or gas produced by bacterial fermentation of indigestible carbohydrates.

Foods included A wide variety of foods from the basic food groups can be selected and a nutritionally adequate diet can be planned. Cooking methods should be boiling, steaming, poaching, or stewing. Fruits and vegetables with coarse skins, rough fibres, and seeds, e.g., guava and jackfruit should be avoided. Strongly flavoured vegetables such as cabbage, cauliflower, onions; Bengal gram, fried eggs, omelettes, all salads, sweetmeats, and masalas and pickles should be avoided.

Mechanical soft diet This is also called a dental diet and is a variation of the soft diet. It includes foods which are easy to chew and swallow. There is no restriction on seasoning or method of preparation. The texture or consistency of food may be modified by mechanical processing such as mashing, blenderizing, or chopping. This diet is nutritionally adequate if well planned and is given to individuals who have difficulty in chewing or swallowing because of teeth and gum problems.

Light diet or the general hospital diet It is similar to the soft diet and also includes simple salads, fruit salads, and *paneer*.

Pureed diet This is given to individuals who have difficulty in chewing and swallowing food. It includes all liquid and semi–liquid foods which require no mastication.
Foods included:

1. Milk and milk beverages, egg nog, *lassi*, cream soups, custard, ice cream
2. All fruit and vegetable purees and juices
3. Soft scrambled egg, boiled mashed dals
4. Soft cooked cereals, oatmeal

Bland diet This diet is prescribed for individuals suffering from gastric or duodenal ulcers, gastritis, and ulcerative colitis. It includes foods which are mechanically, chemically, and thermally non-irritating, Foods low in fibre are recommended. Stimulating beverages and spicy foods increase the secretion of gastric juice which in turn causes pain when in contact with the ulcer.

Foods to avoid include strong tea, coffee, alcoholic beverages, condiments, and spices such as black pepper, red chilli powder, cloves, mustard seeds, and nutmeg. High-fibre foods and hot soups and beverages should be avoided. Fried foods and strongly flavoured sulphur containing vegetables should be avoided.

Foods included

1. Milk and milk-based preparations
2. Refined cereals and rice
3. Cream, butter
4. Cooked fruits and vegetables without peel and seeds
5. Dehusked pulses, boiled, baked, or stewed tender cuts of meat/poultry and fish
6. All egg preparations except omelettes and fried eggs

Modifications in Nutrient Content

The nutrient content of the diet is modified to treat deficiencies, change body weight, or control diseases such as hypertension and diabetes. The type and amount of nutrients need to be modified, e.g., in diabetes not only does the amount of carbohydrate need to be reduced but the type of carbohydrates allowed need to be modified, i.e., complex carbohydrates are included instead of simple sugars.

Table 24.1 lists some of the diseases with nutrient modifications required.

TABLE 24.1   Diseases with nutrient modifications

Disease	Nutrient modification
Atherosclerosis	Fat-controlled, low-cholesterol diet
Hepatitis	Restricted fat diets
Anaemia, high fever, injury	High-protein diet
Hypertension, cardiovascular disease	Sodium restricted diet
Lactose intolerance	Lactose-free diet
Hepatic coma	Low-protein diet
Underweight, malnutrition	High-calorie diet

Modifications in fibre

The terms roughage, residue, bulk, and fibre have been used to describe the indigestible components of food. The term fibre will be used for all the indigestible polysaccharides and lignin which remains after digestion of food.

High-fibre diet   The high fibre diet is used to prevent and treat constipation and diverticulosis. Fibre absorbs water to produce soft, bulky stools and influences faecal transit time. It is also prescribed in obesity to increase the volume of food being consumed without increasing the calorie content of the meal.

Foods included

1. All milk and milk products
2. All body building foods specially whole pulses, nuts, and oilseeds
3. All fruits and vegetables especially with edible skins, seeds, and membranes and those which can be consumed raw, e.g., whole orange segments with white membranes is preferred to orange juice
4. Wholegrain cereals, green leafy vegetables

Low-fibre low-residue diet   This diet is presribed during acute infections of the gastrointestinal tract such as ulcerative colitis, acute diverticulitis, and severe diarrhoea.

This diet includes foods that leave a small faecal mass after digestion and absorption. Only those foods which can be completely absorbed are included.

Foods such as arrowroot kanji, barley water, whey water, and sago kheer are recommended. Foods avoided are fruits and vegetables high in fibre, nuts and oilseeds, and whole grains. Refined cereals, meat, fish, poultry, eggs are permitted. Milk is permitted in limited quantities as it leaves a residue. A maximum quantity of two cups milk/day is permitted in the form of milk, paneer, or curds. Fruits and vegetables with 2 g or less fibre are permitted. All fruit and vegetable juices and cooked vegetables such as bottle gourd and potato are permitted.

Modifications in Quantity

The quantity of food served to the patient needs to be modified to check tolerance, control nutrient levels, and bring about weight loss.

In acute vomiting, the quantity of fluid given is 40–80 ml/hour to check the individuals ability to tolerate oral feeding.

In a diabetic diet, the quantity of carbohydrate in each meal is as important as the quantity of carbohydrate consumed in a day.

Modifications in Method of Feeding

Enteral feedings   It is feeding by way of enteron or intestine but not by mouth. Sometimes oral feeding is not possible, and when swallowing is difficult but the gastrointestinal tract is functional, tube feeding is used to provide food. A wide variety of enteral feeding formulas are available. The proteins in the formula may be natural intact proteins of milk, egg, etc. which need digestion or partially broken down proteins, i.e., protein hydrolysates and amino acids. Carbohydrates are in the form of disaccharides or glucose polymers, which are quickly broken down to glucose. Fats are in the form of vegetable oils, lecithin, mono- and diglycerides, and medium chain triglycerides of 8–10 carbon chains, which are specially manufactured for formula feeding as they are digested and absorbed quickly as compared to long chain triglycerides that occur in nature. Vitamins and minerals are added to make the formula nutritionally complete.

Formulas could be prepared by blending ordinary food into a smooth and free-flowing consistency with less viscosity. Chemical formulas require minimal digestion, are quickly absorbed, and leave little residue, while blended formulas with ordinary food are thick and may block the feeding tube. Feeding tubes are inserted either through the nose or through the abdominal wall. Feeding may be done continuously or it may be intermittent.

Parenteral feeding   This method of feeding is resorted to when the intestine is not functioning and needs rest. Parenteral fluids contain water, glucose, amino acids, fatty acids, minerals, and vitamins to meet the individuals requirements for all nutrients. These fluids are given through the peripheral and central veins., i.e., intravenously.

Sometimes only glucose or glucose and saline is administered if required for a short duration.

DIETS FOR COMMON DISORDERS

Diabetes Mellitus

Diabetes mellitus (mel means honey) is a chronic disorder of carbohydrate metabolism characterized by high blood sugar level or hyperglycemia and a high level of sugar in the urine or glycosuria. Along with carbohydrates, the metabolism of proteins and fats is also affected.

Diabetes occurs due to a lack of insulin. The β-cells of islets of Langerhans in the pancreas secrete the hormone insulin that is required for the uptake and utilization of glucose by the cells. If insulin is deficient, glucose is not oxidized in the cells, resulting in hyperglycemia. The normal fasting level of glucose in blood is 70–110 mg/100 ml blood. When the fasting level of glucose rises above 170 mg/100 ml, the renal threshold is exceeded and sugar begins to appear in the urine. In severe uncontrolled diabetes, blood glucose levels may be as high as 400 mg/100 ml. See Table 24.2 for a sample diet for diabetes patients.

Symptoms of diabetes include

1. Hyperglycemia or high blood sugar level
2. Glycosuria or presence of sugar in urine
3. Polyuria or frequent urination
4. Polydipsia or excessive thirst
5. Polyphagia or excessive hunger
6. Ketosis or accumulation of ketone bodies in the blood due to incomplete oxidation of fats. Fats are rapidly broken down as a source of energy since carbohydrates cannot be utilized. A diabetic diet is mainly modified in carbohydrate content and should not exceed 55 per cent of total calories. The carbohydrate content should not exceed 250 g/day. A minimum level of 100 g should be included to prevent ketosis and protein breakdown and as a source of energy for the nervous system.

Treatment of diabetes includes

1. Educating the patient about the chronic nature of the disease
2. Diet management and carbohydrate distribution
3. Regular exercise to lower blood sugar levels
4. Controlling blood glucose levels by
   (a) Oral hypoglycemic drugs
   (b) Insulin injections

TABLE 24.2   Diet for diabetes mellitus patients

Foods recommended	Foods to be avoided
1. Complex carbohydrates rich in dietary fibre—millets, wheat, pasta, brown bread	1. Simple sugars and refined carbohydrates—sugar, jaggery, sweets, preserves
2. Higher proportion of polyunsaturated fatty acid (PUFA) vegetable oils	2. Saturated fats and cholesterol in moderation—hydrogenated fats, ghee, butter, cream
3. Good quality proteins—lean meat, fish, eggs, pulses, milk	3. Alcohol, soft drinks, sweetmeats, nuts, and oilseeds
4. Salads, leafy vegetables, other vegetables	

Fevers and Infection

Fever is defined as an elevation in body temperature above normal temperature of 98.6°F or 37°C. This increase in temperature may be due to infection caused by microorganisms, body reactions, inflammation, or heat stroke. Fever is a classic sign of infection in the body.

Fever is treated by treating the cause of fever and lowering the body temperature by drugs such as antipyretics and by cold sponging. Symptoms such as bodyache are treated with rest and drugs.

The basal metabolic rate (BMR) increases by 7 per cent for every degree Fahrenheit rise in body temperature. Protein catabolism or breakdown increases and body fluids and electrolytes are lost due to excretion of toxic metabolic wastes and excessive perspiration to bring down fever. The stores of carbohydrate, i.e., glycogen and fat are depleted leading to weight loss. Table 24.3 suggests foods to overcome weight loss.

TABLE 24.3   High-calorie, high-protein diet

Foods recommended	Foods to be avoided
All foods should be liquid to semi-solid consistency; smooth texture with no harsh irritating fibres, strong flavour, or spicy food	Solid foods which are hard or tough, requiring lot of mastication
1. Cereals—refined cereals in the form of *kanji*, custard, or *kheer*, *phulka*, boiled rice	1. Cereals—millets, cereal with bran or irritating dietary fibres such as wholegrain cereals and cereal products
2. Good quality, easy to digest proteins—chicken soup, stew, milk-based beverages, eggnog, sweet freshly set curds, custard, health drinks, soft-cooked *khichdi*, dal rice (*moong* dal), boiled vegetables (bottle gourd, pumpkin, potato), stewed fruits, soft fruits, fruit juices, sugar	2. Fried, spicy pulse, and meat/fish/poultry preparations 3. Leafy vegetables, raw fruits, and vegetables with harsh fibres 4. Pickle, *papad*

Fevers may be due to acute infections, such as influenza, septic wounds or chronic fever, lasting from several days to several months as in the case of tuberculosis, typhoid, etc.

Infection or entry and growth of microorganisms in the body is one of the most common cause of fever. A lowered resistance to infective agents results in their proliferation in the body with production of toxic metabolites that give rise to symptoms of fever accompanied by nausea and loss of appetite.

Diet should progress from a clear liquid diet to a full liquid diet to a soft diet.

Cardiovascular Diseases

Cardiovascular diseases (CVD) are diseases of the heart and blood vessels. They are very common in India, and the incidence of these diseases is increasing rapidly.

Cardiovascular diseases include the following:

Hypertension   Hypertension is an increase in blood pressure (BP) above normal. Normal BP is 80/120 mm mercury (Hg) diastolic/systolic pressure. The diastolic BP is the pressure exerted by blood on arterial walls when the heart is contracting and the systolic blood pressure is the pressure exerted by blood on arterial walls when the heart is expanding.

TABLE 24.4   Risk factors for heart diseases

Personal factors	Diet pattern	Other diseases
Heredity or strong family history	Alcoholic	Hypertension
Males/females after menopause	Consumes rich foods	Atherosclerosis
Smoking	High in fat and cholesterol	Diabetes
Obesity	Low in fibre	Obesity
Age group 30–55 years	Refined carbohydrates and sugars	High blood lipid levels
Workaholic—tension and stress	High salt intake	
Sedentary lifestyle		

This is the most common disease of the circulatory system and many individuals are unaware that they are suffering from hypertension. Many factors contribute to high blood pressure such as atherosclerosis, obesity, and diabetes (see Table 24.4). Atherosclerosis increases the blood pressure by causing resistance to blood flow. The heart has to pump harder due to narrowed arteries, increasing the BP. The increased BP in turn damages the arterial walls. In an obese individual, the amount of tissue which needs blood supply increases, thereby increasing the work of the heart. A loss of weight often lowers BP. Blood pressure can be controlled by the following.

1. Restricting sodium (see Table 24.5)
2. Drug therapy
3. Stress management and exercise.

Ischaemic heart disease   Ischaemia is a deficiency of blood supply to the heart muscle leading to a heart attack.

Angina pectoris   Angina is tightness and severe pain across the chest due to deficient oxygen supply following any exertion.

Myocardial infarction   An infarct is a localized area of heart muscle which dies due to lack of oxygen because blood supply is cut off. Myocardial infarction could be fatal.

TABLE 24.5 Sodium-restricted diet

Foods recommended	Foods to be avoided
Foods low in sodium	Foods rich in cholesterol and fat, foods rich in sodium (as sodium chloride or any other sodium salt used as an additive)
1. Cereals—wheat, rice, oatmeal, millets	1. Baking powder—cakes, cookies
2. All fruits—fresh and canned	2. Soda bicarbonate—*nankhatai*
3. Cabbage, cauliflower, tomato, potato, onion	3. Monosodium glutamate (MSG)—Chinese food and food served in restaurants (MSG is used indiscriminately by some caterers)
4. Sugar, honey, jam, jelly	4. Sodium benzoate—tomato sauce
5. Low sodium seasonings instead of salt	5. Sodium propionate—bread
6. Lime juice	6. Sodium chloride—salted snacks, wafers, nuts, farsan, etc.
7. Mint, parsley, dill, basil	7. Papad, pickles
8. Fresh vegetables	8. Vegetables in brine
9. All other vegetables, root vegetables	9. Celery, beetroot, and spinach
10. Vegetable oil as a cooking medium	10. Foods rich in cholesterol and saturated fats—salted butter and processed cheese
11. Milk in moderation	

Atherosclerosis is a common symptom in all CVDs. It is the chief cause of heart attacks and strokes. Coronary arteries are the arteries which supply blood to the heart muscle. A blockage in any coronary artery can cause a heart attack due to death of part of the muscle. An obstruction in the blood vessels in the brain results in a stroke. It is a term used to describe the thickening and hardening of major blood vessels by deposits of lipids such as cholesterol and triglycerides in the lumen of the blood vessel. Table 24.6 suggests dietary modifications for atherosclerosis. These deposits reduce or stop the flow of blood, and if a major artery is involved it leads to a heart attack. Atherosclerosis begins early in life as soft mushy lipids get deposited in the inner walls or lumen of the artery. The deposits gradually thicken and harden making the space through which blood flows narrower. If a clot forms, the blood vessel is totally blocked and cannot supply oxygen or nutrients to that portion of the heart muscle, leading to necrosis or death of tissue cells which could be fatal. (see Fig. 24.2).

Disorders of the Gastrointestinal Tract

Peptic ulcers An ulcer is a localized erosion of the mucosal lining of those portions of the alimentary canal which come in contact with gastric juice. They occur in the oesophagus, stomach, and duodenum.

TABLE 24.6   Modified fat diet

Foods recommended	Foods to be avoided
Foods low in cholesterol and saturated fats	Cholesterol-rich foods
1. Skimmed milk, *paneer* (skimmed milk)	1. Whole milk, butter, cream, *mawa*, cheese (processed)
2. Cereals (whole grain), pulses	2. Indian sweetmeats, rich puddings, bakery products
3. High fibre and soluble fibre such as oat meal, millets, pectin, gums	3. Organ meat (liver, brain, etc.)
4. Salad vegetables, fruits, green leafy vegetables, other root vegetables	4. Egg yolk, fish roe, shellfish, fatty meat, processed meat
5. Lean meat, egg white, fish	5. Nuts, oilseeds, pickles
6. Vegetable oils, sugar, jaggery	6. Margarine, *vanaspati*, fried food
	7. Alcohol

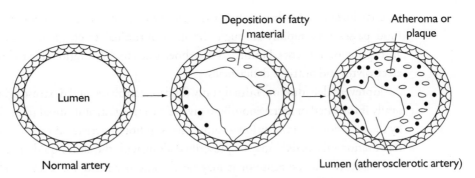

Fig. 24.2   Narrowing of the lumen and hardening of the artery due to deposits of fatty material such as cholesterol and triglycerides

A person suffering from ulcers gets a burning, gnawing, or piercing pain 1–3 hours after a meal. The pain is relieved on taking antacids, or eating food which does not stimulate gastric secretion. It is treated by giving drugs to control acidity, giving bed rest to the patient, and prescribing a bland diet that is mechanically, thermally, and chemically non-stimulating. Ulcers are also known as the disease of hurry, worry, and curry. Cold milk is a good buffer and is recommended to ulcer patients along with cream or ice cream (see Table 24.7).

Diarrhoea   Diarrhoea is the frequent passage of loose watery or semisolid stools of greater than normal volume. When blood and/or mucous is present, the condition is called dysentery. It is often accompanied by abdominal pain, cramps, and vomiting.

The most common cause of diarrhoea is eating contaminated food or overeating, causing indigestion. Other causes are anxiety, nervousness, antibiotic treatment, etc.

TABLE 24.7 Diet for peptic ulcers

Foods recommended	Foods to be avoided
1. Cereals—all refined cereals, bread, rice, pasta	1. All wholegrain cereals
2. Milk—all milk beverages and all milk products, weak tea	2. All stimulating beverages—alcohol, tea, coffee, aerated drinks
3. Eggs, lean meat, fish, poultry as protein to heal ulcers	3. All fatty meat
4. Dehusked pulses, boiled and mashed	4. Whole pulses
5. Stewed fruits, vitamin C for healing	5. Raw fruits
6. Butter, cream, ice cream	6. Spices, condiments, fried foods
7. Cooking methods—boiling, baking, stewing, poaching	7. Frying, barbecuing, salted, smoked foods

Diarrhoea is not a disease, but a symptom of an infection or disease. In this condition, food passes very rapidly through the gastrointestinal tract, giving very little time for absorption of nutrients. Prolonged diarrhoea leads to dehydration due to loss of fluids, and electrolytes and nutrient deficiencies.

To prevent dehydration, initially only fluids, electrolytes, and dextrose (glucose) are given orally if tolerated or intravenously to give rest to the gastrointestinal tract. This is followed by the clear liquid diet, very low-residue diet, soft fibre-restricted diet, and normal diet. Oral rehydration salts (ORS) may be prescribed along with the clear liquid diet.

Diarrhoea may be acute or it may be chronic persisting for a few weeks, resulting in nutritional deficiencies.

Clear liquid diet is recommended for diarrhoea patients.

Constipation Constipation is the infrequent or difficult evacuation of hard stools. It is the opposite of diarrhoea. It is often accompanied by loss of appetite, headache, discomfort, and a coated tongue.

A person may get constipated due to various reasons such as

1. Irregular eating and toilet habits
2. Change in surroundings and food habits
3. Lack of exercise and poor muscle tone
4. Low-fibre diet and inadequate fluid consumption to prevent passing urine at night
5. Chronic use of laxatives

Constipation is treated by drinking adequate fluids and increasing intestinal bulk to stimulate evacuation. Care should be taken to increase the fibre content of the diet gradually to prevent bloating and cramps caused by excessive fibre intake. Regular meal timings and exercise is also necessary (see Table 24.8).

TABLE 24.8   High–fibre, moderate–fat diet for constipation

Foods recommended	Foods to be avoided
1. Fluids—at least 1.5 litres	1. Refined cereals—rice, seived flours
2. Cereals—wholegrain cereals, millets, oats	2. Dehusked pulses
3. Pulses with husk—*rajma*, ground nuts, peas	3. Castor oil
4. Fruits—raw and cooked fruits and vegetables, guavas, figs, pears, apples, citrus fruit	
5. Milk, butter milk, butter, ghee	
6. Soups, tea, coffee	
7. Green leafy vegetables, salads	
Use fruits and vegetables with edible skin and peel	

Liver Disorders

The liver is the main organ associated with our digestive system. It is a complex organ performing hundreds of functions related to nutrient metabolism, bile production and excretion, and detoxification of poisonous substances.

Jaundice, a yellow pigmentation of the skin and tissues, is a common symptom of liver disorders caused due to elevated levels of bile pigments. When the liver cells are damaged due to agents such as microorganisms, toxins, alcohol, and obstruction of bile, the diet needs to be modified to give rest to the organ and protect and repair liver cells.

Common liver disorders are

1. Hepatitis or inflammation and degeneration of liver cells. It is an infectious disease which may be viral or drug induced. Type A hepatitis is caused due to consumption of contaminated food or water mainly due to sewage contamination.
2. Cirrhosis is a chronic liver disease involving destruction of liver cells, often associated with chronic alcoholism.
3. Hepatic coma is a serious liver disease with high levels of ammonia in blood in which liver cells fail to function.

Liver disorders are treated by giving an appetizing protein-rich diet (except in hepatic coma) high in carbohydrate with a moderate restriction in fat. Adequate bed rest is also essential to regenerate damaged liver cells.

Symptoms of liver disorder (hepatitis) are nausea, vomiting, anorexia or loss of appetite, fever, abdominal pain, weight loss, diarrhoea, and jaundice.

Because of these symptoms, the diet should progress in the following manner.

1. Parenteral fluids in case of severe vomiting and diarrhoea
2. Clear fluid diet
3. Full fluid diet

4. Soft low-fibre diet

5. High-protein, high-carbohydrate, low-to-moderate fat diet (see Table 24.9).

TABLE 24.9 High-protein, high-carbohydrate, low to moderate fat diet

Foods recommended	Foods to be avoided
1. Nutritious beverages	1. Strongly flavoured vegetables
2. Soft-cooked cereals and pulses	2. Fried foods
3. Fruits	3. Food with high-fat content
4. Vegetables	4. Nuts and oilseeds
5. Milk and milk products	5. Rich desserts and pastries
6. Lean meat, fish, poultry	6. Spicy and highly seasoned foods
7. Eggs	
8. Jam, jelly, sugar	
9. Simple desserts	

Kidney Disorders

The kidneys are the main organs for excretion of nitrogenous wastes arising from protein metabolism. Urea, which is formed from the breakdown of food and tissue proteins, is excreted by the kidneys via the urine.

The main function of the kidneys is to maintain the normal composition and volume of blood and other body fluids. This is achieved by filtering blood to remove toxic wastes. Blood is filtered through the millions of nephrons which are present in each kidney. The nephron is the functional unit of the kidney and is made up of a glomerulus or a filter and a long winding tubule that opens into a collecting duct where urine is collected. Approximately 150 to 180 litres of blood is filtered by the kidneys.

In kidney disorders, the waste products of protein metabolism, fluids and electrolytes may accumulate in blood, or proteins may get filtered into the urine. Common kidney disorders are as follows:

Nephrosis or nephrotic syndrome   It is a condition in which proteins are filtered into the urine due to injury to the glomerulus. Accumulation of body fluids is also seen.

Renal failure   The kidneys fail to function normally and waste material accumulates in blood resulting in uremia (excess urea in blood) and ultimately coma.

Kidney stone   Kidney stones or calculi form in any part of the kidney or urinary tract causing extreme pain. They form when concentration of salts in urine is high or fluid intake is less resulting in precipitation of salts in the form of crystals or stones.

Foods allowed will depend on the nature of mineral, e.g., calcium oxalate, calcium phosphate, and uric acid stones. If the body loses protein, the protein content of the diet will need to be increased. If urea accumulates in blood, the protein content of the diet will have to be reduced. Fluids and electrolytes need to be controlled if there is water retention.

In kidney disorders, like liver disorders, nutrients have to be modified depending on the symptoms and nature of the disorder.

SUMMARY

A well-planned balanced diet can not only promote and preserve good health but can also act as a therapeutic aid in restoring health. A diet which is planned for treatment of a disease is a therapeutic diet. There are many types of therapeutic diets with modifications in nutrient content, quantity, consistency or texture, and special method of feeding. The aim of diet therapy is to treat deficiency diseases, alter nutrient requirements according to the body's ability to metabolize nutrients, to give rest to the body or to an organ, and to change body weight.

The normal balanced diet is the basis for planning modified diets. Modified diets include the liquid diets (clear liquid and full liquid diets), the soft diet, light diet, pureed diet, mechanical soft or dental soft diet, and bland diet. Nutrient content is modified to treat nutrient deficiencies or adapt to the body's ability to metabolize nutrients. Modifications in quantity and special methods of feeding by a nasogastric tube or by intravenous fluids in case of patients who are too ill to eat or in cases when an organ needs rest are also used as part of the treatment.

Special diets for diabetes mellitus, hypertension, and atherosclerosis—all lifestyle diseases; for fevers and infections; gastrointestinal disorders; cardiovascular diseases; and kidney and liver diseases have also been outlined for ready reference.

KEY TERMS

Clear liquid diet   A diet comprising of clear liquids without milk which provides fluids and electrolytes and few calories.

Convalescence   The period during which the clinical symptoms of disease have gone but the person is not fit to resume normal work and needs rest and proper nourishment.

Diverticulosis   Tiny sacs or pouches in the colon called diverticula which when inflamed cause diverticulitis.

Enteral   Any feeding involving the gastrointestinal tract. Term used specially for tube feeding when swallowing food is difficult due to obstructions in the oesophagus, surgery, etc.

Flatus   Gas produced by bacterial fermentation of indigestible carbohydrate in the colon.

Formula feeding   Feeding the patient a nutritionally adequate meal which is made by blending ordinary foods, or commercial formulas may be purchased. A nasogastric tube is used for feeding. Formulas should be smooth and free flowing.

Full fluid diet   A diet comprising of liquids and solids which liquify at body temperature and is generally milk based.

Gastritis   Inflammation of the stomach.

Nasogastric tube   A flexible plastic tube inserted through the nose into the stomach through which a formula containing nutrients in required amounts is fed. Used for persons who cannot chew or swallow.

Parenteral   Method of feeding via the peripheral veins when the intestine is not functioning.

Protein hydrolysates   Partially broken down proteins in the form of small peptides and amino acids used in formula feeding.

REVIEW EXERCISES

1. Answer briefly
   (a) Why do calorie needs increase when suffering from fever?
   (b) Why is fat restricted in liver disorders
   (c) Why is protein restricted in kidney failure?
   (d) Why does blood sugar increase in diabetes mellitus?
   (e) Why is strong tea or coffee not served to peptic ulcer patients?

2. Describe the following and state when it is prescribed.
   (a) Bland diet
   (b) Clear liquid diet
   (c) Full liquid diet
   (d) Low-residue diet

3. Classify the various types of modified diets and state the basis for classification.

4. Apart from diet, what are the other factors responsible for cardiovascular diseases?

5. What foods need to be restricted in a low-sodium diet. List any ten foods.

6. Define atherosclerosis, hypertension, and diabetes mellitus.

7. How would you modify a diet to prevent constipation? What other advice would you give the person?

8. List 10 popular items on a typical Indian restaurant menu, which are suitable for a diabetic individual.

9. Match the following disease in column I with a suitable answer from column II

I	II
Disease	Symptom
(i) Diabetes	(a) Atheroselerosis
(ii) Hepatitis	(b) Rise in body temperature
(iii) Cardiovascular disease	(c) Dermatitis
(iv) Peptic ulcer	(d) Hyperglycemia
(v) Fever	(e) Pain in the spinal cord
	(f) Jaundice
	(g) Dementia
	(h) Burning, gnawing pain in the stomach

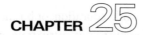

New Trends in Nutrition

Learning Objectives

After reading this chapter, you should be able to
- understand the practices being followed while preparing food in institutions
- identify the measures to be taken to provide nutritional meals
- examine the nutritive value of fast food
- suggest ways to improve the nutrient adequacy of a meal
- know the categories of convenience foods available in the market
- describe the format for a nutrition label
- understand the significance of nutrition labelling

NEED FOR SERVING NUTRITIONAL AND HEALTH-SPECIFIC MEALS

Food provided by residential institutions, such as boarding schools, college hostels, hospitals, and old-age homes, are probably the only source of nutrition for the residents and must be adequate. The list of residential institutes is long, and it is the responsibility and moral obligation of the caterer to provide nutritionally adequate meals to the residents. Sample menus based on the principles of meal planning and recommended dietary allowances (RDAs) should be provided to the caterer to ensure that the meal is balanced as well as attractive, appetizing, and affordable. Correct cooking practices should be followed to prevent losses of heat-labile nutrients, oxidative losses as well as leaching losses. While selecting commodities, fruits and vegetables at the proper stage of maturity, which are fresh and intact, should be purchased. If convenience foods are to be purchased, their cost should be considered. The food standards laid down by the government for various commodities should be checked especially for compulsory standards. For example, the fruit product order for processed fruit and vegetable products such as tomato sauce, pineapple slices in syrup, and sweet corn cream style. Just planning balanced meals is not sufficient. The nutrients present in the food should be conserved while preparing food, and cooking practices which enhance nutrients should be observed.

Eating out has become a way of life. In the past, people ate in restaurants to celebrate a special occassions or it was the weary traveller on the look out for bed and board. Today, practically everybody who steps out of the house for work, education, or business has at least one main meal away from home. A number of food joints to suit every strata of society have mushroomed in towns and cities. Many of these places are unlicenced, with the food handler having little or no knowledge about nutrients and nutrition, health and disease. The purpose of eating is to satisfy the hunger pangs and tickle the taste buds. What the consumer looks for today is cost and convenience, the majority paying little heed to the oil bubbling and frothing in the frying pan, or to the indiscriminate addition of ajinomoto to make vegetarian food more flavourful. To make quick money, hygienic practices are ignored or sufficient investments in proper storage and cooking equipments is not made leading to the vicious cycle of disease and malnutrition affecting work efficiency and productivity.

The need for nutritious meals, each meal meeting one-third of RDA, is necessary for the growth and well-being of the individual and the nation. Different requirements based on age, gender, activity, and physiological state should be provided. Nutritional education and awareness of the community at large is necessary. People should be more particular about what they eat and where they eat. This is particularly necessary to combat the lifestyle diseases to which youngsters are falling prey.

Some common practices which reduce the nutritional value of food and are harmful to health are

1. Buying poor quality fruits and vegetables in bulk because of lower rate
2. Improper storage leading to further loss of nutrients
3. Faulty cooking practices such as using excess water and then evaporating it to get correct consistency; cutting and then washing vegetables
4. Overcooking and discarding cooking water (pot liquor)
5. Soaking vegetables in water
6. Cooking in an open pan
7. Keeping hot food hot over extended service period
8. Repeated reheating of entire food instead of reheating quantity required
9. Adding alkali to hasten softening of pulses and vegetables, and to preserve green colour
10. Discarding water while boiling rice (rice should always be cooked by absorption method)
11. Indiscriminate use of preservatives
12. Re-using oil repeatedly for deep fat frying without adding fresh oil, or straining out food particles in oil
13. Using trans fats for better texture in baked products
14. Frying moist foods in fat without coating the food
15. Using *aji-no-moto* (MSG) in all preparations to bring out the flavour of food. *Aji-no-moto* is used in soups in place of stock. Permitted level in food is 1 per cent
16. Indiscriminate use of food colours not permitted under PFA Act 1954 in products. For example, use of artificial red colour in tandoori chicken is not permitted by law.

17. Switching off the deep freezer at night to save on power consumption can affect the quality of deep frozen foods. This is done by some unscrupulous traders.   Even refreezing food which has once thawed can affect not only the nutritive value and freshness but also the microbiological safety of the food.

Foods served in restaurants are often spicy with little attention to cooking procedures to retain nutrients. Water-soluble nutrients are often discarded along with the water in which vegetables are soaked or boiled. Rice is cooked by the throw-away method, discarding the little vitamin B_1 or thiamine remaining after rice is polished. The Indian gravies are rich in fats apart from the cooking medium such as coconut paste, coconut milk, cashew paste, poppy seeds, sesame seeds, cream, and butter which are used to finish the product. Snacks are mostly deep-fried, and cheese and paneer are popular ingredients in many preparations. There is no doubt that the calorie and fat content of a restaurant meal is very high specially in saturated fats, cholesterol, and monosodium glutamate. Both the chef and the consumer have to be alert and make wise choices from options on the menu, opting for salads, fruit salad, and vegetables with minimal gravy. The method of cooking used also influences the caloric content to a great extent.

NUTRITIVE VALUE OF FAST FOOD AND JUNK FOOD

The fast-food industry is growing rapidly all over the world to provide a quick meal to the customer at an affordable cost and in very little time. In India the fast-food industry comprises mainly of Udupi restaurants serving south Indian and Punjabi snacks and popular regional cuisine as well as the multi-national companies (MNCs) such as McDonalds, Pizza Hut, Kentucky Fried Chicken, Subway, Dominos, and Barista which have franchises in major cities of India. Many products have been modified to suit the Indian palate and respect religious sentiments. Many of these provide take-away or drive-thru services as well as a seating area to eat food on the premises. Modern commercial fast food is often highly processed and prepared in an industrial fashion. Most items on the menu are prepared at a central supply facility and then shipped to individual outlets where they are reheated/cooked or assembled in a short time. The central kitchen ensures consistency in product quality and ability to deliver the order quickly to the customer eliminating labour and equipment costs in the individual restaurants.

Since the fast food concept relies on speed, uniformity, and low cost, fast food items need additives and processing to ensure flavour, consistency, and freshness of the product. This processing often reduces the nutritive value of food. Many popular fast food items are unhealthy and excessive consumption can lead to obesity. Table 25.1 shows us the nutritive value of some fast-food items. These foods adversely affect the eating habits and health of children who prefer burgers, french fries, and soft drinks to a traditional hot meal at the table. Local cuisines are dying a slow death as people are forgetting the richer, more varied,

TABLE 25.1 Nutritive value of some fast-food items

Item	Total calories	Fat calories	Total fat (g)	Sat. fat (g)	Chol-estrol (mg)	Sodium (mg)	Carbo-hydrate (g)	Protein (g)
McDonald's Cheese-burger	330	130	14	6	45	830	36	15
McDonald's Big Mac	590	310	34	11	85	1,090	47	24
McDonald's Filet-O-Fish	470	240	26	5	50	1,200	67	24
McDonald's French Fries (large)	540	230	26	4.5	0	350	68	8
McDonald's Diet Coke	0	0	0	0	0	20	0	0
Pizza Hut Pan Pizza Pepperoni	280	130	14	5	15	610	28	11
Pizza Hut Stuffed Cheese Crust	445	174	19	10	24	1,090	46	22
Pizza Hut Spaghetti with Meat Balls	850	220	24	10	17	1,120	120	37
Pizza Hut Garlic Bread (1 slice)	150	70	8	1.5	0	240	16	3
KFC Chicken Breast	400	220	24	6	135	1,116	16	29
KFC Honey BBQ (6 pieces)	607	343	38	10	193	1,145	33	33
KFC Cole Slaw	230	130	14	2	15	540	23	4
KFC Strawberry Cream Pie (1 slice)	280	130	15	8	15	130	32	4

and nourishing tastes of freshly harvested seasonal food. Some fast food chains are offering healthy alternatives of fresh fruit and salads and low-fat items in their menu. However, these foods are still high in fat and cholesterol and refined cereals. South Indian fast food snacks are fermented food combinations which are more nutritious than their Western counterparts. They are a blend of cereal and pulses and are non-greasy, easy to digest, and safe to eat.

NUTRITIONAL EVALUATION OF NEWLY LAUNCHED PRODUCTS

A wide variety of convenience foods are available and new products in attractive packages are being launched everyday to meet the growing demands of working women, single families, the elderly and commercial establishments who are too busy to invest valuable time and labour in pre-preparations. The newly launched products in the market can be categorized under five heads, namely:

1. Basic product
2. Ready-to-cook product (see Fig 25.1)
3. Ready-to-use product
4. Precooked product (see Fig 25.2)
5. Table-ready product

In short these products are at the basic level cleaned, washed, peeled, and cut or ready-to-use, ready-to-eat, or ready-to-serve (see Table 25.2). Although these products

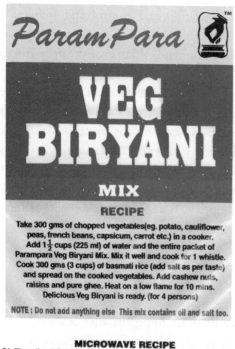

ParamPara™

VEG BIRYANI MIX

RECIPE

Take 300 gms of chopped vegetables(eg. potato, cauliflower, peas, french beans, capsicum, carrot etc.) in a cooker. Add 1½ cups (225 ml) of water and the entire packet of Parampara Veg Biryani Mix. Mix it well and cook for 1 whistle. Cook 300 gms (3 cups) of basmati rice (add salt as per taste) and spread on the cooked vegetables. Add cashew nuts, raisins and pure ghee. Heat on a low flame for 10 mins. Delicious Veg Biryani is ready. (for 4 persons)

NOTE : Do not add anything else This mix contains oil and salt too.

MICROWAVE RECIPE

Take 300 gms (3 cups) of basmati rice in a microwave bowl. Add 6 cups of water and salt (as per taste) and let it remain for half an hour. Cover and cook on micro 800 w for 18 mins. Take another microwave bowl and put in it 300 gms of chopped vegetables (eg. potato, cauliflower, peas, french beans, capsicum, carrot etc.) and the entire packet of Parampara Veg Biryani Mix and 2 cups (300 ml) of water and mix it well. Cover and Cook on micro 800 w for 10 mins. Now spread the cooked rice on it and add cashew nuts, raisins and pure ghee. Cover and keep this on micro 450 w. for 8 mins. Delicious Veg Biryani is ready. (for 4 persons)
NOTE : **Do not add anything else. This mix contains oil and salt too.**

Fig. 25.1 Ready-to-cook product

TABLE 25.2 Types of convenience foods

Category		Example
Category 1:	*Basic product* The product needs some preparation before cooking	Shelled green peas
Category 2:	*Ready-to-cook product* The product needs no further preparation before cooking	Frozen green peas
Category 3:	*Ready-to-use product* The product must be prepared and heated	Instant tomato soup powder
Category 4:	*Precooked product* This is a prepared dish which needs to be heated before consumption	Paneer makhanwala
Category 5:	*Table-ready product* The packet can be opened and consumed as it is	Potato chips

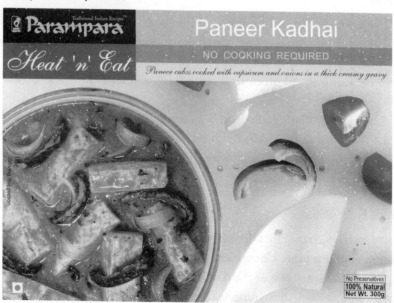

Fig. 25.2 Precooked products, popular abroad, are now gaining market in India

are industrially prepared often under strict regulation and control and sometimes bacteriologically safer than fresh goods, if they are not stored under temperature-controlled storage during retailing, their nutritive value and overall quality can be grossly affected.

Many products launched in the market make health claims which at times could be misleading. Convenience is not the main criteria, but meeting the day's nutritional needs should be checked. Some newly launched products based on soy proteins, flax seeds, carotene, and vitamin E rich oils have distinct benefits while other foods such as non-dairy creams have both advantages because of no cholesterol and disadvantages because of fatty acid composition of vegetable oils used. Bakery shortenings in the market are specifically designed for a particular product and the ready products are of superior quality but the trans-fatty acids present in these fats are harmful to health.

ANTIOXIDANTS

Antioxidants are compounds that prevent oxidation. Oxidation is the process that turns newspaper yellow and cut apples brown. Oxidation leads to degenerative changes in our body, i.e., it contributes to the breakdown of body cells as we age. Antioxidants, such as vitamin C, vitamin E, beta-carotene, and selenium, help protect against free radical damage. They scavenge free radicals and protect body cells against cancer. They prevent atherosclerosis and coronary artery diseases (CAD). The sources of antioxidants are listed below.

1. *Vitamin E* Soya oil, sunflower oil, almonds, spinach, and mint
2. *Vitamin C* Amla, guava, green leafy vegetables, all citrus fruit, papaya, tomato, cabbage, and capsicum
3. *Betacarotene* All green leafy vegetables, and all yellow, orange, and red fruits and vegetables
4. *Selenium* Whole grains, whole pulses, green leafy vegetables, and cauliflower
5. *Non-nutrient antioxidants* Phenolic compounds, flavonoids, and isoflavones present in beans, cloves, oats, tea, coffee, grapes, turmeric, mustard, red wine, etc.

We need to consume much more than the RDA for antioxidant effect.

Trans Fatty Acids

Fatty acids which contain a double bond can exist in either of two geometric isomeric forms: cis form or trans form. Unsaturated fatty acids in foods are usually in the cis configuration, i.e., the hydrogen atoms at the double bond are on the same side of the molecule. In the trans configuration, the hydrogen atoms at the double bond are on the opposite side.

The trans molecule assumes a saturated fatty acid like configuration. The change in configuration alters the physical property of the oils, changing liquid oils into semi-olid to solid fats.

$$CH_3(CH_2)_7 \diagdown \overset{\text{H}}{\underset{\overset{\|}{C}}{C}} \diagup$$
HOOC(CH_2)_7 — C — H

Oleic acid (cis form)

$$CH_3(CH_2)_7 \diagdown \overset{\text{H}}{\underset{\overset{\|}{C}}{C}} \diagup$$
H — C — (CH_2)_7 COOH

Elaidic acid (trans form)

Oleic acid, the cis isomer, is a liquid oil while elaidic acid, its trans isomer is solid.

Trans-fatty acids are commercially introduced agents created by partial hydrogenation of the essential fatty acid, thereby reducing their content in the fat. Their use has been eliminated from retail fats and spreads in many parts of the world, but are still used in baked goods and deep-fat fried fast foods.

They are popular in the food industry because they have a high melting point compared to the cis-form and help in making crisper puff pastry and other baked products. However, clinical studies have demonstrated that they are more atherogenic than saturated fatty acids. They increase the LDL cholesterol or bad cholesterol and decrease the HDL cholesterol or good cholesterol affecting the ratio of LDL to HDL cholesterol thereby increasing the risk of coronary heart diseases. Apart from industrially hardened oils, dairy and meat fats are also a source of trans fatty acids.

The Food and Agriculture Organisation (FAO), World Health Organisation (WHO) joint committee has recommended that less than 1 per cent energy should come from trans fatty acids, i.e., on a 2,000 kcal diet, trans fatty acid intake should be less than 2g per day. The United States Food and Drug Administration (USFDA) has made it mandatory to mention trans fatty acids content on all processed food. The use of trans fatty acids is banned in some countries.

Sources Major source of trans fatty acids are partially hydrogenated vegetable oils. They are preferred because they have a long shef life, are stable at high temperature of baking and frying and the degree of hydrogenation can be customized for different uses in bakeries, Refer the section on commercial uses of fats and oils in Chapter 7.

Trans fats are widely used in bakery products such as biscuits, puff pastry, *kharis*, cakes, cream fillings and crunchy cookies, deep-fried fast foods, packaged savoury snacks.

The type of fats consumed in the diet is more important than the total amount of fat consumed. While the intake of saturated fatty acids need to be reduced in the diet, both mono- and polyunsaturated fatty acids need to be increased and the total fat intake should be restricted to 30 per cent of total energy for greater cardiovascular protection. This can be achieved through appropriate admixtures of different oils or through genetic modification of oilseed crops.

Disadvantages of consuming ready-to-serve and ready-to-cook foods

1. They have high calorie content because of high percentage of fat and carbohydrates.
2. Trans fats and saturated fats (hydrogenated fats) are used for better organoleptic qualities.
3. Sodium content of ready mixes is high. Salt used in imported products is not iodized.
4. The proportion of protective and regulatory nutrients is extremely small as the vegetable content is low. They are deficient in most vitamins, minerals, protein, and fibre.
5. Many foods contain artificial preservatives, colour, and taste enhancers, i.e., additives which may cause allergic reactions in some individuals.
6. Ready-to-use products are often very expensive as compared to fresh, wholesome, and nutritious preparations.
7. Packaging, storage, and damage to container during transport may adversely affect the quality.
8. Most of them do not provide a full meal and are lacking in proteins, vitamin A, vitamin C, B-complex vitamins, vitamin E, and essential minerals and fibre.

If precooked meals or table-ready snacks have to be consumed, check nutrition facts on label before purchasing. Check fat and sodium content as well as adequacy of protein before selecting the meal. Follow manufacturer's instructions and add fresh/processed fruits, vegetables, and low-fat milk or yoghurt to supplement the precooked meal and enhance its nutritional adequacy.

Nutritional and product evaluation of newly launched products

Newly launched products lay emphasis on a low or zero cholesterol content (see Tables 25.3 and 25.4).

TABLE 25.3   Dairy-free whip topping and cooking cream

Product features	Dairy-free whip topping	Fresh cream
Stability	Yes	No
Consistency	Yes	No
Economical	Yes	No
Fresh taste	Yes	No
Design decoration	Yes	No
Calorie content	Low	High
Cholesterol	No	Yes
Curdling	No	Yes

TABLE 25.4 Paneer tikka masala (nutritive value of one precooked serving, 100 g)

Nutrient	Amount	% daily value
Calories (kcal/kJ)	191/802	
Calories from fat	139	
Total fat (g)	15	23
Saturated fat (g)	9	45
Cholesterol (mg)	10	3
Sodium (mg)	310	13
Total carbohydrate (g)	8	3
Fibre (g)	2	8
Sugar (g)	5	
Protein (g)	5	10
Vitamin A		24
Vitamin C		5
Calcium		4
Iron		11

SIGNIFICANCE OF NUTRITIONAL LABELLING

Convenience foods form a significant part of the food supplies which are purchased both for home or commercial foods. They not only save consumer's time in the kitchen and reduce costs due to spoilage but have been developed specifically to preserve the oversupply of agricultural products so as to stabilize the food markets in developed countries.

Because of advances in food preparation technology these foods have a longer shelf life and attractive appearance, they are at a premium among people with little cooking experience, the elderly, single people, and professional women who do not have the time for elaborate pre-preparations and cooking.

Today, even food service establishments depend on convenience foods for quicker service with minimum processing space. Since these foods are being frequently used, it is necessary that apart from the net weight and cost of the pack, the consumer is aware of the nutritive value of the product and the percentage of RDAs received by consuming the product. This is of special importance to people on a weight reduction diet, a diabetic diet, a hypertensive diet, or an atherosclerotic diet. Convenience foods are often high in fat, trans fats, salt, and refined carbohydrates. People who are sensitive or allergic to certain foods or additive must study the labels very carefully, and this is another reason why nutritional labelling is very important.

The consumer purchases a product based on the attractive packaging and cost, the need felt for purchasing a product, and the special information mentioned on the label. The health conscious consumer will focus his attention on the information provided on the label.

Some countries have their own set of standards as far as nutritional labelling is concerned. The USFDA has its own nutritional labelling regulations and if convenience food has to be exported to the United States, the label should specify the nutrients and be in accordance with the standards laid down by USFDA. Nutrition facts and health claims are closely regulated in the United States.

TABLE 25.5 Format for nutrition facts: Paneer kadhai

Nutrition facts			
Serving size:	100 g		
Servings per packet:	3		
Amount per serving			
Calories (kcal/kJ):	176/739		
Calories from fat:	134		
			% **Daily value***
Total fat		15 g	23
Saturated fat		8 g	40
Cholesterol		10 mg	3
Sodium		360 mg	15
Total carbohydrate		3 g	1
Fibre		3 g	12
Sugars		6 g	
Protein		8 g	16
Vitamin A	19%	Vitamin C	5%
Calcium	4%	Iron	28%
Calories			
		2,000	2,500
Total fat	(less than)	65 g	80 g
Saturated fat	(less than)	20 g	25 g
Cholesterol	(less than)	300 mg	300 mg
Sodium	(less than)	2,400 mg	2,400 mg
Total carbohydrate		300 g	375 g
Dietary fibre		25 g	20 g
Proteins		50 g	65 g
Calories per gram			
Fat: 9 Carbohydrates: 4 Proteins: 4			

*Per cent daily values are based on a 2,000 calories diet. Your daily values may be higher or lower depending on your calorie needs.

Nutritional labelling is necessary for foods which are a meaningful source of calories or nutrients. All nutrients need not be mentioned on the label, e.g., B-complex vitamin content need not be mentioned (see Table 25.5). Nutrition facts are required for those foods which supply

1. 2 per cent or more of the RDA per serving, e.g., vitamin A, vitamin C, iron, or calcium
2. More than 40 kcal per serving or more than 0.4 kcal per gram
3. More than 35 mg of sodium per serving.

The format for the nutrition facts is fixed and any other health claim made by the manufacturer should be mentioned on any other part of the label. Nutrition information for any health claim is mandatory.

All nutrients are expressed in their prescribed units and as a percentage of the RDA for a diet providing 2,000 kcal and 2,500 kcal. For example, the total daily value for fat is 65 g on a 2,000 kcal diet or 30 per cent kcalories from fat which is equal to 600 kcal. One standard serving of *paneer kadhai* contains 15 g of fat which means 135 kcal from fat or 23 per cent of the daily value

$$\frac{15g}{65g} \times 100 = 23\%$$

Similarly, one serving of *paneer kadhai* provides 3 g fibre which is 12 per cent of the daily value

$$\frac{3g}{25g} \times 100 = 12\%$$

The daily values are the RDA for nutrients and on the label, the nutrition facts need to be expressed as a percentage of daily values prescribed for a 2,000 and a 2,500 kcalorie diet. The USFDA has fixed the serving size for various food items and the serving size in the packet is no longer at the discretion of the product manufacturer.

Various health claims such as fat-free, cholesterol-free, and sugar-free are made by product manufacturers. In order to use these terms, values have been set for the content of nutrient present and accordingly terms such as free, light, low, and high are used to describe these products (see Table 25.6).

TABLE 25.6   Some health claims

Claim	Nutrient content/serving
Cholesterol-free	Less than 2 mg cholesterol and no claims for fat
Fat-free	Less than 0.5 g fat
Low fat	Less than 3 g fat
Light	One-third calories of reference product
Sugar-free	Less than 0.5 g of sugar
Calorie-free	Less than 5 kcal
High fibre	More than 5 g fibre

Any declaration on the label which is not according to law will be deemed to be misbranded.

If a product is commonly combined with other ingredients, e.g., a biryani masala mix and the directions for preparation and addition of other ingredients is mentioned then the nutritional facts may be mentioned on the basis of the product alone. For example, it can be on the basis of nutrient value of masala mix alone, or on the basis of the final product, i.e., ready biryani with all added ingredients mentioned in the recipe. The additional ingredients and method of cooking on a burner or in a microwave oven should be clearly specified in the recipe.

Some declarations are voluntary such as the declaration of potassium, soluble fibre, insoluble fibre, stearic acid, sugar, alcohol, other carbohydrates, and B-complex vitamins.

Nutrition facts for nutrients present in small quantities can be mentioned as follows:

1. Not a significant source—less than 2 per cent RDA for calcium, iron, vitamins A and C
2. Fibre, carbohydrate sugar, protein

    >0.5 g = to be mentioned as zero

    >1 g = to be mentioned as less than one gram

For labelling a product as fresh would mean it has not been frozen, heat-processed, or otherwise preserved in any way.

NUTRACEUTICALS

It is now a well-known fact that apart from proteins, carbohydrates, fats, vitamins, minerals, and water present in our food, there are a number of important non-nutritive chemical components which play a vital role in maintaining optimal health (see Plate 4).

Traditional forms of medicine have been used all over the world since time immemorial for prevention and treatment of disease and for vitality, and longevity.

The healing effects of food have been advocated by Hippocrates, the father of Western medicine.

Evidence from ancient civilizations have suggested that people were aware of the medicinal benefits of food for healing and curing ailments. Ayurveda has mentioned the benefits of food for therapeutic purpose.

The modern nutraceutical market has its beginnings several thousand years ago. Since the 1980s it has gained momentum because of new research stressing on the preventive and curative properties of food. Today, nutraceuticals form part of the daily diet of people in developed and developing countries worldwide. Let us understand the meaning of this term.

There are many components in food apart from the six nutrients which play a vital role in the link between food and health. An increase in life span and change in lifestyle with the advent of technology have been the two main reasons for interest in non-nutritive components. These chemical components derived from plant sources, our food and microorganism have shown to possess medicinal benefits and can promote long term health and well being. These chemical components which are not classified as nutrients are called nutraceuticals. The term 'nutraceuticals' has been derived from the words 'nutrition' and 'pharmaceutical' and is now used for food or food products that provide health and medical benefits, ie., they are used to prevent and treat disease. Following are types of nutraceuticals.

1. Prebiotics and probiotics
2. Antioxidants
3. Phytochemicals

Definition   Nutraceuticals is, thus, a large umbrella term used to describe any product derived from food sources that provides extra health benefits in addition to the basic nutritive value of the food. They claim to improve health, prevent chronic disease, delay the aging process and increase life expectancy.

Nutraceuticals are available in many different forms (see Fig 25.3). For example, they may be isolated or purified from foods and are generally sold in medicinal forms. They may also be added to foods we consume everyday.

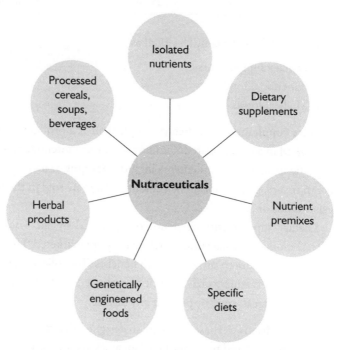

Fig. 25.3   Forms in which nutraceuticals are available

Some examples of nutraceuticals are given in Table 25.7.

TABLE 25.7 Examples of nutraceuticals

Health claim	Chemical component	Source
Antioxidants	Flavonoids resveratrol	Red grapes
	Naringin	Citrus fruits
	Carotenoids	Carrots
	Polyphenols	Tea, wine, dark chocolate
	Alyl sulfides	Onions and garlic
	Anthocyanins	Berries
Cholesterol lowering	Soluble dietary fibre	Psyllium seed husk
Cancer prevention	Sulphoraphane	Broccoli
	Indoles	Cabbage
	Capsaicin	Peppers
	Isoflavonoids	Soya beans
	Saponins	Beans
Anti-inflammatory	Alpha-linolenic acid	Flaxseeds, olive oil
Antibacterial effect	Allicin	Garlic oil
	Proanthocyanidins	Cranberries

Nutraceuticals are broadly classified as

1. Dietary supplements
2. Functional foods
3. Medical foods

Dietary supplement A dietary supplement is a product that contains nutrients derived from food in a concentrated liquid or solid form intended to supplement the diet. Dietary ingredients in these supplements include vitamins, minerals, amino acids, enzymes, herbs, organ tissues, glandulars and metabolites. They are sold in the form of tablets, capsules, soft gels, liquids or powders.

Dietary supplements need not be approved by the Food and Drug Administration (FDA) unlike pharmaceuticals before they are marketed. However they need a label if the supplements claim to provide health benefits. The following needs to be mentioned on the label: 'These statements have not been evaluated by the FDA. This product is not intended to diagnose, treat, cure, or prevent any disease.'

Functional foods These foods are so designed that the additional health claims are added to the food itself and need not be taken as a separate supplement:

These foods have been either enriched, with a deficient nutrient or fortified with extra nutrients, or losses in processing have been restored.

Additional components or ingredients are added to ordinary food to give it a specific medical or physiological benefit. Foods which are consumed daily should be enriched with chemical components which regulate a biological process which can help prevent or control disease.

Medical foods   These foods need a doctor's prescription and are not available over-the-counter to consumers. They are specially formulated foods given either orally or through tube feeding under medical supervision with an aim to therapeutically manage a specific disease or condition. They are always designed to meet certain nutritional requirements. These foods are regulated by FDA unlike dietary supplements and functional foods and need a prescription of a registered medical practitioner.

PREBIOTICS AND PROBIOTICS

While probiotics are the beneficial bacteria found in the intestine, prebiotics are special indigestible carbohydrates known as oligosaccharides that feed probiotic bacteria and support their growth and colonization in our gut.

Prebiotics

Prebiotics are non-digestible food ingredients found in plants, which stimulate the growth and/or activity of bacteria in our digestive system. They mainly include carbohydrates, such as oligosaccharides and soluble dietary fibre, which stay intact during cooking and baking. Because of this property, they can safely be used in cooked and baked food items.

Prebiotics as a functional food are beneficial to health. The non-digestible carbohydrates allow microorganisms to grow, as they reach the intestine unaffected by the digestion process. Prebiotic fibre is selectively fermented in the gut and brings about changes in the composition and activity of microorganisms in our gastrointestinal tract.

The main prebiotics are the fructooligosaccharides (FOS), inulin, and oligofructose and galactooligosaccharides (GOS) which are added to processed foods.

Some are fermented slowly, e.g., the longer chain prebiotic inulin, while others are fermented more rapidly, e.g., oligofructose.

Prebiotics increase the number and activity of Bifidobacteria and lactic acid bacteria in the gut and increase resistance to invading pathogens. These groups of bacteria have several beneficial effects on humans such as improving digestion, enhancing absorption of mineral elements, and strengthening our immune system.

Sources of prebiotics

No plant or food is a prebiotic by itsely. Foods contain prebiotics in varying quantities. Sources include whole grains, specially, oats, wheat bran, barley, psyllium, soya beans, and products, pulses, flax seeds, sunflower seeds, fenugreek seeks, carrots, citrus fruits. Jerusalem artichoke and chicory root are richest sources of inulin, while wheat, almonds and honey contain smaller quantities. Other plant-based foods, such as bananas, onions, leeks, garlic, and tomatoes, contain lesser amount of inulin. Prebiotic fibre supplements are added to processed foods to increase their health benefits.

Everyday foods, such as cereals, biscuits, bread, health drinks, yoghurt, and table spreads, contain prebiotics.

Daily allowances　To maintain good digestion, an intake of 6 g of prebiotic has been suggested for healthy individuals and at least 15 g per day to individuals suffering from active digestive disorders.

Beneficial effects of prebiotic fibre

Prebiotics promote the growth of probiotics or beneficial bacteria. Bacteria such as *Clostridium* and *Bacteroides* species produce short chain fatty acids (SCFA). Prebiotics lead to the increased production of SCFA which creates a medium conducive to good digestive health because SCFAs nourish the colon walls, create a slightly acidic medium which helps in reducing the number of sulphate producing bacteria which form H_2S gas. When the diet is low in fibre over a long period of time, SCFA production reduces. Beneficial effects are as follows:

1. An increase in calcium and other mineral absorption
2. Increased immune system effectiveness
3. Regulation of bowel pH
4. Decrease in risk of colorectal cancers
5. Reduced risk of Crohn's disease and ulcerative colitis
6. Reduction in hypertension

Probiotics

Probiotic bacteria are also known as beneficial bacteria or friendly bacteria and are naturally present in some of our foods or are added to processed foods for their health benefits Probiotics are the live microorganisms present in the food we eat. They are not affected by our digestive process, hence live, healthy bacteria directly reach our large intestine or colon where they grow and form colonies. These healthy bacteria in the intestine can combat harmful bacteria and provide a number of health benefits which have been discussed under prebiotics.

Prebiotics are beneficial because they stimulate the growth of healthy bacteria such as species of *Bifidobacteria* and *Lactobacilli* in the gut. There are many types of probiotic bacteria but *Lactobacilli* and *Bifidobacteria* are present in largest numbers and are also popular probiotics added as a supplement to various foods.

The following bacteriare most commonly found in supplements and capsules.

- *Lactobacillus acidophilus*
- *Lactobacillus rhamnosus*
- *Lactobacillus bulgaricus*
- *Lactobacillus plantarum*
- *Lactobacillus casei*
- *Lactobacillus sporogenes*
- *Clostridium butyricum*
- *Bifidobacteria bifidum*
- *Bifidobacteria longum*
- *Bifidobacteria infantis*
- *Streptococcus thermophilus*
- *Streptococcus faecalis*
- *Bacillus mesentericus*

Antibiotics are administered to destroy pathogenic organisms. Along with pathogens, they also destroy the normal intestinal flora. Probiotic bacteria are administered in the form of capsules along with anti-fungal or antibacterial therapy to restore the proper balance of organisms in the gut. They prevent colonization by other organisms in the gut. Recent research indicates that the gut flora could be related to development of food and airborne allergies and improving the gut flora could reduce the severity and number of allergies as well.

Sources of probiotics

Sources of probiotics include fermented milk products such as curds, yoghurt, and butter-milk and their variations. *Lactobacillus casei* is added to Yakult, a probiotic yoghurt drink.

Probiotics are added along with prebiotics to everyday products as well as special health drinks, powders, and capsules. They work best in combination.

Bifidobacteria They prevent and treat antibiotic induced diarrhoea. Bifidobacteria synthesize B-complex vitamins. They help regulate normal bowel movements and prevent colonization of pathogenic bacteria by producing acids which maintain the pH balance.

Lactobacilli They help in digestion of lactose and dairy products. They acidify the intestinal tract and improve nutrient absorption. The acidic pH prevents pathogens. Like *Bifidobacteria*, they prevent and treat antibiotic induced diarrhoea.

Lactobacilli casei and L. salivarius They sigmificantly inhibit the growth of peptic ulcer causing bacteria *Helicobacter pylori* (*H. pylori*).

ROLE OF PHYTOCHEMICALS

A number of newly launched products have included phytochemicals ('phyto' is a Greek word meaning 'plant') in their composition. Phytochemicals are biologically active, naturally occurring chemical components in plant foods. They are beneficial to health as they reduce the risk of cancer and other chronic diseases. They influence hormonal and enzymatic processes but their exact mechanism is not yet known. These chemical compounds are not proteins, carbohydrates, fats, vitamins, minerals, or fibre but are non-nutrient chemicals found in plants such as the plant pigments flavonoids, carotenoids, anthocyanin, lycopene, indoles, terpenes, sulfides, and phytoestrogens.

These phytochemicals were earlier thought to be 'associated food factors' in plants which might be as nutritionally important as vitamins and minerals. Today these 'associated food factors' are called phyto nutrients. They may provide many added nutritional benefits and can help reduce our risk of developing chronic health conditions such as heart diseases, stroke, cataract, Parkinson's disease, or even cancer (see Fig. 25.3).

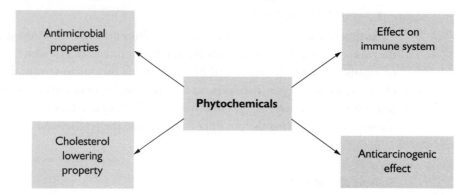

Fig. 25.3 Functions of phytochemicals

They are present in abundance in parsley, broccoli, alfalfa, water cress, spinach, carrots, acerola cherries, kelp, soya beans, turmeric, yellow corn, tomatoes, cranberries, blueberries, garlic, onions, flaxseeds, walnuts, etc.

Since these phytochemicals are found widely distributed in fruits and vegetables, a generous intake of fruits and vegetables containing phytochemicals is a better option instead of consuming phytochemicals in the form of nutrient supplements or added in multivitamin pills.

SUMMARY

Food provided by residential institutions is probably the only source of nutrition for the residents, and needs to meet the RDAs for the residents. If a single meal is served it should provide one-third the RDA, which means food should be selected, stored, prepared, and served keeping nutrient retention in mind, and cooking practices which enhance the nutritive value should be followed. All this is necessary because eating out has become a way of life and more of a compulsion than a choice. The caterer or food manufacturer should know that many nutrients can be lost through faulty cooking practices and it is the moral responsibility of the caterer to ensure that food served is wholesome and safe.

The consumer is gaining awareness about nutrition and health and is making wise choices as far as food is concerned, to keep lifestyle-related diseases away. Fast foods which are highly processed are very convenient for a meal but the health benefits of many such items is limited as they lack essential nutrients and food groups such as vitamins, minerals, and fibre. Most fast foods are rich in fats and refined carbohydrates.

Nutritional evaluation is the need of the hour and many factors should be considered before selecting food products. A wide range of processed foods is available, but reading the nutritive value mentioned on the label should become a matter of habit before making a choice.

The healing effects of food for prevention and treatment of disease and for added vitality and longevity are not new. Apart from the nutritive component, food contains non-nutritive components which are gaining interest especially because of an increase in life span and changes in our lifestyle. Nutraceuticals like antioxidants, phytochemicals, and prebiotics and probiotics, play a vital role in maintaining optimal health and are available off the counter as dietary supplements, functional foods, and medical foods with additional health claims. To give food specific medical or physiological benefits, additional components or ingredients are added to ordinary foods. The health-conscious consumer has a wide array of products to choose from.

KEY TERMS

Acerola cherry   One of the richest source of vitamin C.

Fast foods   These are processed foods available in market that require little or no preparation before consumption.

Junk food   These are processed foods that are low in healthy nutrient content.

Phytochemicals   A large group of chemicals present in plants which are biologically active and affect hormonal and enzymatic processes in the body other than the six nutrients.

Precooked product   A convenience food which is already cooked and only needs to be heated before it is served.

Trans fatty acids   Geometrical isomers of unsaturated fatty acids that assume a saturated fatty acid like configuration giving the fat a higher melting point and making the baked product crisper.

Dietary supplement   A product that contains nutrients derived from food in a concentrated form as tablets, capsules, liquids, or powders intended to supplement the diet.

Functional foods   These are foods which have been enriched or fortified or in which nutrients lost in processing have been restored, e.g., ascorbic acid in fruit juices, so that consumers get benefits through food instead of taking tablets or supplements. Also includes addition of prebiotics and probiotics to food.

Medical foods   Foods specially formulated to be consumed or administered internally under medical supervision for specific dietary management of a disease or condition, to be consumed by mouth or tube feeding.

Probiotics   Beneficial bacteria found in the intestine which combat harmful pathogens and provide additional health benefits.

Prebiotics   Special indigestible soluble fibres present in plant foods that support the growth of probiotic bacteria without being affected by cooking or digestive processes.

Phytochemicals   Non-nutritive biologically active chemical components present in plants proven to prevent and cure disease, increase lifespan and preserve youth.

REVIEW QUESTIONS

1. Why is it necessary to mention nutrient facts on the label?
2. Which are the nutrients that must be disclosed on a food label?
3. Discuss the nutritive value of fast foods and foods served in restaurants.
4. What influence does cooking have on the nutritive value of food?
5. Discuss the concept of fast foods and the factors influencing the growth of this section of the industry.
6. List the various categories of convenience foods giving a suitable example for each category.

7. Why is a knowledge of nutrition and food processing essential for people who prepare or manufacture food?
8. Define the following terms:
   (a) Antioxidant   (e) Functional foods
   (b) Phytochemical   (f) Medical foods
   (c) Probioticcs   (g) Dietary supplements
   (d) Prebiotics   (h) Nutraceuticals
9. Discuss the beneficial effects of prebiotics and probiotics.

ASSIGNMENT

Visit any health food store or website and list nutraceuticals along with the health claims made of any 10 food items.

References

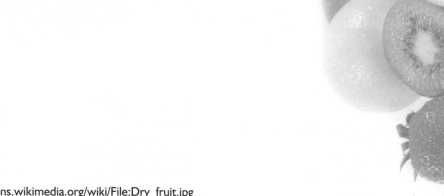

- http://commons.wikimedia.org/wiki/File:Dry_fruit.jpg
- http://commons.wikimedia.org/wiki/File:N2_fruit_salad.jpg
- http://commons.wikimedia.org/wiki/File:Vegan_Gardein_Tofu_Foods_Display.jpg
- http://commons.wikimedia.org/wiki/File:High_Fat_Foods_-_NCI_Visuals_Online.jpg
- http://commons.wikimedia.org/wiki/File:ARS_copper_rich_foods.jpg
- http://commons.wikimedia.org/wiki/File:ARS_-_Foods_high_in_zinc.jpg
- http://commons.wikimedia.org/wiki/File:Fat,_Butter_and_Oil_-_NCI_Visuals_Online.jpg

Index

About the Author

Sunetra Roday is Principal, Maharashtra State Institute of Hotel Management and Catering Technology (MSIHMCT), Pune. She has been teaching food science and nutrition for over 30 years.

A post-graduate in foods and nutrition from Lady Irwin College, New Delhi, she also has a master's degree in tourism management. She has published books on hygiene and sanitation, cookery, and food preservation. She is actively involved in consultancy projects, curriculum development, and nutrition counselling.

INTERNATIONAL CUISINE AND FOOD PRODUCTION MANAGEMENT   (with CD) [9780198073895]

Parvinder Bali, Oberoi Centre of Learning and Development (OCLD), Delhi

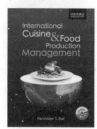

International Cuisine and Food Production Management is a comprehensive textbook specially designed for the final year degree/diploma students of hotel management.

Key Features

- Devotes a complete part to advanced confectionery including cakes, pastries, chocolates, desserts, cookies, and biscuits
- Includes key managerial issues such as production planning and scheduling, production quality and quantity control, forecasting and budgeting, menu costing, yield management, and new product development
- CD that includes over 370 recipes together with formulas to calculate waste percentage and food cost of the dish, recipes divided into cold kitchen, international cuisines, and advanced pastry and confectionery, PowerPoint presentations on step-by-step preparation of terrine and pate

QUANTITY FOOD PRODUCTION OPERATIONS AND INDIAN CUISINE   (with CD) [9780198068495]

Parvinder Bali, Oberoi Centre of Learning and Development (OCLD), Delhi

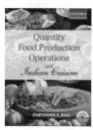

Quantity Food Production Operations and Indian Cuisine is a comprehensive textbook specially designed for students of hotel management. It aims to familiarize the readers with the fundamentals of volume cooking and Indian cuisine.

Key Features

- Concepts supported by suitable photographs including 28 colour plates
- An appendix on internship training in hotels
- Accompanying CD containing 337 recipes

HOTEL HOUSEKEEPING, 2E   (with DVD) [9780198061090]

G. Raghubalan, Hospitality Consulting and Management Group, Mumbai and **Smritee Raghubalan**, Garden City College, Bangalore

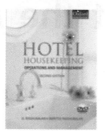

The book explores the key elements of housekeeping as also its theoretical foundations and techniques of operations. It provides an exhaustive coverage of the core concepts of the subject.
Students of hotel management and home science would find the book highly useful.

Key Features

- Provides guidelines on the practical aspects of the operations and management of housekeeping
- Detailed illustrations of cleaning equipment and flower arrangements to aid students requiring to sketch these in their journals
- DVD with videos explaining the exact procedure involved in bed-making, room cleaning, flower arrangement, and organizing the maid's cart.

FOOD AND BEVERAGE SERVICE   [9780198065272]

R. Singaravelavan, SNR Sons College, Coimbatore

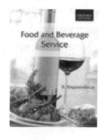

Food and Beverage Service is a comprehensive textbook designed to cater to the needs of the students of degree/diploma courses of hotel management and certificate courses of food craft institutes. It covers all aspects of the food and beverage (F&B), department as required by the syllabi of hotel management courses.

Key Features

- Provides a detailed description of the various types of wines, non-alcoholic beverages, guéridon service, and specialized service skills for breakfast, afternoon tea, brunch, and so on
- Illustrates the key concepts with the help of photographs of various table layouts and other services, colour plates, sample menus, and side bars

Other Related Titles

Visit us at www.oup.co.in and www.oupinheonline.com